NEUROSCIENCE RESEARCH PROGRESS

MOVEMENT DISORDERS: CAUSES, DIAGNOSES AND TREATMENTS

NEUROSCIENCE RESEARCH PROGRESS

Additional books in this series can be found on Nova's website
under the Series tab.

Additional E-books in this series can be found on Nova's website
under the E-books tab.

NEUROSCIENCE RESEARCH PROGRESS

MOVEMENT DISORDERS: CAUSES, DIAGNOSES AND TREATMENTS

BARBARA J. LARSEN
EDITOR

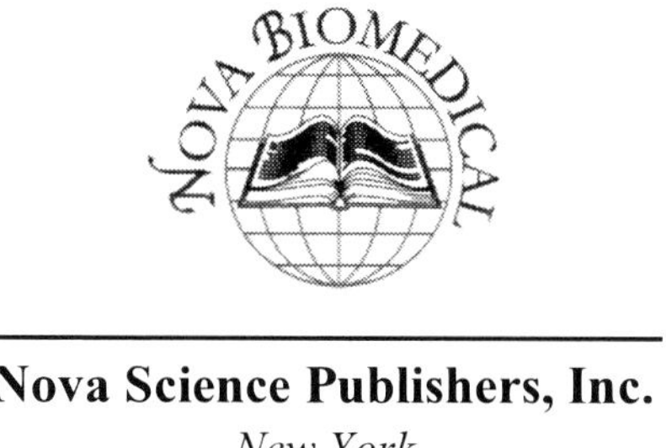

Nova Science Publishers, Inc.
New York

For permission to use material from this book please contact us:
Telephone 631-231-7269; Fax 631-231-8175
Web Site: http://www.novapublishers.com

LIBRARY OF CONGRESS CATALOGING-IN-PUBLICATION DATA

Movement disorders : causes, diagnoses, and treatments / editor, Barbara J.
Larsen.
p. ; cm.
Includes bibliographical references and index.
ISBN 978-1-61209-200-3 (hardcover)
1. Movement disorders. 2. Parkinson disease--Complications. I. Larsen,
Barbara J.
[DNLM: 1. Movement Disorders--etiology. 2. Movement
Disorders--diagnosis. 3. Movement Disorders--therapy. 4. Parkinson
Disease--complications. WL 390]
RC376.5.M6843 2010
616.8'3--dc22
2010047063

Published by Nova Science Publishers, Inc. † New York

Contents

Preface

Movement disorders are neurological conditions that affect the speed, fluency, quality, and ease of movement. This book presents current research in the study of movement disorders, including serotonin dysfunction in Parkinson's Disease; restless leg syndrome and periodic limb movements of sleep; peripheral and central changes induce movement disorders on the basis of disuse or overuse and traditional mirror therapy in the management of movement and postural control problems.

Chapter I - Several recent studies have emphasized a crucial role for the interactions between serotonergic and dopaminergic systems in movement control and the pathophysiology of the basal ganglia. These observations are supported by anatomical evidence demonstrating large serotonergic innervation of all the basal ganglia nuclei. In fact, serotonergic terminals have been reported to make synaptic contacts with both substantia nigra dopamine-containing neurons and their terminal areas such as the striatum, the globus pallidus and the subthalamus. These brain areas contain a high concentration of serotonin (5-HT), with the substantia nigra pars reticulata (SNr) receiving the greatest input. In this review, the distribution of 5-HT different receptor subtypes in the basal ganglia nuclei will be described. Furthermore, evidence demonstrating the serotonergic control of basal ganglia activity will be reviewed, and the contribution of the different 5-HT receptor subtypes examined. The new avenues that the increasing knowledge of 5-HT in motor control has opened for exploring the pathophysiology and pharmacology of Parkinson's disease and other movement disorders will be discussed. It is clear that these avenues will be fruitful, despite the disappointing results so far obtained by clinical studies with selective 5-HT ligands. Nevertheless, these studies have led to a great increase in the attention given to the neurotransmitters of the basal ganglia and their connections.

Chapter II - To gain new insights into the underpinning mechanisms of movement disorders observed with both cerebral palsy and repetitive motion disorders, the authors have investigated the long-term effects of movement disuse or overuse on musculoskeletal tissues and topographical organization of the primary somatosensory and primary motor cortices, using two different rat models. The authors provide strong evidence that experience-dependent movements play a crucial role in shaping normal as well as aberrant movement abilities. Cerebral palsy is a developmental neurological disorder characterized by spasticity of some muscles, but also disuse in other muscles, and motor abnormalities. The data from a rat model of cerebral palsy shows that aberrant sensorimotor inputs during development resulting from prolonged disuse (i.e. hind limb immobilization during the first month of life) induces peripheral tissue changes, such as muscle atrophy and extracellular matrix changes, joint degeneration, and drastic topographical disorganization of primary somatosensory and motor cortical hind limb representations. These peripheral and central tissue changes were associated with increased muscular tone at rest and with active flexion and extension around movement-restricted joints that resulted in abnormal walking patterns. Observed tissue changes and movement disorders were worsened when developmental disuse was combined with neonatal asphyxia. In contrast, repetitive motion disorders, such as carpal tunnel syndrome and focal hand dystonia, are a type of overuse associated with tasks that require prolonged, repetitive behaviors. The data from a rat model of repetitive reaching and grasping shows that peripheral tissue changes are induced with cumulative task exposure, including myofiber fray, fibrotic nerve compression, and increased macrophages and inflammatory cytokines. These tissue changes were associated with declines in reach performance, grip strength and agility. The motor declines also correlated with disorganization of the forepaw representation in the primary somatosensory cortex, including the emergence of large receptive fields, and a drastic enlargement of the overall forepaw map area of the primary motor cortex, in which emerged the representation of joint movements specifically involved in the repetitive task. Peripheral inflammation correlated with signs of central sensitization (mechanical allodynia, myalgia, and increased neurochemicals and cytokines in the spinal cord), and with the reduced amount of current needed in the motor cortex to evoke forelimb movements. The data from a rat model of repetitive motion injuries show that peripheral inflammation, spinal cord neuroplasticity and cortical neuroplasticity jointly contribute to the development of chronic repetitive motion disorders. In conclusion, both prolonged disuse and overuse lead to both peripheral and central changes that are interdependent to drive cerebral plasticity and altered motor output function.

Chapter III - Restless legs syndrome (RLS) is a common, chronic, sensorimotor, hyperkinetic movement disorder, which is characterized by significant uncomfortable creeping, crawling or cramping sensations at rest and irresistable urge to move for alleviating the symptoms focused primarily on the lower extremities and sometimes also other parts of the body. RLS symptoms may occur intermittently or daily. Symptoms begin or are exacerbated in the evening or at night and also interfere with sleep and may result in reduced sleep efficiency and even serious insomnia. PLMS are brief jerks (repetitive stereotypic movements), a flexion at the ankle, knee, and hip with an extension of the toes during sleep lasting between 0.5 to 5.0 seconds, typically occur at 20- to 40-second intervals. PLMS affect one or both legs and rarely involve the arms. PLMS usually occur during non-REM sleep and may be associated with awakening. In addition, PLMS that reduce sleep quality are common with a prevelance of 80% during sleep in patients with RLS. RLS affects about 3% to 12% of the general population, and is more common in females with a female-to-male ratio of 2:1. Although RLS could be seen from 2 to >80 years of age, the mean age at the diagnosis time is 35–40 years. RLS can be primary (idiopathic) or secondary (sporadic or symptomatic) as a result of iron deficiency (with or without anemia), chronic renal and hepatic failure, pregnancy, rheumatic diseases (especially rheumatoid arthritis and fibromyalgia), neuropathies and radiculopathies, neurodegenerative diseases such as Parkinson's disease and drugs such as antihistamines, dopamine antagonists, mirtazapine, tricyclic antidepressants, serotonergic reuptake inhibitors. Idiopathic RLS is suggested to be a complex polygenic disorder with possible genetic heterogeneity because of variations in penetrance and anticipation. Genomewide linkage analysis studies showed at least 3 major susceptibility loci on chromosomes 12q13-23, 14q13-21 and 9p24-22 regions in large families. Genes and loci associated with RLS on 2q, 20p and 16p have also been identified. While the pathophysiology of RLS and PLMS has not yet been fully understood, dopamine dysfunction locally within the central nervous system appears to have a central role in the pathophysiology of both conditions. Moderate aerobic exercise, hot baths, massage, and stretching are nonpharmacologic treatment options with some benefit. Carbidopa/levodopa, dopamine agonists particularly ropinirole and pramipexole, opioids, benzodiazepines, antiepileptic drugs (carbamazepine, gabapentine, pregabaline) and iron supplements are recommended with nonpharmacologic treatment options as primary treatments.

Chapter IV - Besides the classical motor symptoms, Parkinson's disease (PD) also leads to cognitive, behavioral and mood symptoms. Among them, impulsiveness disorders or addictive behaviors such as addiction to antiparkinsonian medications, compulsive behaviors, pathological gambling, hypersexuality and compulsive shopping have been reported. Hypersexuality in PD was first described in 1983 and Molina et al. reported in 2000 pathological gambling (PG). The same year, Giovannoni et al. described Hedonistic Homeostatic Dysregulation (HHD), the original term for Dopamine Dysregulation Syndrome (DDS). Many recent studies have reported this syndrome suggesting that it could be more frequent than assumed. Recently in the field of impulsive disorders spectrum, binge-eating has also been described. Some patients may even develop addiction problems or behavioral symptoms in association with DDS and this co-occurrence has been already demonstrated by Laurence et al. in 2003. Depression, anxiety, apathy, anhedonia, mania/hypomania and hallucinations are among psychiatric disorders that also constitute the dark side of PD. Specific scales in each domain can be helpful in detecting not only severe but early cases.

Concerning the risk factors for addiction, several studies have now demonstrated an association with antiparkinsonian medications and behavioral disorders such as HS, PG and DDS. L-dopa in monotherapy and more specifically in higher doses can induce or worsen these disorders. Dopamine agonists were also associated with DDS, PG and HS. The predominant role of dopamine agonists has been emphasized by Mamkinian et al. Recent studies show that dopamine agonists increase the sensation of a "better than expected" outcome and impair the negative reinforcing effect of losing. However, controversy exists over the role and importance of L-dopa in relation to addiction/repetitive behaviors/impulse control disorders. Risk factors for depression, anxiety, apathy, anhedonia, mania/hypomania and hallucinations have been much debate and only recently considered to be a whole part of the disease. Global approach of psychiatric comorbidities in PD can be a good strategy for good management of this disease resulting in an improvement in the quality of life and suitable conditions for treatment by neurosurgery when indicated.

Chapter V - Parkinson syndrome (PS) has been repeatedly described as a clinical feature of mitochondrial disorders (MIDs). PS may be mild and only one of several other phenotypic features or PS may dominate the phenotype. PS manifestations may precede the other MID manifestations or may develop after onset of the non-PS MID manifestations. Evidence for an association between PS and MID comes also from a number of patients with PS or Parkinson disease (PD), who developed clinical or instrumental features of a MID in the absence of an immunhistochemical, biochemical or genetic defect indicative of a MID. Repeatedly, it has been also shown that some of the PD patients have an increased number of various mtDNA mutations in the nigrostriatal area. It has been also shown that mutations in genes causing hereditary PD, such as parkin, PINK1, alpha-synuclein (SCNA), leucine-rich kinase-2 (LRRK2), or DJ1, cause mitochondrial dysfunction, for which the term "mitochondrial nigropathies" has been coined. This mini-review wants to give an overview about the close relation between mitochondrial dysfunction and PS/PD at least in some of these patients.

Chapter VI - The concept of awareness of illness refers to the ability that people have in recognizing their disturbances. The presence of a possible unawareness of illness is well described in different clinical pathologies. The awareness of deficits may be sometimes altered in patients suffering from Parkinson's disease (PD). In order to have a greater clinical utility, theoretical models of unawareness, should allow for the possibility of integrating neurobiological and neuropsychological levels of explanation and should comprehend convergent analyses of these levels. With the aim of integrating such levels of explanations, a series of variables of interest will be considered from a convergent perspective at the neurobiological, neuropsychological and psychological-psychiatric levels.

In particular, this chapter will focus on a specific analysis of awareness of movement disorders in non-demented patients with PD and motor fluctuations. So far, only one study has analyzed differences in the awareness of deficits in PD patients by comparing the *on* and *off* states using an extensive battery of cognitive and behavioral functioning. The results of this study demonstrated that PD patients have a selective reduced awareness of dyskinesias when in the *on* state, while being aware of their hypokinesias in the *off* state. Interestingly, such a reduced awareness of dyskinesia-related movement disorders was associated with executive functions in the *on* state. In contrast, no association with executive functions was found in the *off* state.

The authors believe that this study together with more in depth analysis of the phenomenon of unawareness of deficits may add important elements to the literature on neuropsychological impairments observed in unaware - non-demented patients with PD - in terms of executive dysfunctions. Besides, such elements may significantly contribute to the management of this particular class of pathology.

The explanatory hypothesis is that the disruption of prefrontal-subcortical connections may cause impaired insight, independently of cognitive deterioration. Our model will also critically discuss the role that motivation may have in the unawareness of symptoms in the *on* medication state.

Chapter VII - Mirrors have a long history as an 'essential' piece of rehabilitation equipment, and can be found in many physical therapy treatment areas. Traditionally one of their main uses is to provide patients with a reflected body image of themselves, usually as (a component of) a therapeutic strategy aimed at retraining movement control and posture. For example, when as a result of central nervous system (CNS) damage such as stroke, people have impaired postural control, then therapists might provide them with a reflected mirror image of themselves to deliver augmented visual feedback during treatment sessions where motor training is occurring.

There has recently been much interest in the therapeutic use of mirrors placed perpendicular to the patient's coronal plane; i.e mirrors able to reflect an image of one limb onto the limb of the opposite body side. Recent works by researchers such as Ramachandran, and Sutbeyaz and Yavuzer, have indicated that this may be a useful therapeutic strategy in instances where CNS pathology has resulted in unilateral instances of paresis, neglect or phantom pain. So for example, a mirror might be used to reflect the left (sound) arm onto the right (paralysed) arm following a stroke, as part of a therapeutic strategy aiming to rehabilitate movement on the affected side. One proposed mechanism is that reflection creates an illusion of normal movement/sensation on the affected side of the body, thus facilitating voluntary production of movement and/or normal sensory processing on that side.

Whilst this newer work, now often referred to as 'mirror therapy', is advancing, the original more traditional and (possibly) simpler therapeutic use of mirrors described at the start appears to be being somewhat overlooked and neglected. In this more traditional context (hereafter referred to as 'Traditional Mirror Therapy' or TMT), a full length body mirror is typically placed in front of the person (i.e. parallel to their coronal plane), thus providing them with a full frontal image of their body and its movements. In this way the person is provided with augmented (visual) feedback of their postural alignment and/or bodily movement. This might typically be carried out in conjunction with corrective instructions from the therapist.

One of the puzzles regarding TMT is the apparent absence of any evidence base or instructional advice for what is in effect a fairly simple and straightforward training strategy with a seemingly long history. The notion of therapist/educator-provided augmented feedback during (motor) learning is a well established one; in a recent narrative review for example, van Vliet and Wulf identified a reasonably substantial (albeit nascent) evidence base for this general strategy for motor skills training following stroke. They identified verbal, visual, video and kinematic feedback strategies as the main ones which have been used and evaluated by therapists working with this very common patient group. Interestingly however, this overview did not identify any literature relating to TMT. Similarly, if one accesses key physical therapy instructional texts, there is usually a very limited amount of information on TMT. For example, in a fairly seminal UK text, Howe and Oldham state that "*Full length mirrors are frequently used in physiotherapy departments to make patients more aware of their static posture either in sitting or standing and dynamic posture during movement. Mirrors are also employed in gait retraining...*". Howevere no further details are provided.

It is perhaps not difficult to explain this dearth of information regarding TMT. Despite its longstanding presence in the physical therapist's armamentarium, it is easily conceivable that the approach has yet to receive the level of investigation and exploration which it deserves. The physical therapy evidence base is still in its relative infancy and the majority of existing therapeutic strategies await appropriate formal evaluation; TMT is probably no exception in this respect.

The aim of this chapter is to provide an overview of several aspects of TMT. Specifically, the chapter covers 3 topics, these being:

- Literature: what is known about TMT from published peer-reviewed reports of formal investigations of this strategy
- Recent research: an overview of 3 pilot projects conducted by the author and colleagues which each evaluate an aspect of TMT
- Clinical perspectives: a report of a pilot evaluation of how practising UK clinicians utilise TMT

In: Movement Disorders: Causes, Diagnoses and Treatments ISBN 978-1-61209-200-3
Editor: Barbara J. Larsen

Chapter I

Serotonin Dysfunction in Parkinson's Disease

Giuseppe Di Giovanni*

Department of Physiology and Biochemistry, University of Malta,
Msida MSD 2080, Malta

Abstract

Several recent studies have emphasized a crucial role for the interactions between serotonergic and dopaminergic systems in movement control and the pathophysiology of the basal ganglia. These observations are supported by anatomical evidence demonstrating large serotonergic innervation of all the basal ganglia nuclei. In fact, serotonergic terminals have been reported to make synaptic contacts with both substantia nigra dopamine-containing neurons and their terminal areas such as the striatum, the globus pallidus and the subthalamus. These brain areas contain a high concentration of serotonin (5-HT), with the substantia nigra pars reticulata (SNr) receiving the greatest input. In this review, the distribution of 5-HT different receptor subtypes in the basal ganglia nuclei will be described. Furthermore, evidence demonstrating the serotonergic control of basal ganglia activity will be reviewed, and the contribution of the different 5-HT receptor subtypes examined. The new avenues that the increasing knowledge of 5-HT in motor control has opened for exploring the pathophysiology and pharmacology of Parkinson's disease and other movement disorders will be discussed. It is clear that these avenues will be fruitful, despite the disappointing results so far obtained by clinical studies with selective 5-HT ligands. Nevertheless, these studies have led to a great increase in the attention given to the neurotransmitters of the basal ganglia and their connections.

* Corresponding author: Prof. Giuseppe Di Giovanni, Department of Physiology and Biochemistry, Faculty of Medicine and Surgery, University of Malta. Msida MSD 2080, Malta. Tel.: +356 23402776 (direct) +356 21316655 (department) +356 21310577 (fax); giuseppe.digiovanni@um.edu.mt

Keywords: *serotonergic receptors, basal ganglia, Parkinson's disease, motor disorders, dyskinesia, selective 5-HT drugs.*

Introduction

Since the 1950's, when serotonin (5-HT) was discovered in the mammalian central nervous system (CNS), an enormous amount of experimental evidence has revealed the pivotal role of this biogenic amine in a bewildering diversity of behavioural and physiological processes. This is not surprising, considering the almost ubiquitous distribution of 5-HT-containing axon terminals throughout the CNS, although 5-HT is synthesized by a small group of neurons within the raphe nuclei of the brain stem. Despite this broad axon-terminal domain of 5-HT neurons, a closer examination reveals a preferential targeting of motor areas in the CNS (Steinbusch, 1981). For example, in the rat there is a very dense innervation of the ventral horn of the spinal cord, the motor nucleus of the trigeminal, the facial motor nucleus and all components of the basal ganglia circuitry (Lavoie and Parent, 1990). It is thus likely that 5-HT plays a role in regulating the appropriate selection of voluntary movements by the basal ganglia, and abnormalities in 5-HT transmission might contribute to the neural mechanisms underlying disorders of basal ganglia origin, such as Parkinson's disease (PD), Tourette's syndrome and obsessive compulsive disorder (Ring and Serra-Mestre 2002). Indeed, biochemical evidence suggests that 5-HT transmission is abnormal in the basal ganglia of patients with PD (Hornykiewicz, 1998) and, moreover, in the movement abnormalities generally associated with the use of L-3,4-dihydroxyphenylalanine [levodopa (L-DOPA)] and classical antipsychotic drugs' (APDs) motor side-effects (Blackburn, 2004; Bezard et al., 2001, Di Giovanni et al., 2006a).

During the last decades, advances in the understanding of receptors mediating the effect of 5-HT have represented one of the success stories of neuropharmacology. Many of the 5-HT receptors are found within the basal ganglia and are most likely involved in the modulation of basal ganglia circuitry and in the pathology of their correlated disorders. Of particular interest with respect to the development of new treatments for PD and other motor disorders are the 5-$HT_{1A/B}$ and 5-$HT_{2A/C}$ receptor subtypes. This will be the subject of further discussion in the remainder of this review. First, the 5-HT innervations of the basal ganglia and the distribution of 5-HT receptors throughout the various nuclei will be summarized. Thereafter, several aspects of 5-HT control of pathophysiology of basal ganglia nuclei will be discussed.

Therefore, it is clear that a detailed understanding of the neurotransmitter function in each condition is not merely academic but can lead to a rationale for drug design and treatment strategies appropriate for that group of patients.

Serotonin Innervation of Basala Ganglia

More than fifty years have passed since Twarog and Page (1953) isolated an indole, identified as serotonin (5-HT), in the mammalian brain. Subsequently, Brodie and colleagues (1955) suggested that 5-HT might serve as a neurotransmitter in the CNS.

In vertebrates, the majority of the neurons containing 5-HT are grouped in 9 nuclei named B1 to B9, located in the medial part of the brainstem, generically called the raphe nuclei (Dahlström and Fuxe, 1964). These midline clusters can be divided into two major groups. The caudal or inferior group, localized in the medulla, contains the three nuclei projecting essentially to the grey matter of the spinal cord: the nucleus raphe magnus (NRM, cell group B5), nucleus raphe obscurus (NRO, cell groups B1-B2-B3), and nucleus raphe pallidus (NRP, cell group B4). The rostral or superior group, located in the pons/ mesenchepalon, contains the dorsal raphe nucleus (DRN, cell groups B6 and B7) and the medial raphe nucleus (MRN, cell group B8). These nuclei supply about 80% of the serotonergic innervation to the forebrain. Even if in many brain areas, the innervation coming from the two nuclei overlaps, in certain regions the innervation comes exclusively or prevalently from one nucleus only. For example, the dorsal hippocampus receives a serotonergic innervation only from MRN; other areas innervated preferentially from this nucleus are: the medial preoptic area, the suprachiasmatic nucleus, the olfactory bulb and the medial septum nucleus. The dorsal raphe nucleus innervates all the basal ganglia circuitry, sending projections to the corpus striatum, the globus pallidus (GP), the subthalamic nucleus (STN), substantia nigra (SN) and the pedunculopontino nucleus (PPN), and provides most of the innervation of the prefrontal cortex, including the motor cortices. Serotonin-containing cell bodies of the raphe send projections to both dopamine (DA)-ergic and GABAergic cells in the SN, and to their terminal fields (Moukhles et al., 1997; Van Bockstaele et al., 1993; Hervé et al., 1987). Moreover, electron microscopy demonstrates the presence of synaptic contacts of (^{3}H)5-HT labeled terminals with both dopaminergic and non-dopaminergic dendrites in the SN pars compacta (SNc) and reticulate (SNr) (Hervé et al., 1987; Moukhles et al., 1997; Lee et al., 2000). The DRN innervates, together with the MRN, the ventral part of the hippocampus, the nucleus accumbens and various nuclei of the thalamus, among them the ventral lateral nuclear group that processes motor information and the hippocampus (Azmitia and Segal, 1978; Jacobs and Azmitia, 1992; McQuade and Sharp, 1995). Moreover, extensive serotonergic connections between the DRN and the MRN also exist (Jacobs and Azmitia, 1992).

Serotonin Receptors' Distribution within the Basal Ganglia Nuclei

A vast amount of research has led to the discovery and characterisation of a plethora of 5-HT receptor subtypes. At present, seven classes of 5-HT receptors (5-HT$_{1-7}$ receptors) have been identified which comprise at least a total of 15 subtypes (Hoyer et al, 2002). This is not surprising, since with so many potential targets distributed throughout all the CNS, 5-HT is a major neurotransmitter involved in such a large number of physiological and pathological processes.

The distribution of 5-HT receptors among the various basal ganglia structures has been widely investigated. Autoradiographic, in situ hybridization and binding studies, as well as functional and pharmacological investigations, showed a differential distribution of the various 5-HT receptors subtypes both within the basal ganglia nuclei and between the different mammalian species that were used in these studies (Waeber et al., 1990a).

Strikingly, the described pattern of distribution and expression of these receptors is modified in the animal model of pathologies involving basal ganglia circuitry as well as in human patients. Nevertheless, this could be no more than an epiphenomenal effect.

Striatum

High concentrations of both receptors mRNA and protein of different 5-HT receptor subtypes have been found in the striatum of various species.

5-HT_{1A} was one of the first serotonin receptor subtypes that was identified and pharmacologically characterized and its distribution among different species of mammals has been widely investigated. So far, most of receptor autoradiography, radioimmunohistochemistry and *in situ* hybridization studies have reported low or barely detectable levels of labelling for both 5-HT_{1A} receptor protein and mRNA in the caudate-putamen of the rat (Miquel et al., 1991; Riad et al., 1991; Kung et al., 1995; Wright et al., 1995), mouse (Schiller et al., 2003) and primate brain (Mengod et al., 1996). The same regional distribution has been found in the caudate and putamen nuclei of human brain using *post-mortem* radiolabelling and *in vivo* PET with various radio tracers (Pike et al., 1995; Pasqualetti et al., 1996; Hall et al., 1997; Duncan et al., 1998; Ito et al., 1999). However, a recent study reported a patchy distribution of 5-HT_{1A} receptors confined to striosomes of the primate striatum characterized by poor calbindin immunostaining. In these compartments, the receptor density was equal to other enriched brain areas, such as some hippocampal fields, and it was increased in a 1-methyl 4-phenyl 1,2,3,6-tetrahydropyridine (MPTP)-lesioned primate model of Parkinson's disease, suggesting a key role for this receptor subtype in the control of movement by the basal ganglia (Frechilla, 2001).

The 5-HT_{1B} receptor subtype localization in the striatum has been widely demonstrated in various mammal brains. In rats and mice, early [^{3}H]5-HT binding studies, using selective ligands as displacing agents for the 5-HT_{1A} receptors subtype, showed intermediate to low concentration of 5-HT_{1B} binding or immunoreactivity sites in the caudate-putamen (Pazos and Palacios, 1985; Blurton and Wood, 1986; Verge et al., 1986; Waeber et al., 1989; Middlemiss and Hutson, 1990; Sari et al., 1999). In a first attempt to characterize the distribution of 5-HT receptors in the brain of different mammal species, autoradiographic data seemed to indicate a lack in cats, guinea-pigs, monkeys and humans, of receptors with a similar pharmacological profile to the rat and mouse 5-HT_{1B} (Hoyer et al., 1986; Pazos et al., 1987a; Waeber et al., 1989). Similarities in the 5-HT_{1D} brain distribution in these species to that of 5-HT_{1B} in rats and mice led to the hypothesis that these two receptors subtypes were species homologues (Waeber et al., 1989; del Arco et al., 1993). Subsequent findings, relative to the molecular cloning of 5-HT_1 receptor subtypes, showed the presence in human brains of two genes expressing different receptors displaying the pharmacology of the originally described 5-HT_{1D} sites, named 5-$HT_{1D\alpha}$ and 5-$HT_{1D\beta}$ (77% sequence homology in the transmembrane domain), the latter of which (5-$HT_{1D\beta}$) showed a 96% homology to the cloned rodent 5-HT_{1B} receptor. Following this new experimental evidence, the 5-$HT_{1B/1D}$ receptor nomenclature underwent a reassessment (for reviews see Barnes and Sharp, 1999; Hoyer et al., 2002). According to the new classification, comparative studies showed binding sites for this receptor, as well as high hybridization signals for its mRNA, in the caudate-putament of rodent brain (Bruinvels et al., 1994; Bonaventure et al., 1998) and in the corresponding caudate and putamen in humans (Varnas et al., 2001, 2005); moreover, some authors showed a dorsoventral gradient in the distribution of both this receptor and its mRNA, with higher levels in the ventral as compared to the dorsal striatum (Compan et al., 1998; Varnas et al., 2001, 2005) in both rats and humans. According to the authors, this evidence, together with the complete lack of mRNA in both the SN and ventral pallidum, seems to indicate a localization of the 5-HT$_{1B}$ receptor subtype on axon terminals arising from medium spiny neurons of the ventral striatal regions, thus confirming previous immunoreactivity and in situ hybridization studies in mouse and rat brain (Boschert et al., 1994; Sari et al., 1999). On the other hand, binding sites in the striatum may reflect both a somatodentritic and presynaptic localization of this receptor on striatal neurons (projection neurons and/or interneurons) or on thalamic/cortical afferents respectively (Bonaventure et al., 1998).

The presence of 5-HT$_{1D}$ (namely 5-HT$_{1D\alpha}$) receptor and mRNA in the striatum of rodents, primates and humans has been reported, even if weaker levels of both protein binding and hybridization signals were observed with respect to the 5-HT$_{1B}$ (Bruinvels et al., 1993a). Similarly to 5-HT$_{1B}$ receptors, some authors described a discrepancy in the distribution pattern of 5-HT$_{1D}$ mRNA and its protein in mouse brain between the striatum, SN and GP hypothesizing, therefore, a presynaptic localization of 5-HT$_{1D}$ receptors in the last two areas (Boschert et al., 1994). Finally, regarding the 5-HT$_1$ receptor family, Bruinvels et al. (1993b) reported the presence of the 5-HT$_{1E}$ receptor subtype mRNA, in both the caudate nucleus and putamen of primate, showing stronger hybridization signals in monkey brain than that obtained in human brain.

Both 5-HT$_{2A}$ receptor subtype and its mRNA have been extensively demonstrated to be present in the striatum of various mammal species. Moreover, the described distribution pattern showed increasing gradients for this receptor in the rostrocaudal and mediolateral directions (Pazos et al., 1985; Pazos et al., 1987b; Mengod et al., 1990; Pompeiano et al., 1994; Wright et al., 1995; Lopez-Gimenez et al., 1997). In human brain, using the high affinity radioligand [^{3}H]MDL 100907, high density of labelling has been shown to be distributed in patches throughout the caudate nucleus and putamen (Lopez-Gimenez et al., 1999). Regarding cellular distribution, the 5-HT$_{2A}$ receptors showed a somatodendritic localization, as demonstrated also by the correlation between the distribution of 5-HT$_{2A}$ protein and its mRNA (Cornea-Hébert, 1999). Furthermore, a more prominent localization in dendrites than in cell bodies was found in the dorsolateral caudate-putamen of rat brain using immocytochemistry (Rodríguez, 1999).

A number of studies have demonstrated a widespread distribution 5-HT$_{2C}$ receptor subtype in rat, monkey and human brains, particularly among the different basal ganglia structures. Moreover, marked differences have been revealed in the distribution of 5-HT$_{2C}$ mRNA and its level of expression within the different subregions of the basal ganglia (Hoffman and Mezey, 1989; Mengod et al., 1990; Wright et al., 1995; Eberle-Wang et al., 1997). Most labelled neurons in the striatum were efferent medium-sized neurons but not cholinergic interneurons, although recently PCR evidence revealed instead high expression of 5-HT$_{2C}$, 5-HT$_6$, and 5-HT$_7$ mRNAs in cholinergic interneurons (Bonsi et al., 2007).

Neurons expressing 5-HT$_{2C}$ mRNA have been found in discrete areas of the caudate-putamen showing no preferential localization with either substance P, dynorphine or enkephalin, thus indicating that 5-HT$_{2C}$ receptors are not differentially expressed on the two major striatal output pathways (striatonigral and striatopallidal projection neurons). On the other hand, with regard to patch/matrix striatal structures, 5-HT$_{2C}$ mRNA showed a preferential localization in the patch compartment areas, suggesting a role for this receptor in the modulation of striatal projections to the SNc (Gerfen, 1984, 1985; Ward and Dorsa, 1996).

Using various radioligands, some authors have reported the presence of 5-HT_3 receptors in the striatum of different mammals, albeit higher receptor densities have been found in the human caudate nucleus and putamen than in the correspondent structures of the rat brain (Barnes et al., 1990; Gehlert et al., 1991; Laporte, 1992; Abi-Dargham et al., 1993; Bufton et al., 1993; Parker et al., 1996; Morales, 1998; Fletcher and Barnes, 1999; Marazziti et al., 2001). Binding studies on homogenates of human putamen suggested a localization of these receptors on neurons that have their cell bodies within this region, such as GABAergic projection neurons, and not on DAergic neurons. Indeed, patients with diagnosed Huntington's disease showed decreased binding densities in the striatum, unlike those affected by DAergic cell loss associated with Parkinson's disease (Steward et al., 1993). Moreover, as for other brain areas, data obtained using synaptosomes isolated from rat striatum showed the presence in this area of functional presynaptic 5-HT_3 receptors, besides the known postsynaptic localization (Nichols and Mollard, 1996; Ronde and Nichols, 1998; Nayak et al., 1999).

Analysis of the distribution of the 5-HT_4 receptor showed its presence in several components of the basal ganglia of different mammal species. Generally, the distribution pattern of 5-HT_4 receptor binding sites in the striatum matched that observed for its mRNA in all the different species used in binding and *in situ* hybridization studies. However, some species' differences have been shown. Thus, a ventromedial to dorsolateral increasing gradients of labelling densities have been observed in the rat and mouse brain caudate-putamen (Waeber et al., 1994; Vilaro et al., 1996), while it was less pronounced in the same structure of guinea-pig brain; similarly, monkey and human caudate nucleus and putamen showed very high densities of receptor and mRNA binding sites but without any apparent gradient in their distribution (Bonaventure et al., 2000; Vilaro et al., 2005). The decrease in binding densities following selective lesion of rat caudate-putamen indicated a somato-dendritic localization of 5-HT_4 receptors on GABAergic projection neuron and on cholinergic/GABAergic interneurons in this structure; on the other hand, following 6-hydroxydopamine (6-OHDA) lesion of nigrostriatal pathway there were no changes in striatal levels of receptor binding, clearly indicating that this receptor is not localized on DAergic terminals (Compan et al., 1996; Vilaro et al., 2005). These data are in agreement with *post-mortem* studies on brains of patients with Huntington's or PD showing a decrease in receptor binding only in the first group of patients (Reynolds et al., 1995; Vilaro et al., 2005).

Only moderate to low expression of 5-HT_{5A} receptor protein and mRNA has been found in the striatum of mouse, rat and human brain (Boess and Martin, 1994; Rees et al., 1994; Wesolowska, 2002). In particular, 5-HT_{5A} immunoreactivity was detectable at low levels in medium spiny neurons of rat caudate-putamen (Oliver et al., 2000).

On the other hand, the 5-HT_6 receptor subtype has been shown to be particularly abundant in this area of the basal ganglia. High levels of both protein and mRNA expression have been found in the caudate-putamen of the rat and pig brain (Monsma et al., 1993; Ruat et al., 1993a; Ward et al., 1995; Kohen et al., 1996; Yoshioka et al., 1998; Hirst et al., 2000) as well as in the caudate nucleus and putamen of human brain (Kohen et al., 1996; Hirst et al., 2003), thus demonstrating a similar distribution pattern for this receptor in the brain of these species. In contrast, only low levels of both 5-HT_6 receptor protein and mRNA have been found in the same brain areas of two different strains of mice (Hirst et al., 2003). As the regional distribution of 5-HT$_6$ receptor generally matched that found for the 5-HT$_6$ receptor mRNA, it is likely that the former is mainly localized on somas and/or dendrites of neurons. This conclusion is further supported by light and electron microscopy immunoreactivity data clearly showing the localization of this receptor on dendritic processes of spiny neurons in the striatum (Gerard et al., 1997; Hamon et al., 1999). Finally, selective lesion of 5-HT neurons by injection of 5,7-dihydroxytryptamine in the DRN has been shown to not affect levels of 5-HT$_6$ mRNA in the striatum of rat brain, thus confirming the postsynaptic localization of this receptor with respect to 5-HT neurons innervating this area (Gerard et al., 1996) Similarly, the lack of any difference in the levels of protein binding following 6-OHDA selective lesion of the nigrostriatal pathway demonstrated that the 5-HT$_6$ is also not located on membranes of dopamine neurons (Roberts et al., 2002).

Finally, the presence of the 5-HT$_7$ receptor subtype has been reported in the *striatum* of rodents as well as in the caudate nucleus and putamen of human brain with a protein distribution pattern generally matching that of its mRNA. In addition, some species' differences in receptor densities were reported between human and rodent brain (Ruat et al., 1993b; Wesolowska, 2002; Martin-Cora and Pazos, 2004; Varnas et al., 2004).

Substantia Nigra and Globus Pallidus

Very low levels of binding have been found in the SN or GP of mouse, rat and human brain for both 5-HT$_{1A}$ receptor protein and its mRNA (Khawaja, 1995; Kung et al., 1995; Wright et al., 1995; Hall et al., 1997; Schiller et al., 2003). Interestingly, some authors showed high binding of ^{3}H-zolpidem in the rat SN in contrast to low binding observed in the same region of human brain (Duncan et al., 1998). By contrast, among the basal ganglia nuclei, the highest levels of 5-HT$_{1B}$ protein bindings were found in both SN and GP of different mammal species. Unlike the striatum, in situ hybridization studies failed to reveal the presence of 5-HT$_{1B}$ mRNA in these structures. Taken together, therefore, these data seem to suggest a presynaptic localization of this receptor subtype, presumably on terminals of striatal afferents (Pazos et al., 1987a; Boschert et al., 1994; Bruinvels et al., 1994; Bonaventure et al., 1998; Sari et al., 1999; Varnas et al., 2001, 2005), where it acts as heteroreceptor (Barnes and Sharp, 1999). Moreover, the levels of 5-HT$_{1B}$ binding sites in these areas after selective lesion of nigral dopaminergic cells or striatal neurons, as well as radioligand studies on post mortem human brain of patients who had suffered degenerative movement disorders, clearly demonstrate the localization of this receptor on striatonigral and striatopallidal GABAergic afferents (Waeber et al., 1990b; Castro et al., 1998; Compan et al., 1998). Similarly to the 5-HT$_{1B}$ subtype, radiolabelled sites fot 5-HT$_{1D}$ receptors were found in these structures, despite of the lower densities as compared to the previous receptor (partially due to the lack of specific radioligand), while in situ hybridization studies showed a lack of its mRNA (Bruinvels et al., 1993a, 1994). Again, these data, together with receptor and mRNA distribution in the striatum previously reported, are in line with a putative localization on axon terminals in these areas.

Regarding the 5-HT$_2$ family, intermediate levels of 5-HT$_{2A}$ receptor mRNA were found in the SNc, SNr and *pars lateralis* of rat brain (Mengod et al., 1990; Pompeiano et al., 1994; Wright et al., 1995). Regarding receptor distribution, as mentioned above, there is a general concordance between the distribution of 5-HT_{2A} protein and its mRNA. Early studies found high concentrations of [^{3}H]ketanserin binding in the SNc and SNr in rats while only very low concentrations for this receptor have been showed in the GP (Pazos et al., 1985; Pazos et al., 1987b). Nevertheless, some recent immunohistochemistry and autoradiography studies found lower levels of 5-HT_{2A} receptors expressed in these areas (Cornea-Hébert, 1999; Lopez-Gimenez et al., 1999; Bubser et al., 2001). These discrepancies in receptor concentrations in the SN could be explained by the use in previous studies of some radioligands such as [^{3}H]ketanserin that has been shown to have a high affinity for non-serotoninergic sites, as well as its known selectivity for the 5-HT_2 receptor family (Lopez-Gimenez et al., 1997). Finally, the presence of this receptor subtype in the GP of rat brain has been confirmed by recent immunohistochemistry data showing that about 70% of neurons expressing the 5-HT_{2A} receptor project to the striatum (Bubser et al., 2001). Neither 5-HT_{2C} mRNA nor receptor protein has been found in the globus pallidus or in the entopeduncular nucleus (EPN) while neurons showing labelling for this receptor have been found in both the SNc and SNr. Furthermore, the distribution pattern of the 5-HT_{2C} in this area showed a marked rostro-caudal labelling gradient, characterized by higher receptor densities in caudal regions of both nuclear subdivisions. Finally, with regard to cellular localization, receptor expression seems to be confined to GABAergic neurons but not to DAergic cell bodies (Van Bockstaele et al., 1994; Van Bockstaele and Pickel, 1995; Steffensen et al., 1998; Di Giovanni et al., 2001).

The 5-HT_3 receptor subtype has been detected by membrane binding essays and immunolabeling in the SN of both rat and human brain (Laporte, 1992; Bufton et al., 1993; Gehlert et al., 1993; Doucet et al., 1999). Nevertheless, only lightly detectable receptor densities have been shown for this area.

The presence of 5-HT_4 receptor protein, but not its mRNA, has been reported in both the GP and SN of different mammal species, with the highest densities in the latter area, thus supporting the idea of a localization of this receptor on striatopallidal and striatonigral terminals (Compan et al., 1996; Ullmer et al., 1996; Vilaro et al., 1996; Bonaventure et al., 2000). Moreover, 5-HT_4 receptor binding sites in the rat SN were confined to the *pars lateralis* while in guinea pig brain a wider distribution was observed in the same area, with most of the SNr being strongly labelled (Waeber et al., 1994; Vilaro et al., 2005); in human and monkey brain, the distribution pattern resembled that of guinea pig brain.

Finally, with regards to the last three serotonin receptor families, only moderate to low concentrations of both receptor proteins and mRNA have been found in the SN and GP of rat and human brain for the 5-HT_{5A} (Rees et al., 1994; Oliver et al., 2000), 5-HT_6 (Kohen et al., 1996; Gerard et al., 1997; Hamon et al., 1999; Roberts et al., 2002; Hirst et al., 2003) and the 5-HT_7 (Ruat et al., 1993b; Martin-Cora and Pazos, 2004; Varnas et al., 2004) receptors subtypes.

Subthalamic Nucleus

So far, little evidence exists regarding the presence of moderate to low concentrations of 5-HT_{1A}, 5-HT_4, 5-HT_5 and 5-HT_6 receptors and/or their mRNA in the STN (*Pompeiano et al., 1992*). By contrast, high hybridization signals were found for both 5-HT_{1B} and 5-HT_{2C} receptors mRNA in the rodent brain (Bruinvels et al., 1994; Eberle-Wang et al., 1997).

Serotonin Modulation of Basala Ganglia Circuitry

The 5-HT modulates dopaminergic nigrostriatal function, in term of control of DA SNc neurons firing discharge and DA release in the striatum (see Alex and Pehek, 2007).

Serotonin Modulation of Striatal Activity

In agreement with anatomical data, most of the reports on this subject indicate that striatal cells are predominantly affected by dorsal raphe stimulation, the median raphe stimulation being unable to alter striatal cell activity directly (olpe and koella, 1977; Davies and Tongroach, 1978). In addition, it has been found that suppression of spontaneous firing activity is the main response of cultured striatal cells (yakel et al., 1988) and *in vivo* following dorsal raphe stimulation, excitation being observed in only about 10% of them. Nevertheless, a rebound excitation was observed in some cells that were initially inhibited. Local application of 5-ht was found to produce similar changes to that caused by raphe stimulation and most of the cells responsive to the raphe stimulation were also affected by nigral stimulation (Davies and Tongroach, 1978). However, using intracellular recording techniques, Kitai and co-workers (Vandermaelen et al., 1979) found that dorsal raphe stimulation was consistently capable of generating excitatory postsynaptic potentials. These findings were subsequently repeated in the kitai laboratory, and it was indicated that non-5-ht dorsal raphe-striatal neurons could be involved in striatal responses to 5-HT. They also showed that the increase of the firing frequency in rat neostriatal medium-spiny neurons induced by 5-ht depended on reducing voltage-dependent potassium currents (Park et al., 1982; Stefani et al., 1990; Wilms et al., 2001).

Stimulation of postsynaptic 5-HT$_{1A}$ receptors by 8-OHDPAT induced an increase in locomotor activity (Mignon and Wolf, 2002). Moreover, Gerber et al. (1988) and Matsubara et al. (2006) reported that 5-HT$_{1A}$ receptor stimulation has an anti-Parkinsonian effect in 6-OHDA lesioned rats, inducing a robust contralateral rotational behavior. Current theories of circling behaviour hypothesize that the animal turns away from the basal ganglia output, where activity has been reduced. Moreover, the stimulation of 5-HT$_{1A}$ receptors has been shown to be capable of inducing controlateral-rotation also following degeneration of DRN (Blackburn et al., 1984; Gerber et al. 1988). This rotational behaviour has been explained by a supersensitivity of 5-HT$_{1A}$ receptors in the snc of the DA lesioned rats, resulting in an increase of DA in the striatum (Blackburn et al., 1984; Gerber et al. 1988). In agreement with this theory, tandospirone, a highly potent and selective 5-HT$_{1A}$ receptor agonist, remarkably potentiated the contralateral turning induced by apomorphine (Matsubara et al., 2006). Nevertheless, it has been shown that 8-OHDPAT can also induce ipsilateral turning in unilateral 6-OHDA-lesioned rats (Mignon and Wolf, 2002, 2007).

The discrepancies notwithstanding, these findings are valuable in demonstrating the potential utility of drugs that possess 5-HT$_{1A}$ in the symptomatic treatment of PD. The 5-HT$_{1A}$ agonists might inhibit 5-HT release acting presynaptically (Gerber et al., 1988) or have a postsynaptic action (Lucas et al., 1997; Matsubara et al., 2006) decreasing striatal glutamate release from corticofugal projections, without involving direct activation of D_2 receptors (Antonelli et al., 2005; Mignon and Wolf 2005, 2007). Similarly, WAY100135, increased glutamate outflow in the striatum of rats (Dijk et al., 1995). These findings suggest that 5-HT_{1A} receptor stimulation could give rise to a decrease in the corticofugal glutamate drive (e.g., to the striatum or subthalamic nucleus) that could ultimately be manifested as decreased activation of the output nuclei of the basal ganglia (medial globus pallidus and substantia nigra pars reticulata). A reduction in excitatory drive to these output nuclei would lead to a disinhibition of the motor thalamus, thereby ameliorating the motor deficits of PD (Mignon and Wolf, 2007). These results suggest that 5-HT_{1A} agonists could have therapeutic potential for the treatment of PD by modulating neuronal activities of non-dopaminergic pathways, such as the excitatory amino acid pathways in the basal ganglia.

Serotonin released from 5-HT-ergic terminals in the striatum exerts a negative feedback on its own neuronal activity via 5-HT_{1B} auto-receptors, as well as of 5-HT_{1A}. Indeed, stimulation of 5-HT_{1B} receptors, localised on the terminals of 5-HT neurons, reduced 5-HT release and also modulated L-DOPA metabolism to DA in the striatum (Knobelman et al., 2000; Carta et al., 2007). Several *in vivo* electrophysiological and neurochemical studies suggest an important role of the 5-HT_{1B} receptor in modulating the activity of mesostriatal DA-ergic neurons. Indeed, 5-HT_{1B} receptor stimulation enhances striatal DA-ergic activity, generally attributed to an inhibition of GABA release and a consequent disinhibition of DA neuronal activity (see Di Matteo et al. 2008). Rats with unilateral DR lesions showed contralateral turning in response to the putative $5HT_{1B}$ agonist RU 24969, while a much weaker effect in 6-OHDA-lesioned rats was revealed (Gerber et al., 1988). 5-HT_{1A} and 5-HT_{1B} receptors appear to act synergistically in reducing 5-HT transmission in the basal ganglia and it is important to note that low doses of agonists for these receptors are able to suppress dyskinesia, without affecting the anti-Parkinsonian effect of L-DOPA in the presence of spared dopamine terminals, suggesting an early use of these drugs to counteract the development of dyskinesia in PD patients (Carta et al., 2007).

The 5-HT_2 family has been intensively investigated in the striatum. Compelling data by blier and colleagues (el mansari et al., 1994; el mansari and blier, 1997) concerning single-unit recordings coupled with microiontophoresis *in vivo*, in rats, guinea pigs and in 5-HT_{2C} receptor mutant mice, support the hypothesis of an inhibitory action of the 5-HT system on the neuronal activity of the striatum [presumably striatal medium spiny projection neurons (MSNS)] that trough the activation of 5-HT_2 receptors. These authors investigated only in the head of the caudate nucleus and reported an inhibitory effect of 5-HT, mimicked by the 5-HT_{2A} receptor agonist doi and the 5-HT_{2C} receptor agonist m-CPP (El Mansari et al., 1994; El Mansari and Blier, 1997). It is noteworthy that significantly less quisqualate was required to activate neurons in the caudate nucleus of 5-HT_2 mutant mice than in the wild-type mice, suggesting that 5-HT_{2C} receptors serve a tonic inhibitory role in membrane excitability (rueter et al., 2000). Strikingly, neither the selective 5-HT_{2A} agonist mdl 100907 nor clozapine antagonized doi or m-CPP in the caudate nucleus in mice. The authors suggested that doi and m-CPP might be acting in the caudate nucleus through an atypical 5-HT_2 receptor yet to be characterized, and hypothesis that has not been investigated by successive studies. More likely, this lack of antagonism depends on the pharmacological design of the experiments. Indeed, in rats, El Mansari and Blier (1997) showed that the inhibitory effect of doi, but not that of mCPP, was antagonized by a 4-day treatment with metergoline and ritanserin, indicating that the suppressant effect of doi may be mediated by 5-HT_{2A} receptors in the head of the caudate nucleus. Contrary evidence has been shown by an *in vivo* study in which only excitation of the striatal neurons induced by microintophoretical application of 5-HT was revealed, while the DOI caused a preferential inhibitory response, highlighting diverse effects of 5-HT in different parts of the stiatum (wilms et al., 2001).

Recently, the role of serotonergic control on striatal cholinergic interneurons has been explored *in vitro* (Blomeley and Bracci, 2005; Bonsi et al., 2007a). Striatal acetylcholine (ACh), and its interplay with DA has long been recognized as playing a crucial role in voluntary movement (Duvoisin, 1967). In the striatum, ACh is mainly released by a population of large aspiny interneurons (LAIS) (Phelps et al., 1985; Zhou et al., 2002; Tepper and Bolam, 2004). Pakhotin and Bracci (2007) have shown that LAIS exerted a strong inhibitory control over the neighboring striatal MSNS via inhibition of their glutamatergic input. These effects are presynaptic and mediated by both M_2 and M_3 muscarinic receptors, both present on corticostriatal terminals. Serotonin strongly and reversibly increased LAIS spontaneous firing rates *in vitro* via a reversible reduction of two pharmacologically and kinetically distinct after-hyperpolarizations (AHPS) that play an important role in limiting the excitability of cholinergic interneurons (Blomeley and Bracci, 2005). Blomeley and Bracci (2005), furthermore, showed that 5-HT_2 receptors were responsible for the excitatory effects of serotonin in cholinergic interneurons, although they could not identify the 5-HT receptor subtype involved since they used α-methyl-5-HT and ketanserin, highly unspecific ligands. Recently, Bonsi et al., (2007a) managed to rule out the role of 5-HT_{2A} showing that only the pretreatment with the selective 5-HT_{2C} antagonist RS 102221 caused a significant reduction in the 5-HT-induced depolarization of cholinergic interneurons. This evidence was strongly supported by PCR analysis data showing that the 5-HT_{2C} receptors are expressed by about 80% of lais in contrast to a sporadic expression of the 5-HT_{2A} subtypes. Accordingly, the response of striatal cholinergic interneurons to the 5-HT was partially blocked by phospholipase C (PLC) inhibitor, the transduction pathways linked to the 5-HT_{2C} receptor subtypes. Thus, 5-HT induces cell depolarization and increase in firing frequency acting through postsynaptic 5-HT_{2C} receptors, probably causing inhibition of K^+ currents, or increase of a cationic conductance in striatal cholinergic interneurons. In light of these recent results, 5-HT_{2C} agonists might reduce striatal msns activity indirectly via an increase of the inhibitory cholinergic tone. Moreover, 5-HT_6 and 5-HT_7 receptor subtypes are also involved on 5-HT potent excitatory effect but not on that of 5-HT_3 and 5-HT_4 (Bonsi et al., 2007a). Therefore, modulating the activity of cholinergic striatal interneurons by 5-HT_{2C}, 5-HT_6 or 5-HT_7 receptors may have positive therapeutic benefits for motor diseases.

In concordance with these inhibitory 5-HT effects on MSNs through the activation of 5-HT_{2C} receptors, there is the behavioural evidence that caudate injections of 5-HT provoked contraversive turning, while conversely, intracaudate methysergide induced ipsiversive circling (James and Starr, 1980). In addition, the facilitation by hyoscine and the attenuation by eserine of the 5-HT induced contraversive circling, together with the converse effects of these drugs on methysergide-evoked ipsiversive rotations, are consistent with raphe-caudate 5-HT fibres synapsing directly with, and exciting, striatal cholinergic neurons. Given that motor behaviour recruits multiple striatal neurotransmitter systems, recent attention has focused on the interaction between DA and 5-HT receptors. In the intact striatum, several studies have consistently demonstrated that intrinsic 5-HT_2 receptors can modify DA function, and have postulated divergent roles for 5-HT_{2A} and 5-HT_{2C} receptor subtypes (Lucas et al., 2000; Porras et al., 2002). 5-HT_{2A} antagonists reduce hyperlocomotion induced by cocaine, amphetamine and 3,4-methylenedioxymethyamphetamine (MDMA) (Kehne et al., 1996; O'Neill et al., 1999), whereas, 5-HT_{2C} receptor antagonists have been shown to enhance or reduce these effects depending upon which compounds and neuronal sites are studied (Filip and Cunningham, 2002; Fletcher et al., 2002; Filip et al., 2004). Recent studies from Walker's group have shown that following DA depletion D1-induced locomotor activity can be reduced by antagonism of striatal 5-HT$_{2A}$, but not 5-HT$_{2C}$ receptors (Bishop et al., 2005). This preferential involvement of the 5-HT$_{2A}$ subtype is confirmed by the evidence that intrastriatal injections of the selective 5-HT$_{2C}$ antagonist RS 102221 had no effect on motor activity, conversely the 5-HT$_{2A}$ agonist DOI induced motor behaviour in neonate 6-OHDA-lesioned rats which was attenuated by the 5-HT$_{2A}$ receptor antagonism (Bishop et al., 2004).

Interestingly, recent pharmacological data and lesion studies have established that the biosynthesis of neuropeptides in the striatum is regulated by the 5-HT innervation originating from the DRN suggesting that 5-HT in the striatum might exert a metabolic regulatory function on the biosynthesis of neuropeptides rather than acting as an ion channel modulator (D'Addario et al., 2007; Horner et al., 2005).

Serotonin Modulation of Substantia Nigra Pars Reticulata Activity

The SNr neurons receive the largest 5-HT innervation from the DRN of all brain regions (Fibiger and Miller, 1977; Corvaja et al., 1993), and express a high level of 5-HT receptors which are both post-synaptic and located on the somato-dendritic region of SNr neurons and post-synaptic on terminals of SNr inputs. It has been calculated that the density of 5-HT-immunoreactive varicosities in the SNr is in the order of $9x10^6/mm^3$, of which about 74% form synaptic specializations with GABAergic projection neurons (Moukhles et al., 1997). This picture gives an idea of the great influence that 5-HT could exert on the activity of SNr neurons. Early studies have revealed a primarily inhibitory action of serotonin on SNr neurons. Electrical stimulation of the DRN caused mostly inhibitory responses in the SNr, as measured by single-unit extracellular recording *in vivo* (Fibiger and Miller, 1977). Similarly, the iontophoresis of 5-HT into the SN produced mixed, although mostly inhibitory, effects in the SNr (Dray et al., 1976; Collingridge et al., 1981). The inhibition of SNr neurons by 5-HT is supported by the finding that unilateral injection of 5-HT, 5-HT$_{1D}$ agonist, and SSRIs, into the SNr of freely moving rats elicited a contraversive circling behaviour (James and Starr, 1980; Oberlander et al., 1981; Blackburn et al., 1981; Higgins et al., 1991; Bata-Garcia et al., 2002) as muscimol does (Oberlander et al., 1981). In spite of this evidence, Lacey and co-workers have shown, by using *in vitro* electrophysiological methods, that 5-HT not only excites SNr neurons directly but also disinhibits them by reducing GABA release from striotonigral terminals acting on presynaptic 5-HT$_{1B}$ receptors (Rick et al., 1995; Stanford and Lacey, 1996). On the other hand, a subsequent electrophysiological *in vitro* study, demonstrated also a direct inhibitory action of 5-HT on SNr neurons (Góngora-Alfaro et al., 1997). 5-HT and the 5-HT-uptake inhibitor duloxetine reduced the firing rate of the majority of SNr neurons recorded, suggesting that synaptically released endogenous 5-HT act directly on 5-HT$_{1B}$ receptors located in these neurons, in that agonists that mimicked that effect were only of the 5-HT$_{1B}$-class (CP 93129 and TFMPP). Neither the 5-HT$_2$-antagonist ritanserin nor the GABA$_A$-antagonist, bicuculline were able to block that inhibition, suggesting that, in addition to an indirect action (Stanford and Lacey, 1996), some SNr neurons may be directly inhibited by 5-HT.

The 5-HT-induced excitation observed in the majority of the SNr neurons recorded is most probably mediated by a direct action on 5-HT_2 receptors being blocked by ketanserin and ritanserin and mimicked by α-methyl-5-HT, unselective antagonists and agonist of the 5-HT_2 receptor subtype, respectively (Rick et al., 1995; Stanford and Lacey, 1996). In addition, Góngora-Alfaro and colleagues' *in vitro* study revealed that 5-HT can excite about half of SNr neurons tested; this effect was seen in the neurons and blocked by methysergide, thus confirming the involvement of 5-HT_2 receptors (Gongora-Alfaro et al., 1997). The above experimental evidence, although underlining a pivotal role for the 5-HT_2 receptor subtype in the modulation of SNr neurons, does not discriminate the involvement of different subtypes. We have tried to answer this question, and consistent with the aforementioned evidence, we showed that selective 5-HT_{2C} activation excites SNr neurons *in vivo* (Di Giovanni et al., 2001, Invernizzi et al., 2007). This effect was evident both after systemic administration and local microiontophoretic application of m-CPP, RO 60-0175 (Di Giovanni et al., 2001; Invernizzi et al., 2007). As further confirmation of a selective activation of 5-HT_{2C} receptors, m-CPP and RO 60-0175 excitatory effects were blocked by pretretment with SB 242084 and SB 243213, two potent and selective 5-HT_{2C} antagonists. An interesting finding of our first study was the differential effect exerted by mCPP on subpopulations of SNr neurons. Thus, mCPP caused a marked excitation of the so-called P(0) non-DA neurons in the SNr, whereas it did not affect the P(+) neurons. These neurons are identified on the basis of the presence P(+) or the absence P(0) of an excitatory response to a noxious stimulus (footpinch). There is evidence that P(+) neurons in the SNr are GABAergic interneurons that exert a direct inhibitory influence on DA neurons in the SNc, whereas P(0) cells represent SNr projection neurons. Thus, mCPP caused a marked excitation of presumed SNr projection neurons but did not modify the SNr interneurons firing discharge (Di Giovanni et al., 2001). These data have been confirmed using RO 600175, the most selective agonist to date, that caused excitation only in half of SNr neurons recorded, although no information about the territory of their innervations was investigated (Invernizzi et al., 2007). Nevertheless, it is most likely that the SNr neurons excited by the 5-HT_{2C} agonist RO 600175 are the P(0) projecting neurons that responded to m-CPP treatment (Di Giovanni et al., 2001) Consistent with these electrophysiological data, both systemic and intranigral administration of RO 60-0175 and m-CPP, markedly increased extracellular GABA levels in the SNr, while glutamate levels were not affected. The stimulatory effect of systemic and local RO 60-0175 on GABA release was dependent on ongoing neuronal activity (TTX sensitive) and completely prevented by systemic administration of SB 243213. On the other hand, local application of SB 243213 into the SNr only partially blocked RO 60-0175-induced GABA release. This suggests that the control exerted by 5-HT_{2C} receptors on extracellular GABA in the SNr involves both intra- and extra-nigral components, such as the striotonigral pathway (Invernizzi et al., 2007). Based on our *in vivo* (Di Giovanni et al., 2001; Invernizzi et al., 2007) and *in vitro* (Rick et al., 1995; Stanford and Lacey, 1996; Gongora-Alfaro et al., 1997) evidence it is possible to speculate that 5-HT released *in vivo* elicits a direct excitatory response in a discrete population of SNr neurons, probably resulting in the expression of 5-HT_{2C}, which in turn inhibits a greater number of neighbouring SNr cells through GABA release from their extensive axon collaterals (Mailly et al., 2003; Invernizzi 2007). The source of GABA in the SNr might have, therefore, many different origins: i.e., it might derive from a subpopulation of GABAergic neurons in the SNr that are excited by 5-HT_{2C} agonists and from release of GABA by the somatodendritic regions and their recurrent collaterals; and/or from the GPe neurons excited, in turn, by the STN. We can exclude a striatal GABA source since its neurons are principally inhibited by 5-HT_{2C} receptor agonists.

The overall effect of activation of 5-HT_{2C} receptors, therefore, would be the overinhibition of nigrothalamic GABAergic neurons and consequent decrease of GABA levels in the motor thalamus. According to the current model of basal ganglia functional organization (DeLong et al., 1990), reduction of the subthalamonigral GLUergic excitatory drive and/or increase of the GABAergic inhibitory influence on nigrothalamic GABAergic neurons lead to disinhibition of thalamocortical GLUergic projections and movement initiation (Deniau and Chevalier, 1985). Thus, drugs acting at 5-HT receptors might be useful in treating akinesia and other Parkinsonian symptoms characterized by an overactivity of the nigral-thalamic pathway (Deniau and Chevalier, 1985; DeLong et al., 1990).

Strikingly, under physiological conditions, 5-HT_{2C} receptors do not exert any tonic control upon the basal ganglia activity, although blocking these receptors in the striatum leads to an increase of DA release. Indeed, there is evidence that a number of selective 5-HT_{2C} antagonists, i.e. SB 200646A, SB 206553 and SB 242084, do not elicit locomotory activity when given alone (Kennett et al., 1994; Kennett et al., 1996; Kennett et al., 1997). Moreover, intranigral infusion of the antagonist SB 206553 into the SNr on the unlesioned side of a 6-OHDA-lesioned rat did not elicit a significant rotational response (Fox et al., 1998).

On the other hand, it has been shown that 5-HT_{2C} receptor transmission may be a key determinant in the activity of SNr in Parkinsonism basal ganglia. Accordingly, infusion of SB 206553 into the SNr on the 6-OHDA-lesioned side elicited a marked rotational response, contraversive to the injection (Fox et al., 1998). Such behaviour represents a reduction in activity of basal ganglia outputs and can be taken as representing a potential anti-Parkinsonian action. Moreover, systemic administration of SB 206553 enhanced the action of D_2 agonist quinpirole and D_1 agonist SKF 82958 in eliciting a rotational response contraversive to the lesioned side (Fox et al., 1998; Fox and Brotchie, 2000a). The mechanism whereby 5-HT_{2C} receptor antagonists enhance the anti-Parkinsonian action of DA receptor agonists may involve reducing the overactivity of the SNr. When given alone, 5-HT_{2C} receptor antagonists may be capable only of reducing the activity to a certain degree following systemic administration. Therefore, there may not be sufficient reduction in the activity of the SNr to restore the normal thalamo-cortical output and have an overt anti-Parkinsonian effect.

From these findings it is clear that in the 6-OHDA PD model the antagonists at 5-HT_{2C} receptors show anti-Parkinsonian effects, and are probably decreasing SNr activity, an effect that in normal rats is obtained with the agonists instead. We explained this paradox suggesting that under pathological conditions, when the basal ganglia circuitry is impaired by DA depletion, the 5-HT_{2C} receptor transmission is also altered. The overexpression of 5-HT_{2C} receptors in the SNr could lead to a clear-cut excitatory effect on the output structures, since the indirect collateral inhibition is totally overcome. Thus, the consequence is a contribution to the SNr overactivity that is known to be a hallmark of PD and related disorders (Di Giovanni et al., 2006b). 5-HT_{2C} receptor transmission may be a key determinant in the activity of the SNr in Parkinsonism basal ganglia and its selective activation in this condition might have a surprising opposite effect compared to that which it has on the "normal" circuitry. Studies are currently underway in my laboratory to verify this supposition.

In addition, the blockade of 5-$HT_{2A/2C}$ receptors is determinant in the effect of clozapine and rispridone in inhibiting the discharge of SNr neurons (Bruggeman et al., 2000).

Bruggeman et al., (2000) showed, indeed, that concurrent 5-$HT_{2A/2C}$ and moderate DA D_2 receptor antagonism can mimic the *in vivo* effects of these atypical antipsychotics on the firing rate of SNr neurons. Therefore, the inhibitory effect of the atypical antipsychotics clozapine and risperidone and of concurrent 5-HT_2/D_2 antagonism on the SNr may reflect a mechanism to counteract motor side effects [extrapyramidal symptoms (EPS)] by disinhibiting thalamocortical circuits.

On the other hand, it could also be a mechanism to alleviate negative symptoms. This is based on the fact that the SNr, aside from prominent innervations from the dorsolateral striatum, also receives afferents from the nucleus accumbens, innervating subfields of the mediodorsal and ventromedial thalamic nuclei mainly affiliated to the prelimbic area and the prefrontal cortex. Therefore one must consider that changes in SNr activity may reflect not only motor activity -and in that sense EPS-, but also emotional and motivational processes, which may be involved in negative symptoms.

Serotonin Modulation of Subthalamic Nucleus Activity

The subthalamic nucleus is an important mediator of the output circuits subserving basal ganglia motor function and a potent link between the serotonergic system, the STN and motor behaviour has been highlighted. It is interposed in the direct pathway between the external segment of the GP (GPe) and the the internal segment of the GP (GPi)/SNr. The STN also has projections that interact with the other primary output pathway from the striatum, the direct pathway, at the level of the GPe (Kita and Kitai, 1987; Shink et al., 1996). This connectivity provides the STN with a unique ability to mediate basal ganglia motor function, and accordingly, the STN has a strong influence on motor behaviour related to basal ganglia DAergic neurotransmission. For instance, the STN has been implicated in the mediation of Parkinsonian movement disorders. An increase in the basal activity of the excitatory glutamatergic afferent neurons of the STN, associated with the loss of DA terminals in the striatum, may play a role in the hypokinetic symptoms of this condition (Smith and Grace, 1992). Indeed, STN lesion as well as its inactivation by deep brain stimulation has shown to have anti-Parkinsonian effects in primate experimental PD model and in PD patients (Krack et al., 1998; Charles et al., 2004; Sturman et al., 2004). Under normal DA function, in both humans and primates, unilateral lesions of the STN result in hemiballism and chorea which are characterised by involuntary, hyperkinetic movements of the contralateral limbs (Mitchell et al., 1985; Bhidayasiri and Truong, 2004). During the past decade, patients suffering from PD have undergone modulation of this STN hyperactivity by high frequency stimulation (HFS) (Limousin et al., 1995). HFS of the STN has dramatic therapeutic effects on locomotor symptoms (Krack et al., 2003). The mechanism by which STN HFS improves locomotor symptoms is not well understood, but some evidence suggests that HFS modulates the pathological activity within the STN (Garcia et al., 2005) lowering GABA release in the motor thalamus (Stefani et al., 2006).

On the other hand, it is known that 5-HT neurons, mainly from the DRN, innervate the STN, and clearly modulate its neuronal activity. 5-HT may have multiple actions in the STN. Whole-cell patch-clamp and extracellular single-unit recordings on rat brain slices with selective 5-HT agonists and antagonists indicated both inhibitory mediated 5-HT_{1A} receptor and 5-HT_{2C} and 5-HT_4 receptor-mediated excitatory responses of 5-HT in subthalamic neurons (Stanford et al., 2005; Shen et al., 2007). In addition, 5-HT inhibits synaptic transmission in the STN by activating presinaptic 5-HT_{1B} receptors. Indeed, in a recent electrophysiological study in slices of rat brain, 5-HT reduced the amplitude of both glutamatergic excitatory postsynaptic currents (EPSCs) and GABAergic inhibitory postsynaptic currents (IPSCs) on the STN neuron's membrane (Shen and Johnson, 2008). The 5-HT-induced inhibition of synaptic currents was associated with a significant increase in the paired-pulse ratios of evoked EPSCs and IPSCs, suggesting that 5-HT acts presynaptically to suppress both glutamate and GABA release. However, 5-HT was more potent for reducing EPSCs compared with IPSCs (Shen and Johnson, 2008). This inhibitory effect was mediated via activation of 5-HT_{1B} receptors because selective 5-HT_{1B} antagonists blocked 5-HT-induced inhibition of EPSCs and IPSCs (Shen and Johnson, 2008). Consistent with its presynaptic location, 5-HT_{1B} receptor activation has been shown to cause presynaptic inhibition of GABA-mediated transmission in the substantia nigra also (Johnson et al., 1992; Stanford and Lacey 1996). According to a widely used model of basal ganglia function, a reduction in excitatory glutamate input to the STN would be expected to improve symptoms of PD (Bonsi et al., 2007b). Indeed, injection of 5-HT_{1B} agonists systemically (Oberlander et al., 1987; Rempel et al., 1993) or into the STN (Martinez-Price and Geyer, 2002) has been reported to increase locomotion in rats. However, 5-HT_{1B} receptor stimulation has also been reported to reduce L-DOPA induced dyskinesia in a rat model of PD (Carta et al., 2007), which is not what one would predict based upon inhibition of excitatory input to the STN. Moreover, 5-HT_{1B} agonists have also been reported to interfere with the benefit of L-DOPA in a marmoset model of PD. Activation of 5-$HT_{1B/1D}$ receptors induced motor deficits and inhibited the motor response to L-DOPA, whereas blockade of 5-HT_{1B} receptors had no observable effects on motor behaviours (Jackson et al., 2004). These data suggest that neither stimulation nor blockade of 5-HT_{1B} receptors will be therapeutically beneficial in the treatment of PD or in the treatment of drug-induced dyskinetic syndromes.

The 5-HT_{2C} receptors are most likely to be involved in 5-HT effects, since they are present in a relatively high concentration in this nucleus. The most frequent response to 5-HT seems to be an excitation of STN neurons (Flores et al., 1995; Xiang et al., 2005; Stanford et al., 2005; Shen et al., 2007). This effect is mediated by the activation of the 5-HT_{2C} and 5-HT_4 receptors being reversed by the combined use of selective antagonists for 5-HT_4 and 5-HT_{2C} receptors (Xiang et al., 2005; Stanford et al., 2005). In addition, Shen et al., (2007) found that STN neuron burst firing was facilitated by 5HT_{2C}- and 5HT_4-dependent currents, and since excessive burst firing of STN neurons has been implicated in the expression of symptoms of PD, suggested that antagonists at 5HT_{2C} or 5HT_4 receptors might be useful in the treatment of PD. Moreover, an inhibitory action of 5-HT over a small subpopulation (about 20%) of STN neurons has been also shown (Stanford et al., 2005, Shen et al., 2007), and it seems to be mediated by 5-HT_{1A} receptors activation (Stanford et al., 2005). Thus, this electrophysiological evidence indicates that 5-HT-induced excitation or inhibition in the STN are separate entities and most likely to arise as a consequence of independent, direct post-synaptic effects mediated by 5-HT_{2C}, 5-HT_4 and 5-HT_{1A} subtypes. The excitatory 5-HT effect through the activation of 5-HT_{2C} receptors is in accordance with the results of a recent study that investigated the effect of subthalamic DBS, using clinically relevant stimulation parameters, on DOI-induced hypomobility (Hameleers et al., 2007) These authors found that administration of DOI decreased the locomotor activity, as evidenced by a net decrease in distance moved, velocity and the time spent moving. This decrease in locomotion was reversed by DBS of the STN. Varying results of DOI administration on locomotion have been obtained in the past. Some studies showed an increase in locomotor activity after DOI administration (Darmani et al., 1996) and (Granoff and Ashby Jr., 1998); some authors found no effects (Hawkins et al., 2002) and others demonstrated hypomobility in rats treated with DOI (Krebs-Thomson and Geyer, 1996). It is probably the concentration of DOI that is contributing to the difference in these studies. In their study, Xiang et al. (2005) found a clear reduction of locomotor activity, which was reversed by STN HFS. It is known that injection of 5-HT_{2A} and 5-HT_{2C} agonists can increase the firing rate of STN neurons (Xiang, et al., 2005). Since DOI activates these receptors, it is likely that DOI excites STN neurons and induces increased STN activity. Increased STN activity is thought to be responsible for the hypokinesia in PD. In addition, these findings support the hypothesis that 5-HT_2 receptors may mediate the therapeutic effects of STN HFS on locomotor symptoms.

However, this evidence is not in accordance with a large body of behavioural evidence which shows an inhibitory action of 5-HT over the STN by acting on 5-HT_{2C} receptors. As a result, a decrease in the excitatory input from the STN to GPe/SNr occurs, which in turn enhances the activity of the ipsilateral motor thalamus. Indeed, the unilateral injection of 5-HT into the STN induces a contralateral dose-dependent turning behaviour which is blocked by a non selective 5-HT_2 antagonist mianserin. The contribution of the 5-HT_{2C} receptor in 5-HT-induced behaviour was revealed by the intrasubthalamic injection of the 5-HT_{2C} receptor agonist MK 212, that in concordance, increased the net turns (Belforte and Pazo, 2004). In addition, the blockade of subthalamic 5-HT_{2C} receptors suppressed the stereotypic behaviour induced by apomorphine administration (Barwick et al., 2000) while both systemic administration and local unilateral infusion of m-CPP into the STN induced an increase in oral movements in rats (Eberle-Wang et al., 1996; Mehta et al., 2001; De Deurwaerdere and Chesselet, 2000), that resemble the orofacial dyskinesias occurring as a severe side effect of prolonged treatment with antipsychotic drugs in humans (Waddington et al, 1986; Ellison, 1991). Oral dyskinesia observed after peripheral injections of m-CPP was enhanced by 5,7-dihydroxytryptamine (5,7-DHT)-induced lesion of the serotonergic neurons, probably due to an altered sensitivity to 5-HT_{2C} receptor stimulation in the STN (Mehta et al., 2001). Interestingly, these authors observed m-CPP induced seizure-like behaviours in a subset of lesioned rats that were never observed in sham-lesioned animals, thus demonstrating a pivotal role for the 5-HT_{2C} receptor in the control of the normal neuronal excitability, a phenomenon already noted by others (Mehta et al., 2001). Despite the fact that the mechanism by which serotonergic inputs to the STN contribute to its normal functioning remains controversial, the behavioural data discussed above clearly suggest that excess stimulation of 5-HT_{2C} receptors in this region may lead to hyperkinetic movement disorders. Thus 5-HT_{2C} antagonists can be useful to treat the side effects of long-term administration of neuroleptics in schizophrenia (Tarsy and Baldessarini, 1984; Reynolds, 2004). Serotonergic projections from the dorsal and medial raphe nuclei innervate all components of the basal ganglia circuitry; thus, there is evidence that endogenous 5-HT induces excitations of the STN neurons through several types of 5-HT receptors (Belforte and Pazo, 2004; Stanford et al., 2005; Xiang et al., 2005). Since this nucleus is considered to be a major driving force in the basal ganglia circuit (Albin et al., 1989; Utter and Basso, 2008), it is important to understand the role of the various 5-HT receptor subtypes in the control of this area. With regard to the other 5-HT receptors, besides 5-HT_{1A}, 5-HT_{1B}, 5-HT_{2A} and 5-HT_{2C}, there is evidence that only the 5-HT_3 and 5-HT_4 receptors are involved in the control of the subthalamic neurons. Unilateral injection of 5-HT into the STN induced a contralateral dose-dependent turning behaviour, attributed to a decreased excitatory imput from the STN to the SNr, which in turn enhanced the activity of the ipsilateral motor thalamus (Belforte and Pazo, 2004). Similar results were also observed with microinjections of quipazine, a mixed 5-$HT_{2B/2C/3}$ agonist, MK-212, a 5-$HT_{2B/2C}$ agonist and m-chlorophenylbiguanidine, a 5-HT_3 agonist (Belforte and Pazo, 2004). Furthermore, kainic acid lesion of the SNr suppressed the contralateral rotations elicited by the stimulation of 5-$HT_{2B/2C}$ and 5-HT_3 subthalamic receptors (Belforte and Pazo, 2004). Taken together, these data suggest that 5-HT tonically stimulates the subthalamic-nigral pathway, through 5-HT_{2C} and 5-HT_3 receptor subtypes, without involving the dopaminergic innervation of the nucleus, because stimulation of subthalamic 5-HT receptors in animals bearing a lesion of the nigrostriatal pathway did not modify this motor response (Belforte and Pazo, 2004).

The stimulating action of 5-HT on the STN is further confirmed by electrophysiological investigations. Endogenous applied 5-HT in mouse and rat brain slices increased the firing frequency of subthalamic neurons (Flores et al., 1995; Stanford et al., 2005; Xiang et al., 2005).

The increased firing rate of these neurons was attributed to the depolarization of membrane potential caused by a reduction of potassium conductance mediated by 5-HT_{2C} and mainly by 5-HT_4 receptor subtypes (Stanford et al., 2005; Xiang et al., 2005). Using several 5-HT-ergic agonists and antagonists Xiang et al. (2005) found that only α-methyl-5-HT, a 5-HT_2 agonist with good affinity for 5-HT_4 receptors, and cisapride, a 5-HT_4 agonist, mimicked the action of 5-HT. Furthermore, the 5-HT action was partially reversed by the 5-HT_4 antagonist SB 23597-190, the 5-HT_2 antagonist ketanserin, and the 5-HT_{2C} receptor antagonist RS 102221; in addition, the effect of RS 102221 was comparable with that of ketanserin. Therefore, it was concluded that 5-HT_4 and 5-HT_{2C} receptor subtypes are involved in the excitatory action of 5-HT in STN neurons and that these receptors may be co-localized in a single neuron (Xiang et al., 2005). These data were replicated by Stanford et al. (2005) who showed that the pre-infusion of RS 102221 and GR 113808, another 5-HT_4 antagonist, reduced excitations of STN neurons induced by local application of 5-HT. On the basis of these results, it was concluded that when there is the cortical activation for a specific movement, a group of raphe serotonergic neurons that project to the STN and STN neurons itself might be simultaneously activated, this amplify subthalamic activity, and consequently facilitate the excitation of the output structures in the basal ganglia, which in turn inhibits the thalamic motor area (Xiang et al., 2005). In the classical rate model of basal ganglia function, the neural mechanisms underlying the generation of Parkinsonian symptoms are thought to involve reduced activation of primary motor and premotor cortex and supplementary motor areas, secondary to an over activation of the output regions of the basal ganglia, i.e. SNr and GPi (Albin et al., 1989), largely because of excessive excitatory drive from the STN, consequent to dopamine loss in the striatum (Nicholson and Brotchie, 2002; Utter and Basso, 2008). Hence, it is theoretically possible that antagonists at the 5-HT_{2C} and 5-HT_4 receptors, which act directly to reduce STN neural activity, may have positive therapeutic benefits in PD.

Serotonin Modulation of Globus Pallidus Activity

Anatomical and experimental evidence support a pivotal role for 5-HT in the control of neuronal activity of both GPe and GPi segments of GP which express several 5-HT receptors. Perkins and Stone (1983) found that typical high-frequency firing GPe neurons in anaesthetized rats were not responsive to iontophoretically applied 5-HT, and 5-HT inhibited a small number of low-frequency firing GPe neurons. In contrast, Querejeta et al. (2005) found that local application of a 5-HT receptor agonist, or fluoxetine excites most of the GPe neurons in anaesthetized rats, showing the presence of a serotonergic excitatory tone on GP neurons. This evidence was further confirmed by a recent patch-clamp recording study (Chen et al., 2008). In reality the effect of 5-HT is more complex because of the existence of various receptor subtypes on presynaptic and postsynaptic membranes in the pallidum. In fact, recent electrophysiological evidence has shown that 5-HT exerts strong modulation on inhibitory and excitatory responses to cortical stimulation in the GPe and GPi (Kita et al., 2007; Hashimoto and Kita, 2008). 5-HT suppressed GABA-ergic inhibitory responses to cortical stimulation in monkeys, through presynaptic 5-HT_{1B} receptors, densely expressed on axons and axon terminals in the pallidum (Kita et al., 2007). On the other hand, 5-HT_{1A} receptors are involved in the suppression of glutamatergic excitations of the globus pallidum, because local application of WAY100635, a 5-HT_{1A} selective antagonist, blocked the effect of subsequent applications of 5-CT in suppressing cortical stimulation-induced excitations (Kita et al., 2007). Hence, 5-HT may reduce ionotropic glutamatergic excitation, probably through 5-HT_{1A} receptors located at presynaptic and/or postsynaptic sites. On pallidal neurons slices, 5-HT and 5-carboxamindotryptamine (5-CT) presynaptically reduce glutamate release in GPe, and the antagonistic effect of GR55562 suggested an involvement of 5-$HT_{1B/1D}$ receptors in this effect (Hashimoto and Kita, 2008).

In according with these findings, an *in vivo* electrophysiological study reported that local application of the 5-HT_{1B} receptor agonist L-694,247 excited most GPe neurons, which can be due to presynaptic suppression of GABA-ergic inhibitions, in anaesthetized rats (Querejeta et al., 2005). In addition, the effect of 5-HT in the electrical activity of GP neurons of rats with unilateral quinolinic acid striatal lesions was severely attenuated, indicating that presynaptic 5-HT_{1B} receptors modulate GABA release from striato-pallidal terminals (Querejeta et al., 2005). Taken together, these data indicate that the tonic activation of 5-HT_{1B} receptors significantly contributes to the decrease of GABA release from striato-pallidal GABA-ergic terminals facilitating GP neurons spiking, and, on the other hand, the blockade of these receptors causes a significant decrease on the spiking frequency of GP neurons due to the augmented GABA release from striato-pallidal terminals (Querejeta et al., 2005). In line with these studies, $5HT_{1B}$ receptor activation with CP-93129, inhibited the release of (^{3}H)-GABA from pallidal slices and intrapallidal injection of CP-93129 alleviated akinesia in the reserpine-treated rat model of PD, indicating that some $5HT_{1B}$ receptors can function as heteroreceptors in the GP, reducing the release of GABA from striatopallidal neurons, this cellular mechanism underlying the anti-akinetic activity of CP-93129 seen in the reserpine-treated rat model of PD (Chadha et al., 2000).

The application of 5-HT into the superfusion medium of brain slices containing globus pallidus neurons, directly stimulated the receptors of the recorded neurons and produced a reversible depolarization of their membrane which consequently increased the firing rate of these neurons (Chen et al., 2008). 5-HT postsynaptic excitation of pallidal neurons occurs through activation of 5-HT_4 or 5-HT_7 receptors but not via 5-HT_{2C} and 5-HT_3 receptors (Bengtson et al., 2004; Chen et al., 2008; Kita et al., 2007; Hashimoto and Kita, 2008).

These findings support the hypothesis that the increase of 5-HT tone, which mainly excite pallidal neurons directly and counteract the inhibition from the striatum selectively, will exert an anti-Parkinsonian effect.

Serotonin in Parkinson's Disease and Other Motor Disorders

Parkinson's Disease

Parkinson's disease is the second most common neurodegenerative disease in the elderly population with an inevitable *exitus*. The idiopathic form is a progressive disorder, the impact of which reaches far beyond the clinical signs and symptoms exhibited by those afflicted. Clinical features at presentation include the asymmetric onset of cardinal motor symptoms such as tremor at rest, bradykinesia, muscular rigidity, stooped posture and instability (Sian et al., 1999).

Since Hornykiewicz's pioneering work in identifying the SNc as the site of major pathological change in PD, reduced DAergic innervation of the striatum has been thought to be central to its pathogenesis (Hornykiewicz, 1973). Hitherto, the underlying mechanisms of neuronal loss in patients are not known, therefore current therapies work mainly to alleviate symptoms rather than to halt the progression of the disease (Di Giovanni, 2008). There have been major advances in understanding the etiopathogenesis of PD, the modalities whereby the neurodegenerative process begins and progresses, therefore the development of drugs to slow and halt DAergic neuronal degeneration or even to prevent the disease, now seem realistic goals (Esposito et al., 2007a,b,c; Di Giovanni 2008).

The modulation of 5-HT of the basal ganglia nuclei has obvious implications for the treatment of a range of motor diseases most notably including PD, L-DOPA-induced dyskinesia and antipsychotic-induced extrapiramidal effects. It has become axiomatic that manipulation of 5-HT transmission may be pivotal in treating the symptoms, and of key importance in improving symptomatologies in this patient-set (Nicholson and Brotchie, 2002; Di Giovanni et al., 2006a,b; Scholtissen, et al., 2006).

Although 5-HT involvement in PD has long since been known (Scatton et al., 1983; Miyawaki et al., 1997), the neuropathological literature on the status of the DRN in PD is not entirely clear. In fact, loss of 5-HT cells bodies and no modification in their number in PD have both been reported (Sawada et al., 1985; Jellinger, 1987; Halliday et al., 1990; Paulus and Jellinger, 1991; Kim et al., 2003). Notwithstanding, in primates, surgical lesion of upper brainstem producing contralateral resting tremor, and bradykinesia were associated with reduced homolateral striatal 5-HT (Goldstein et al., 1969). Compelling evidence instead exists about damage of the ascending pathways limited to the nerve terminal of 5-HT neurons in different regions in PD brains (Chase and Ng, 1972; Chase, 1974; Chinaglia et al., 1993). Indeed, post-mortem examinations have shown a reduction of up to 50% of 5-HT in some areas of the cortex and the basal ganglia (Scatton et al., 1983; Birkmayer and Riederer 1986; Birkmayer and Birkmayer, 1987). Unlike the preferential loss of DA in the putamen, the caudate is affected more than the putamen by loss of all 5-HT markers: serotonin (-66%), the major 5-HT metabolite, 5-hydroxy-indolacetic acid (5-HIIA) (-42%), 5-HT transporter (5-HTT) (-56%) and tryptophan hydroxylase (TPH; the marker synthetic enzyme) (-59%) (Kish et al., 2008). Reduced brain levels of all of the key markers for the serotonin neurotransmitter system provide compelling evidence for a striatal serotonergic abnormality in PD. This evidence has been confirmed by antemortem studies and imaging investigations that showed reduced cerebrospinal fluid levels of 5-HIIA and decreased activity of 5-HTT, not only in the caudate nucleus and the putamen, but also in the thalamus and medial frontal areas, indicating a pathophysiological involvement of 5-HT in the PD pathophysiology (Haapaniemi et al., 2001; Kerenyi et al., 2003; Kim et al., 2003). It is, however, very likely that the degree of serotonergic degeneration depends on the stage of the disease (Scholtissen, 2006). Nevertheless, Björklund's group recently showed that serotonergic innervation of the striatal complex remains relatively intact in most PD patients (Carta et al., 2007).

5-HT Receptors' Expression in PD Animal Models and in Patients

Animal models are important tools in experimental medical science to better understand pathogenesis of human diseases such as PD. However, preclinical research on these animal models has provided inconsistent results, highlighting that these experimental models represent only an imperfect replica of human disorders (Scholtissen et al., 2006).

The first PD animal model developed is the 6-OHDA; this agent selectively disrupts catecholaminergic systems and reproduces specific features of PD in rodents, apparently via oxidative damage (Simola et al., 2007 and references therein). 6-OHDA-lesioned animals have been exploited to test therapeutic approaches for treating functional disturbances observed in this disease and will aid the future development of rational therapeutic strategies. The 6-OHDA lesion can be performed in adult or in neonatal rats, producing different changes in behavior and neurochemistry of these animals, according to the age of the lesion (Breese et al., 2005).

Although independently of the age in which the SNc is injured, 6-OHDA leads to permanent DA ablation while the serotonergic projection to the striatum remains intact. Contrasting results about the activity of DRN serotonergic neurons in 6-OHDA-lesioned rats exist; increase in frequency and burst firing activity (Chu et al., 2004; Zhang et al., 2007) or a decrease (- 60%) of discharge rate (Guiard et al. 2008) have been in fact reported.

Both neonatal and adult lesions actually lead to a 5-HT axonal hyperinnervation within the dorsal striatum (Stachowiak et al., 1984; Breese et al., 1985; Zhou et al., 1991; Molina-Holgado et al., 1994; Mrini et al., 1995; Balcioglu et al., 2003; Maeda et al., 2003). Consistently, striatal 5-HT levels and 5-HTT binding have been reported to be increased in this animal model of PD (Commins et al., 1989; Zhou et al., 1991; Guerra et al., 1997; Mendlin et al., 1999; Balcioglu et al., 2003). Interestingly, it has been proposed that striatal "reactive" serotonergic hyperinnervation in lesioned animals occurs to compensate for the lost function of DAergic terminals and this might 'mask' the true extent of the serotonin loss in PD.

This suggests that 5-HT neurotransmission is impaired and the clarification of the pathophysiological mechanism can provide unique information regarding the treatment of Parkinsonism from a point of view that differs from conventional therapy.

In addition to DA depletion a discrete modification in the regulation of postsynaptic 5-HT receptors in different areas of the basal ganglia circuitry and in other brain areas has been observed in animals and humans (Kienzl et al., 1981; Radja et al., 1993). Therefore alterations of 5-HT-binding constants in PD might reflect an imbalance in serotoninergic activity.

5-HT_{1A} binding is not altered in the basal ganglia nuclei of neonatally 6-OHDA-lesioned rats. In contrast, there is a considerable increase in binding for 5-HT_{1B} receptors. The highest increase of 5-HT_{1B}-binding sites is observed in the SN (54%), GP (33%) and the two portions of neostriatum. The most likely explanation for the present increases in the neostriatal, nigral and pallidal is therefore an augmented production (upregulation) of these receptors by the neostriatal projection neurons and concomitant increase of their axonal transport to both territories of projection. In view of its widespread distribution in the neostriatum, it also seemed likely that the neostriatal increase in 5-HT_{1B} binding was somehow related to the DA denervation of this brain region rather than to its subsequent 5-HT hyperinnervation, suggesting a possible role for DA in the regulation of 5-HT receptor expression during ontogenesis. A significant increase in the density 5- HT_{2C} was also revealed throughout the neostriatum (40%) and in the SN (50%), but unchanged in the globus pallidus, as if this up-regulation preferentially involved striatonigral as opposed to striatopallidal neurons (Radja et al., 1993).

Consistently, enhanced responses of spontaneously firing units to iontophoresed 5-HT and both a 5-HT_{2C} and 5-HT_{2A} agonist have been demonstrated in the 5-HT-hyperinnervated neostriatum after neonatal 6-OHDA lesion (el Mansari et al., 1994). 5-HT_{2A} binding showed an even greater increase (60%), which was restricted to the rostral half of the neostriatum and also seemed imputable to an up-regulation as heteroreceptors. 5-HT_{2A} receptor expression increases significantly on direct pathway neurons (Laprade et al., 1996; Basura and Walker, 1999), even though 5-HT_{2A} receptors are expressed on both direct and indirect striatal projecting neurons (Ward and Dorsa, 1996).

The intracellular mechanisms that mediate the effects of 5-HT within the neonatal lesioned striatum are poorly understood. Neonatal lesions result in altered expression of preprotachykinin (decrease) and preproenkephalin (increase) in direct and indirect striatal pathway neurons, respectively (Sivam et al., 1987). It has been showed that 5-HT acting via 5-HT_2 receptors could regulate preprotachykinin expression selectively in direct pathway neurons and ultimately motor function, after neonatal DA depletion (Basura and Walker, 2001). Recently, it has been shown that neonatal but not adult 6-OHDA lesions result in a novel coupling of 5-HT_{2A} receptors to the ERK1/2/MAP Kinase pathway, a signaling cascade known to regulate neuronal plasticity that is not typically active in these neurons. Because DA-mediated signaling is redundant after 6-OHDA lesions, 5-HT-mediated stimulation of the ERK1/2/MAP Kinase pathway may provide an alternative signaling route allowing the regulation of neuronal gene expression and neuronal plasticity in the absence of DA (Brown and Gerfen, 2006).

In adult rats, destruction of the nigrostriatal dopamine projection by 6-OHDA has not been found to modify (^{3}H)5-HT binding in the neostriatum (Quirion and Richard, 1987).

Consistently, in situ hybridization and autoradiographic radioligand studies from lesioned rats and human postmortem tissue from patients with PD have revealed that striatal 5-HT_{1A} (Numan et al., 1995) and 5-HT_{1B} (Zhang et al., 2008) are not influenced by DA depletion. In the striatum, 5-HT_{2A} receptors appear to be up-regulated (Numan et al., 1995) and 5-HT_{2C}

receptors down-regulated (Numan et al., 1995; Zhang, et al., 2007) or not affected (Basura and 1999; Fox and Brotchie, 2000b). Striatal 5-HT_{2A} and 5-HT_{2C} are therefore differently regulated in 6-OHDA-lesioned animals. There are no significant difference in 5-HT_{2C} binding level for control versus PD tissue in the GPi and GPm (Fox and Brotchie, 2000b), and in the levels of 5-HT_{2C} mRNA between the intact and the 6-OHDA-lesioned hemispheres in the nucleus subthalamicus in rats (Zhang, et al., 2007). Conversely, 50% increase in 5-HT_{2C} receptor binding was observed in 6-OHDA-lesioned rats, strictly in accordance with the evidence that 5-HT_{2C} receptor binding in the SNr of aged-matched control tissue was less than half that in the SNr of patients with PD (Radja et al., 1993; Fox and Brotchie, 2000b).

This evidence highlights a selective change in 5-HT_{2C} receptor activity only in the output regions of the basal ganglia. 5-HT_{2C} receptors up-regulation might be compensatory, being a consequence of a decreased level of 5-HT in this nuclei and thus potentially underlie a role for them in the neuronal mechanisms involved in PD (Fox and Brotchie, 2000b).

It is noteworthy that L-DOPA/benserazide treatment not only reversed the 6-OHDA-induced levels of 5-HT_{2A} mRNA in the striatum, but caused a highly significant reduction in the levels of this receptor. In contrast, 5-HT_{2C} mRNA was not affected by L-DOPA/ benserazide treatment (Zhang et al., 2007). It can be concluded from these findings that the regulation of 5-HT_{2A} is highly dependent upon alterations in DA levels. In contrast, striatal 5-HT_{2C} appears to be regulated by nigrostriatal cell loss and the reduced level(s) of factor(s), other than DA, such as BDNF and cholecystokinin, which are normally expressed in nigrostriatal neurons. Similarly, numerous studies conducted in patients with PD and in animal models of this disease, such as 6-OHDA-lesioned rats and MPTP-treated primates, have shown that L-DOPA-treatment does not adequately reverse the effects of DA cell loss, but rather creates a new functional and neurochemical state, which differs both from the normal and the lesioned states (Bezard et al., 2003). The fact that 5-HT_{2A}, but not 5-HT_{2C}, are responsive to L-DOPA treatment predicts that pharmacological manipulations at 5-HT_{2C}, but not at 5-HT_{2A}, will result in similar effects in PD patients whether they are treated or not with DA replacement. This data therefore support the notion that 5-HT_{2C} receptor antagonists may be useful as an adjuvant treatment to dopamine agonists to treat motor complications of PD (Fox et al., 1998; Di Giovanni et al., 2006a; Zhang, Q.J. et al., 2007).

Consistent with these findings, systemic administration of the selective 5-HT_{2C} antagonist SB 206553 was showed to enhance the action of the anti-Parkinsonian action of the dopamine D_1 and D_2 agonists in 6-OHDA-lesioned rats (Fox et al., 1998; Fox and Brotchie, 2000a), suggesting that the use of a 5-HT_{2C} receptor antagonist in combination with a DA receptor agonist may reduce the reliance upon DA replacement therapies. Hitherto, no studies have been conducted in either non-human primates or humans to address this issue.

5-HT_3 binding is reduced in the entorhinal and prefrontal cortex on the 6-OHDA-lesioned side of the rat brain while no changes in the amygdala and hippocampus were observed (Cicin-Sain and Jenner, 1993). Unfortunately these authors did not measure the 5-HT_3 binding in the basal ganglia. Nevertheless, it has been suggested that the 5-HT_3 blockade might be important in the effect of the anti-Parkinsonian agent talipexole (Nishio et al., 1996).

No modification of the distribution and density of 5-HT_4 receptor binding sites was observed in 6-OHDA-lesioned guinea pig basal ganglia; neither in the caudate-putamen nor in the SN itself (Vilaró et al., 2005). On the other hand, following lesion of DA neurons by intranigral injection of 6-OHDA, an increased 5-HT_4 receptor binding was instead observed in the caudal (59%), but not the rostral part of caudate-putamen, as well as in the GP (93%)

(Compan et al., 1996). Since no decreases in 5-HT_4 receptor density have been detected in both studies (Compan et al., 1996; Vilaró et al., 2005) after the DA lesion, it is likely that these receptors are not expressed in DA neurons but they are located on terminals of striatal projection neurons. Kainic acid lesions of the caudate-putamen were associated with dramatic local decreases in 5-HT_4 receptor binding on the injected side (-89%), which suggested that striatal neurons express 5-HT_4 receptors. Corresponding decreases of 72 and 20% in receptor density were detected in the GP and SN, consistent with a presumed localization of 5-HT_4 receptors on striatal GABA neurons projecting to these regions. In the SN, the decrease in (^{3}H)GR113808 binding was localized to the pars lateralis, indicating that striatal neurons belonging to the cortico-striato-nigro-tectal pathway, and containing GABA and dynorphin, express 5-HT_4 receptors. As yet no experimental evidence has been given about the modification in expression of 5-HT_5 5-HT_6 and 5-HT_7 receptors in the basal ganglia of animal model of PD.

Role of Serotonin in L-DOPA-Induced Dyskinesia

The abnormal involuntary movements, or dyskinesia, generated by prolonged administration of L-DOPA represent one of the major challenges facing current therapy for PD. These debilitating motor disturbances are all the more problematic because L-DOPA, in spite of its introduction several decades ago, still represents the therapy of choice for the treatment of PD. The discovery of pharmacological interventions able to counteract L-DOPA-induced dyskinesia (LID) would therefore represent an important breakthrough in the therapy for PD. The design of novel agents for the prevention and treatment of LID requires the elucidation of the adaptive changes produced in the Parkinsonian brain by repeated administration of L-DOPA and the assessment of their role in the development and expression of this condition. Recently, compelling evidence has been produced about the causative role of 5-HT in LID developing in both animal models and in PD patients suggesting a use of serotonergic agents in reducing LID in PD patients (Jackson et al., 2004; Johnston and Brotchie, 2006; Carlsson, et al., 2007; Carta et al., 2007). In fact, 5-HT neurons have been shown to be able to convert exogenous L-DOPA to DA, and store and release DA in an activity-dependent manner but without the fine control that occurs in DA release by DA neurons (Carta et al., 2007). Therefore, activation of the two autoreceptors, 5-HT_{1A} and 5-HT_{1B}, localized on the soma and terminals of 5-HT neurons, respectively, have been shown to be highly effective in counteracting L-DOPA-induced dyskinesias in the 6-OHDA rat model (Carta et al., 2007). The rationale for the use of these agonists consists in a possible modulation of DA release from 5-HT neurons in a way that resembles the physiological DA release from DA neurons. Hitherto, this attractive hypothesis has not been validated by a human study.

In addition, 5-HT_{2C} receptors might be involved in LID. The changes in 5-HT_{2C} receptor binding reported by Fox and colleagues (1998) were seen in PD patients with LID. It is thus possible that they could be ascribed to the process underlying dyskinesia rather than Parkinsonism (Fox et al., 1998). Thus, reduced stimulation of 5-HT_{2C} receptors would lead to decreased activity of the basal ganglia output nuclei and increased levels of abnormal movements. This hypothesis may predict an efficacious use of 5-HT_{2C} agonists for alleviating the side-effects of long-term treatment with L-DOPA. This seems unlikely since clozapine and quetiapine, antagonists for this receptor subtype, have been used successfully for this purpose (Durif et al., 2004). On the other hand, systemic administration of the selective 5-HT_{2C} antagonist SB 206553 was shown to enhance the anti-Parkinsonian action of the dopamine D1 and D2 agonists in 6-OHDA-lesioned rats (Fox et al., 1998; Fox and Brotchie, 2000a), suggesting that the use of a 5-HT_{2C} receptor antagonist in combination with a dopamine receptor agonist may reduce the reliance upon dopamine replacement therapies. Hitherto, no studies have been conducted in either non-human primates or humans to address this issue.

Role of Serotonin in Parkinsonian Resting Tremor

Furthermore, convincing evidence has indicated a pivotal role of 5-HT in Parkinsonian resting tremor. The most common tremor seen in patients with PD is a "pill-rolling" movement of the hands (Sethi, 2003). Despite a number of clinical and basic studies, the neural substrate for this motor complication remains unclear. The 5-HT causative role in tremorgenesis has been strengthened by a recent PET study in PD patients (Doder et al., 2003). Interestingly, these authors showed that severity of Parkinsonian tremor, but not rigidity or bradykinesia, is correlated significantly with this decrease in midbrain raphe 5-HT_{1A} binding, likely reflecting a dysfunction and loss of serotonergic cell bodies early in the disease process (Doder et al., 2003). This evidence is in agreement with the suggested hypothesis of "disequilibria" in the serotonin-histamine system responsible for tremor-akathisia, whereas "disequilibria" in the dopamine-ACh system might lead to rigidity-akinesia (Barbeau, 1962). A glimmer of light was recently thrown on the potential of subtype selective serotonergic agents for the relief of Parkinsonian tremor by Carlson and colleagues (Carlson et al., 2003). Local injections of a mixed 5-$HT_{2A/2C}$ receptor antagonist into the SNr block tremulous jaw movements in cholinomimetic-model of Parkinsonian tremor in rats (Carlson et al., 2003). This result is consistent with previous studies showing that the jaw movement activity was suppressed potently by clozapine, olanzapine and risperidone (Ikeguchi et al., 1995; Trevitt et al., 1997; Trevitt et al., 1998) and with clinical reports demonstrating serotonergic involvement in the generation and treatment of Parkinsonian symptoms and other motor dysfunction (Ikeguchi et al., 1995).

Role of Serotonin in Psychiatric Complications in PD

Besides being a movement disorder, PD is also associated with numerous non-motor symptoms. Mood disturbance, and especially major depressive disorder, has an average prevalence of 25-40% in outpatient settings (Leentjens, 2004; Veazey et al., 2005; Miller et al., 2007). According to the serotonergic hypothesis of depression in PD (Mayeux, 1990) 5-HT seems to play a central role. Indeed, it has been suggested that the reduced DA activity in PD can lead, as physiological adaptation, to a reduction of serotonergic tone and at the same time constitute a risk factor for depression (Mayeux, 1990). The presence of this biological risk factor for depression may explain the high prevalence of this condition in patients with PD (Leentjens, 2004). Nevertheless, a recent double-blind, randomized study provided no support for the serotonergic hypothesis of depression in PD using the acute tryptophan depletion (ATD) paradigm (Leentjens et al., 2006). Co-morbid depression in PD is usually treated with selective serotonin reuptake inhibitors (SSRIs) or tricyclic antidepressants (TCAs) although these drugs should be used with caution in patients with PD because can exacerbate orthostatic hypotension and anticholinergic adverse effects (Veazey et al., 2005).

We have recently suggested that 5-HT_{2C} receptor antagonists prove useful in addressing depression and also, in PD patients, increasing ventrotegmental area (VTA) DA neurons' activity and accumbal DA release (Di Giovanni et al., 2006a,b). In accord with this, nefazodone, a 5-HT_2 antagonist/reuptake inhibitor has showed a dual activity as an antidepressant and as an agent capable of reducing the EPS in depressed Parkinsonian patients (Avila et al., 2003). Given these desirable motor side effects, nefazodone should be chosen over SSRIs for the treatment of depression in PD patients, if the patient tolerates its use (Avila et al., 2003).

Apart from depression, dementia and psychosis are also common psychiatric problems associated with PD. Psychotic complications are associated with the use of anti-Parkinsonian drugs and make PD management more difficult given the need for antidopaminergic therapy, which worsens motor functioning in patients with PD. For psychosis, clozapine is the only atypical antipsychotic that has proven effective without worsening motor function in PD patients. However, its use requires the monitoring of agranulocytosis. Newer atypical ADPs such as quetiapine have been claimed to be safe in terms of motor functioning, but evidence about their effectiveness is not compelling. The efficacy of the atypical ADPs in treating psychosis in PD patients is likely to be due to their ability in blocking 5-HT receptors. In fact, antagonists or inverse agonists of the 5-HT_{2A} and 5-HT_{2C} receptor are potential therapeutic agents for treatment-induced psychosis of PD (Weiner et al., 2003; Di Giovanni et al., 2006a).

Role of Serotonin in APDs-Induced Extrapyramidal Side Effects

In addition to the neurodegenarative, idiopathic form, Parkinsonian symptoms are also produced by typical APDs therapy such as haloperidol, a mixed DA antagonist. In fact, EPS are common neurological side effects of APDs medication. More than 60% of the people who take conventional antipsychotic medications experience some form of EPS. These side effects can occur within the first few days or weeks of treatment, or it can appear after months and years of antipsychotic medication use. EPS is more common among patients taking conventional antipsychotic medications, compared to the newer atypical drugs. EPS can cause a variety of symptoms, e.g. involuntary movements, tremors and rigidity, body restlessness, muscle contractions and changes in breathing and heart rate. Drug-induced EPS are categorized into acute (acute dystonia, Parkinsonism, and akathisia) and delayed [tardive dyskinesia, (TD)] syndromes based on the time of occurrence during antipsychotic treatment. Neuroleptic-induced Parkinsonism is characterized by the triad of tremor, rigidity, and bradykinesia; it can closely resemble idiopathic PD caused by nigro-striatal degeneration. TD is the major limitation of long-term APDs therapy being potential irreversible. This condition occurs in 15-30% of patients, and results in abnormal, unintentional choreoathetoid movements of the head, limbs, and trunk. The incidence of akathisia, Parkinsonian syndromes and TD, which are relatively frequent in patients treated with classical antipsychotic agents, is also similar with TCAs and SSRIs. Amitriptiline, clomipramine, doxepine, trazodone and fluoxetine induce tardive dyskinesia in patients not previously treated with neuroleptics

(Mander et al., 1994; Clayton, 1995; Barucha and Sethi, 1996) and akathisia, acute dystonia and pseudoparkinson have been induced by some of these drugs, although not all share the same risk for the development of movement disturbances.

It has been proposed that DA receptors' supersensitivity, arising from up-regulation of DA_2 receptors following ADPs, is the base for the development of TD. In addition to DA, 5-HT receptors are also important in the etiology of schizophrenia and in the elicitation of EPS. Particularly 5-HT_{1A}, 5-$HT_{2A/2C}$ and 5-HT_3 receptor signalling seems to be altered in TD. Recently, a possible genetic predisposition to develop TD exists, and association between TD and receptor gene polymorphisms of 5-HT_{2A} and 5-HT_{2C} genes has been indeed shown (Gunes et al., 2007; Gunes et al., 2008).

5-HT_{1A} receptors may be important since postsynaptic 5-HT_{1A} receptor density in the prefrontal and temporal cortices of patients with schizophrenia is elevated (Tauscher et al., 2002). Probably a resultant decrease in the normal inhibitory serotonergic influence on motor activity may be involved in the precipitation of TD in patients on haloperidol therapy, since chronic administration of haloperidol increased the responsiveness of presynaptic and postsynaptic 5-HT_{1A} receptors and reduced 5-HT turnover (Haleem and Khan, 2003). Consistently, repeated administration of low doses of buspirone, a partial agonist at 5-HT_{1A} receptors, decreased the responsiveness of 5-HT_{1A} receptors (Okazawa et al., 1999) and reversed haloperidol-induced deficits of exploratory activity (Haleem et al. 2007a,b). In a widely accepted rat model of TD obtained with chronic treatment by neuroleptics (Ellison and See, 1989) 8-OH-DPAT (Naidu and Kulkarni, 2001a) and sarizotan, a 5-HT_{1A} agonist/D_3/D_4 ligand (Rosengarten et al., 2006) treatment inhibited haloperidol-induced vacuous chewing movements (VCMs). Consistently, buspirone reversed reserpine-induced dyskinetic movements in rats (Queiroz and Frussa-Filho, 1999) and completely reversed the induction of tardive VCMs (Haleem et al., 2007a,b).

The evidence that buspirone at low doses preferentially acts at the somatodendritic 5-HT_{1A} receptors further supports the hypothesis of impaired somatodendritic 5-HT function (Haleem et al., 2003, 2007a,b). These compelling experimental data support an impairment of 5-HT transmission as a possible important contributing factor in the onset of TD and other Parkinsonian-like effects of neuroleptics. Repeated administration of haloperidol elicits an increase in the responsiveness of somatodendritic and postsynaptic 5-HT_{1A} receptors. An increase in the effectiveness of somatodendritic 5-HT_{1A} receptors in rats treated with haloperidol would be expected to decrease the 5-HT input to DA nuclei. Buspirone and 8-OHDPAT might act in reversal of haloperidol-induced dyskinesia by desensitization of 5-HT_{1A} receptors, suggesting that prior administration of buspirone may be of help in the improvement of EPS induced by haloperidol and other antipsychotic drugs (Haleem et al., 2004; Samad et al., 2007).

5-HT_{2C} receptor signaling is also deeply implicated in the development of VCMs and 5-HT_{2C} receptors, which become supersensitized during long-term haloperidol treatment and remain supersensitized even after withdrawal of haloperidol as a treatment (Wolf et al., 2005; Ikram et al., 2007). In fact, m-CPP enhances the oral activity response to a greater extent than the DA D_1 receptor agonist SKF 38393 in neonatal 6-OHDA-treated rats (Gong and Kostrzewa, 1992). It is likely that m-CPP produces its effect at 5-HT_2 receptors (probably 5-HT_{2C} receptors) being blocked by the largely 5-HT_2 receptor antagonist mianserin (Gong et al., 1992). Moreover, DA D1-induced VCMs also appear to be mediated ultimately by 5-HT_{2C} receptors and as a result are attenuated by mianserin (Gong et al., 1992). It is significant that various 5-HT_2 receptor antagonists such as seganserin, ketanserin and ritanserin are able to effectively reduce the number of spontaneous VCMs in a rat model of TD (Naidu and Kulkarni, 2001a).

Concordantly, clozapine and other atypical APDs, that also have a high affinity to 5-HT_{2C} receptors (Altar et al., 1986), reduced motor side-effect liability because of the same degree of intrinsic anti-Parkinsonian characteristics, which act to counteract the pro-Parkinsonian effects of DA blockade. This was suggested by early clinical studies indicating that the 5-$HT_{2A/2C}$ receptor antagonist ritanserin (Leysen et al., 1985; Bersani et al., 1990) can ameliorate negative symptoms as well as attenuate exciting EPS in schizophrenics treated with classical APDs (Bersani et al., 1990; Miller et al., 1990). The relevance of 5-HT_{2C} receptor blocking in the effect of atypical APDs was shown by Canton and colleagues (1990), who revealed the high affinity of clozapine and risperidone for 5-HT_{2C} sites in the rat choroid plexus. These findings were subsequently confirmed (Kuoppamäki et al., 1993; Schotte et al., 1993; Canton et al., 1994; Kuoppamäki et al., 1995) and extended to brain sections (Roth et al., 1992; Roth et al, 1998). Antagonism at 5-HT_{2C} receptors by several atypical antipsychotics was also observed *in vivo*. Indeed, clozapine produces an increase in extracellular levels of DA in the nucleus accumbens (Di Matteo et al., 2002; Shilliam and Dawson, 2005), reverses the inhibition of accumbal DA release induced by the 5-HT_{2C} agonist RO 60175 (Di Matteo et al., 2002) and blocks the hypolocomotion induced by the 5-HT_{2C} agonist m-CPP (Prinssen et al, 2000).

It is worth noting that clozapine, like several atypical APDs, behaves as a 5HT_{2C} inverse agonist in heterologus expression systems *in vitro* (Herrick-Davis et al., 2000; Rauser et al., 2001; Navailles et al., 2006) and *in vivo* (Navailles et al., 2006). Thus, the 5-HT_{2C} receptor inverse agonist might underlie the unique clinical properties of atypical APDs, such as low EPS profile and good antidyskinetic efficacy (Herrick-Davis et al., 2000; Durif et al., 2004; Navailles et al., 2006).

Despite different chemical structures and pharmacodynamic signaling pathways, a variety of antipsychotics inhibit ion fluxes through 5-HT_3 receptors in a noncompetitive manner with the exception of the known competitive antagonists mirtazapine, olanzapine and clozapine (Bymaster et al, 2001; Rammes et al., 2004; Eisensamer et al., 2005). In accord with these findings, it has been shown that 5-HT_3 receptor antagonists ondansetron and tropisetron dose-dependently reversed the haloperidol-induced VCMs and reduced haloperidol-induced wet dog shakes, further supporting the possibility of an alteration in the serotonergic system after chronic haloperidol treatment (Naidu and Kulkarni, 2001b). It can be concluded that these 5-HT receptors can serve as potential therapeutic targets for the development of novel molecules for the treatment and prevention of tardive dyskinesia.

Catalepsy

The neuroleptic-induced state of catalepsy is generally considered as an animal model of the akinesia and rigidity seen in PD and it is predictive of EPS for ADPs. Serotonin is also implicated in ADPs-induced catalepsy (Wadenberg, 1996). For example, different SSRIs attenuate haloperidol-induced catalepsy in mice (Pires et al., 2005). In addition, the 5-HT_{1A} receptor agonists 8-OH-DPAT and buspirone, and the 5-$HT_{2A/2C}$ receptor agonists DOI and DOB, attenuate D2-receptor-mediated catalepsy (Invernizzi et al., 1988; Hicks, 1990; Neal-

Beliveau et al., 1993; Lucas et al., 1997). Moreover, the anti-cataleptic effects of 8-OH-DPAT and DOI are antagonized by WAY 100635, a selective 5-HT$_{1A}$ receptor antagonist (Bartoszyk et al., 1996) and mianserin, a 5-HT$_{2A/2C}$ receptor antagonist (Neal-Beliveau et al., 1993), respectively. In addition, 5-HT$_{1A}$ receptor activation reduces the cataleptogenic potential of novel antipsychotic agents as such as ziprasidone, aripiprazole, bifeprunox, SLV313, SSR181507 and sarizotan (Kleven et al., 2005). These findings strongly indicate that the serotonergic system is involved in the onset of catalepsy. There is strong evidence to suggest that (1) the catalepsy produced by dopamine D1 or D2 receptor antagonists can be completely antagonized by the administration of 5-HT$_{1A}$ receptor agonists acting at 5-HT$_{1A}$ autoreceptors in the DRN; (2) the catalepsy produced by a dopamine D2 receptor antagonist can be completely antagonized by treatment with a 5-HT$_{2A/2C}$ receptor agonists.

On the other hand, it has been shown that clozapine inhibits the cataleptic response to loxapine and olanzapine but does not induce catalepsy by itself (Kalkman et al., 1997). In addition, behavioural evidence shows that SB 228357, a selective 5-HT$_{2B/2C}$ receptor antagonist, and ACP-103, 5-HT$_{2A}$ receptor inverse agonist, attenuated catalepsy produced by haloperidol or risperidone (Reavill et al., 1999; Gardell et al., 2007). On the other hand, the 5-HT$_{2A}$ and 5-HT$_{2B}$ receptor antagonists, MDL 100907 and SB 215505 did not reverse haloperidol-induced catalepsy. This data suggests a role for 5-HT$_{2C}$ receptors in the anti-cataleptic action of SB 228357. Thus, the blockade of 5-HT$_{2C}$ receptors instead of their activation, would play a role in relieving the neuroleptic EPS disturbance. This hypothesis is further reinforced by the observation that the 5-HT$_{2C}$ receptor activation by RO 600175 *per se* induces catalepsy (Grottick et al., 2000).

Therefore, another interesting application of the data regarding the functional role of 5-HT in the basal ganglia is the possible use of 5-HT receptor ligands in the treatment of drug-induced Parkinsonian syndromes in relation to present efforts to develop new atypical neuroleptics with affinity for brain 5-HT receptor subtypes.

Hitherto, only one piece of research has investigated the effect of 5-HT$_6$ receptor antagonism on catalepsy and in rats with unilateral 6-OHDA lesions (Bourson et al., 1998) RO 04-6790, a 5-HT$_6$ selective antagonist, did not induce catalepsy nor did it have any effect on either haloperidol- or SCH 23390-induced catalepsy. Administration of RO 04-6790 was instead able to reverse rotational behaviour induced by the muscarinic antagonists scopolamine and atropine in the 6-OHDA unilaterally lesioned rat. These data suggest that the 5-HT$_6$ receptor is involved in the control of cholinergic neurotransmission in the striatum that is distal to DA transmission. A possible mechanism could be an increase in ACh release induced by 5-HT$_6$ receptor blockade directly or through modulation of GABA neurotransmission in the striatum, since 5-HT$_6$ receptors are expressed on GABA spiny neurons. In addition, RO 04-6790 alone did not induce turning behaviour in the unilaterally lesioned rat nor did it potentiate or inhibit ipsilateral rotations induced by amphetamine. Furthermore, RO 04-6790 had no effect on the contralateral rotations induced by L-DOPA. Therefore, 5-HT$_6$ receptor affinity does not account for the lack of EPS-effects characteristic of clozapine-like compounds (Bourson et al., 1998).

Conclusions and Implications

From the large amount of literature here reviewed it appears evident that the serotonergic neurotransmitter system plays a pivotal role in the modulation of basal ganglia circuitry, and its dysfunction is involved in the pathophysiology of PD and other motor disorders.

Among all the 5-HT receptors present in the basal ganglia nuclei, the 5-$HT_{1A/1B}$ and 5-$HT_{2A/2C}$ receptors are particularly important, because of their localization and their regulatory role on neurotransmitter release in many basal ganglia circuitry, including glutamatergic terminals in the SNc (Pineyro and Blier, 1999). 5-HT_{1A} receptor agonists have the potential for being useful at different stages of PD progression, since they may provide symptomatic relief in early PD, and anti-dyskinetic efficacy in late stage. Moreover, it has been shown (Bezard et al., 2006) that 5-HT_{1A} receptor agonists could also present (partial) neuroprotection, partially blocking the excitotoxic cycle of circuit-driven degeneration caused by the overactivity of the STN afferents of DA neurons, decreasing the hyperactivity of the remaining DA neurons through opening of potassium conductances, and suppressing activity of the vulnerability factor, caspase-3, in the remaining DA neurons.

Although several selective agents for 5-HT receptors have been discovered, none have reached the market for the treatment of motor disorders as yet. However, several companies are very active in 5-HT receptors research in PD, though they have concentrated on different receptor subtypes. Nevertheless despite the promising findings, last year Merck KGaA decided to stop further development of its late-stage development drug sarizotan as a treatment for PD. The company made the decision after examining the results of two Phase III studies of sarizotan in advanced PD patients suffering from dyskinesia. A statement from Merck said that the Phase III studies did not confirm earlier Phase II findings or the results from preclinical studies. The two trials, PADDY 1 and PADDY 2, investigated twice-daily dosing of sarizotan 1mg tablets to investigate whether the drug could achieve a 25% improvement in dyskinesia symptoms, but it failed to meet this efficacy threshold.

From the data here reviewed it should clear that drugs acting at the 5-$HT_{2A/2C}$ receptors might be an important feature of the treatment of PD, drug-related motor disturbances, and the psychiatric symptoms often associated with these neurological disorders. Nevertheless, as happened for the 5-HT_{1A} receptors, no compounds selective for 5-$HT_{2A/2C}$ receptors have been released for the treatment of the major motor disturbances such as PD. A glimmer of hope comes from the pharmaceutical company Acadia that in 2007, initiated the first Phase III pivotal trial with pimavanserin, a 5-HT_{2A} inverse agonist in patients with PD psychosis, after having positively concluded Phase II.

NS-2330, a triple monoamine reuptake inhibitor, has showed therapeutic potential in PD. In 2006, NeuroSearch's global partner Boehringer Ingelheim has concluded that the results from three completed phase II clinical studies in PD did not meet the company's efficacy criteria to proceed with phase III clinical development.

5-HT research is now more than 50 years old, and it has generated a wealth of therapeutic agents, some of which have had a major impact on disease management. The SSRIs are among the most widely prescribed drugs for treating depression and a variety of other disorders including anxiety and social phobia. But we are a long way from a serotoninergic therapeutic intervention for PD.

5-HT receptors research has generated detailed information on the molecular biology and regional and cellular localization of these receptors. A major challenge now is to utilise this knowledge to develop receptor-specific drugs and use the information gained to better treat central nervous system disorders. In addition, further clarification of the role of 5-HT transmission in the pathophysiology of basal ganglia disorders is required, since the overall picture is still confusing. Furthermore, most of the data came from animal studies and animal models of PD that yield contrary results compared to clinical studies. This leaves room for speculation about the real value of preclinical research for clinical PD. Moreover, there are also many avenues that remain unexplored, so there are undoubtedly further advances to be made.

References

Abi-Dargham, A., Laruelle, M., Wong, D.T., Robertson, D.W., Weinberger, D.R. and Kleinman, J.E. (1993) Pharmacological and Regional Characterization of [3H]LY278584 Binding Sites in Human Brain. *J. Neurochem.*, 60, no. 2, 730-737.

Albin, R.L., Young, A.B. and Penney, J.B. (1989) The functional anatomy of basal ganglia disorders. *Trends Neurosci.*, 12, no. 10, 366-375.

Alex, K.D. and Pehek, E.A. (2007) Pharmacologic mechanisms of serotonergic regulation of dopamine neurotransmission. *Pharmacol. Ther.*, 113, n. 2, 296-320.

Altar, C.A., Wasley, A.M., Neale, R.F. and Stone, G.A. (1986) Typical and atypical antipsychotic occupancy of D2 and S2 receptors: an autoradiographic analysis in rat brain. *Brain Res. Bull.*, 16, no. 4, 517-525.

Antonelli, T., Fuxe, K., Tomasini, M.C., Bartoszyk, G.D., Seyfried, C.A., Tanganelli, S. and Ferraro, L. (2005) Effects of sarizotan on the corticostriatal glutamate pathways. *Synapse*, 58, no. 3, 193-199.

Avila, A., Cardona, X., Martin-Baranera, M., Maho, P., Sastre, F. and Bello, J. (2003) Does nefazodone improve both depression and Parkinson disease? A pilot randomized trial. *J. Clin. Psychopharmacol.*, 23, no. 5, 509-513.

Azmitia, E.C. and Segal, M. (1978) An autoradiographic analysis of the differential ascending projections of the dorsal and median raphe nuclei in the rat. *J. Comp. Neurol.*, 179, no. 3, 641-667.

Balcioglu, A., Zhang, K. and Tarazi, F.I. (2003) Dopamine depletion abolishes apomorphine- and amphetamine-induced increases in extracellular serotonin levels in the striatum of conscious rats: a microdialysis study. *Neuroscience*, 119, no. 4, 1045-1053.

Barbeau, A. (1962) The pathogenesis of Parkinson's disease: a new hypothesis. *Can. Med. Assoc. J.*, 87, no., 802-807.

Barnes, J.M., Barnes, N.M., Champaneria, S., Costall, B. and Naylor, R.J. (1990) Characterisation and autoradiographic localisation of 5-HT3 receptor recognition sites identified with [3H]-(S)-zacopride in the forebrain of the rat. *Neuropharmacology*, 29, no. 11, 1037-1045.

Barnes, N.M. and Sharp, T. (1999) A review of central 5-HT receptors and their function. *Neuropharmacology*, 38, no. 8, 1083-1152.

Bartoszyk, G.D., Roos, C. and Ziegler, H. (1996) 5-HT1A receptors are not involved in clozapine's lack of cataleptogenic potential. *Neuropharmacology*, 35, no. 11, 1645-1646.

Barwick, V.S., Jones, D.H., Richter, J.T., Hicks, P.B. and Young, K.A. (2000) Subthalamic nucleus microinjections of 5-HT2 receptor antagonists suppress stereotypy in rats. *Neuroreport*, 11, no. 2, 267-270.

Basura, G.J. and Walker, P.D. (1999) Serotonin 2A receptor mRNA levels in the neonatal dopamine-depleted rat striatum remain upregulated following suppression of serotonin hyperinnervation. *Brain Res. Dev. Brain Res.*, 116, no. 1, 111-117.

Basura, G.J. and Walker, P.D. (2001) Serotonin 2A receptor regulation of striatal neuropeptide gene expression is selective for tachykinin, but not enkephalin neurons following dopamine depletion. *Brain Res. Mol. Brain Res.*, 92, no. 1-2, 66-77.

Bata-Garcia, J.L., Heredia-Lopez, F.J., Alvarez-Cervera, F.J., Arankowsky-Sandoval, G. and Gongora-Alfaro, J.L. (2002) Circling behavior induced by microinjection of serotonin reuptake inhibitors in the substantia nigra. *Pharmacol. Biochem. Behav.*, 71, no. 1-2, 353-363.

Belforte, J.E. and Pazo, J.H. (2004) Turning behaviour induced by stimulation of the 5-HT receptors in the subthalamic nucleus. *Eur. J. Neurosci.*, 19, no. 2, 346-355.

Bengtson, C.P., Lee, D.J. and Osborne, P.B. (2004) Opposing electrophysiological actions of 5-HT on noncholinergic and cholinergic neurons in the rat ventral pallidum in vitro. *J. Neurophysiol.*, 92, no. 1, 433-443.

Bersani, G., Grispini, A., Marini, S., Pasini, A., Valducci, M. and Ciani, N. (1990) 5-HT2 antagonist ritanserin in neuroleptic-induced parkinsonism: a double-blind comparison with orphenadrine and placebo. *Clin. Neuropharmacol.*, 13, no. 6, 500-506.

Bezard, E., Brotchie, J.M. and Gross, C.E. (2001) Pathophysiology of levodopa-induced dyskinesia: potential for new therapies. *Nat. Rev. Neurosci.*, 2, no. 8, 577-588.

Bezard, E., Gross, C.E. and Brotchie, J.M. (2003) Presymptomatic compensation in Parkinson's disease is not dopamine-mediated. *Trends Neurosci.*, 26, no. 4, 215-221.

Bezard, E., Gerlach, I., Moratalla, R., Gross, C.E. and Jork, R. (2006) 5-HT1A receptor agonist-mediated protection from MPTP toxicity in mouse and macaque models of Parkinson's disease. *Neurobiol. Dis.*, 23, no. 1, 77-86.

Bharucha, K.J. and Sethi, K.D. (1996) Complex movement disorders induced by fluoxetine. *Mov. Disord.*, 11, no. 3, 324-326.

Bhidayasiri, R. and Truong, D.D. (2004) Chorea and related disorders. *Postgrad. Med. J.*, 80, no. 947, 527-534.

Birkmayer, W. and Birkmayer, J.D. (1987) Dopamine action and disorders of neurotransmitter balance. *Gerontology*, 33, no. 3-4, 168-171.

Birkmayer, W. and Riederer, P. (1986) Biological aspects of depression in Parkinson's disease. *Psychopathology*, 19, no. 2, 58-61.

Bishop, C., Tessmer, J.L., Ullrich, T., Rice, K.C. and Walker, P.D. (2004) Serotonin 5-HT2A receptors underlie increased motor behaviors induced in dopamine-depleted rats by intrastriatal 5-HT2A/2C agonism. *J. Pharmacol. Exp. Ther.*, 310, no. 2, 687-694.

Bishop, C., Daut, G.S. and Walker, P.D. (2005) Serotonin 5-HT2A but not 5-HT2C receptor antagonism reduces hyperlocomotor activity induced in dopamine-depleted rats by striatal administration of the D1 agonist SKF 82958. *Neuropharmacology*, 49, no. 3, 350-358.

Blackburn T.P. (2004) Serotonergic agents and Parkinson's disease. *Drug Discov. Today: Therapeutic Strategies*, 1, 35-41.

Blackburn, T.P., Cox, B., Heapy, C.G., Lee, T.F. and Middlemiss, D.N. (1981) Supersensitivity of nigral serotonin receptors and rat rotational behaviour. *Eur. J. Pharmacol.*, 71, no. 2-3, 343-346.

Blackburn, T.P., Kemp, J.D., Martin, D.A. and Cox, B. (1984) Evidence that 5-HT agonist-induced rotational behaviour in the rat is mediated via 5-HT1 receptors. *Psychopharmacology (Berl)*. 83, no. 2, 163-165.

Blomeley, C. and Bracci, E. (2005) Excitatory effects of serotonin on rat striatal cholinergic interneurones. *J. Physiol. (Lond)*. 569, no. Pt 3, 715-721.

Blurton, P.A. and Wood, M.D. (1986) Identification of multiple binding sites for [3H]5-hydroxytryptamine in the rat CNS. *J. Neurochem.*, 46, no. 5, 1392-1398.

Boess, F.G. and Martin, I.L. (1994) Molecular biology of 5-HT receptors. *Neuropharmacology*, 33, no. 3-4, 275-317.

Bonaventure, P., Hall, H., Gommeren, W., Cras, P., Langlois, X., Jurzak, M. and Leysen, J.E. (2000) Mapping of serotonin 5-HT(4) receptor mRNA and ligand binding sites in the post-mortem human brain. *Synapse*, 36, no. 1, 35-46.

Bonaventure, P., Voorn, P., Luyten, W.H., Jurzak, M., Schotte, A. and Leysen, J.E. (1998) Detailed mapping of serotonin 5-HT1B and 5-HT1D receptor messenger RNA and ligand binding sites in guinea-pig brain and trigeminal ganglion: clues for function. *Neuroscience*, 82, no. 2, 469-484.

Bonsi, P., Cuomo, D., Ding, J., Sciamanna, G., Ulrich, S., Tscherter, A., Bernardi, G., Surmeier, D.J. and Pisani, A. (2007a) Endogenous serotonin excites striatal cholinergic interneurons via the activation of 5-HT 2C, 5-HT6, and 5-HT7 serotonin receptors: implications for extrapyramidal side effects of serotonin reuptake inhibitors. *Neuropsychopharmacology*, 32, no. 8, 1840-1854.

Bonsi, P., Cuomo, D., Picconi, B., Sciamanna, G., Tscherter, A., Tolu, M., Bernardi, G., Calabresi, P. and Pisani, A. (2007b) Striatal metabotropic glutamate receptors as a target for pharmacotherapy in Parkinson's disease. *Amino Acids*, 32, no. 2, 189-195.

Boschert, U., Amara, D.A., Segu, L. and Hen, R. (1994) The mouse 5-hydroxytryptamine1B receptor is localized predominantly on axon terminals. *Neuroscience*, 58, no. 1, 167-182.

Bourson A, Boess F.G., Bös M. and Sleight A.J. (1998) Involvement of 5-HT6 receptors in nigro-striatal function in rodents. *Br. J. Pharmacol.*, 125, no. 7, 1562-1566.

Breese, G.R., Baumeister, A., Napier, T.C., Frye, G.D. and Mueller, R.A. (1985) Evidence that D-1 dopamine receptors contribute to the supersensitive behavioral responses induced by L-dihydroxyphenylalanine in rats treated neonatally with 6-hydroxydopamine. *J. Pharmacol. Exp. Ther.*, 235, no. 2, 287-295.

Breese, G.R., Knapp, D.J., Criswell, H.E., Moy, S.S., Papadeas, S.T. and Blake, B.L. (2005) The neonate-6-hydroxydopamine-lesioned rat: a model for clinical neuroscience and neurobiological principles. *Brain Res. Brain Res. Rev.*, 48, no. 1, 57-73.

Brodie, B.B., Pletscher, A. and Shore, P.A. (1955) Evidence that serotonin has a role in brain function. *Science*, 122, no. 3177, 968.

Brown, P. and Gerfen, C.R. (2006) Plasticity within striatal direct pathway neurons after neonatal dopamine depletion is mediated through a novel functional coupling of serotonin 5-HT2 receptors to the ERK 1/2 map kinase pathway. *J. Comp. Neurol.*, 498, no. 3, 415-430.

Bruggeman, R., Heeringa, M., Westerink, B.H. and Timmerman, W. (2000) Combined 5-HT2/D2 receptor blockade inhibits the firing rate of SNR neurons in the rat brain. *Prog. Neuropsychopharmacol. Biol. Psychiatry*, 24, no. 4, 579-593.

Bruinvels, A.T., Palacios, J.M. and Hoyer, D. (1993a) Autoradiographic characterisation and localisation of 5-HT1D compared to 5-HT1B binding sites in rat brain. *Naunyn Schmiedebergs Arch. Pharmacol.*, 347, no. 6, 569-582.

Bruinvels, A.T., Palacios, J.M. and Hoyer, D. (1993b) 5-hydroxytryptamine1 recognition sites in rat brain: heterogeneity of non-5-hydroxytryptamine1A/1C binding sites revealed by quantitative receptor autoradiography. *Neuroscience*, 53, no. 2, 465-473.

Bruinvels, A.T., Landwehrmeyer, B., Gustafson, E.L., Durkin, M.M., Mengod, G., Branchek, T.A., Hoyer, D. and Palacios, J.M. (1994) Localization of 5-HT1B, 5-HT1D alpha, 5-HT1E and 5-HT1F receptor messenger RNA in rodent and primate brain. *Neuropharmacology*, 33, no. 3-4, 367-386.

Bubser, M., Backstrom, J.R., Sanders-Bush, E., Roth, B.L. and Deutch, A.Y. (2001) Distribution of serotonin 5-HT(2A) receptors in afferents of the rat striatum. *Synapse*, 39, no. 4, 297-304.

Bufton, K.E., Steward, L.J., Barber, P.C. and Barnes, N.M. (1993) Distribution and characterization of the [3H]granisetron-labelled 5-HT3 receptor in the human forebrain. *Neuropharmacology*, 32, no. 12, 1325-1331.

Bymaster, F.P., Falcone, J.F., Bauzon, D., Kennedy, J.S., Schenck, K., DeLapp, N.W. and Cohen, M.L. (2001) Potent antagonism of 5-HT(3) and 5-HT(6) receptors by olanzapine. *Eur. J. Pharmacol.*, 430, no. 2-3, 341-349.

Canton, H., Verriele, L. and Colpaert, F.C. (1990) Binding of typical and atypical antipsychotics to 5-HT1C and 5-HT2 sites: clozapine potently interacts with 5-HT1C sites. *Eur. J. Pharmacol.*, 191, no. 1, 93-96.

Canton, H., Verriele, L. and Millan, M.J. (1994) Competitive antagonism of serotonin (5-HT)2C and 5-HT2A receptor-mediated phosphoinositide (PI) turnover by clozapine in the rat: a comparison to other antipsychotics. *Neurosci. Lett.*, 181, no. 1-2, 65-68.

Carlson, B.B., Wisniecki, A. and Salamone, J.D. (2003) Local injections of the 5-hydroxytryptamine antagonist mianserin into substantia nigra pars reticulata block tremulous jaw movements in rats: studies with a putative model of Parkinsonian tremor. *Psychopharmacology (Berl).* 165, no. 3, 229-237.

Carlsson, T., Carta, M., Winkler, C., Bjorklund, A. and Kirik, D. (2007) Serotonin neuron transplants exacerbate L-DOPA-induced dyskinesias in a rat model of Parkinson's disease. *J. Neurosci.*, 27, no. 30, 8011-8022.

Carta, M., Carlsson, T., Kirik, D. and Bjorklund, A. (2007) Dopamine released from 5-HT terminals is the cause of L-DOPA-induced dyskinesia in parkinsonian rats. *Brain*, 130, no. Pt 7, 1819-1833.

Castro, M.E., Pascual, J., Romon, T., Berciano, J., Figols, J. and Pazos, A. (1998) 5-HT1B receptor binding in degenerative movement disorders. *Brain Res.*, 790, no. 1-2, 323-328.

Chadha, A., Sur, C., Atack, J. and Duty, S. (2000) The 5HT(1B) receptor agonist, CP-93129, inhibits [(3)H]-GABA release from rat globus pallidus slices and reverses akinesia following intrapallidal injection in the reserpine-treated rat. *Br. J. Pharmacol.*, 130, no. 8, 1927-1932.

Charles, P.D., Padaliya, B.B., Newman, W.J., Gill, C.E., Covington, C.D., Fang, J.Y., So, S.A., Tramontana, M.G., Konrad, P.E. and Davis, T.L. (2004) Deep brain stimulation of the subthalamic nucleus reduces antiparkinsonian medication costs. *Parkinsonism and related disorders*, 10, no. 8, 475-479.

Chase, T.N. (1974) Serotonergic-dopaminergic interactions and extrapyramidal function. *Adv. Biochem. Psychopharmacol.*, 11, no. 0, 377-385.

Chase, T.N. and Ng, L.K. (1972) Central monoamine metabolism in Parkinson's disease. *Arch. Neurol.*, 27, no. 6, 486-491.

Chen, L., Yung, K.K., Chan, Y.S. and Yung, W.H. (2008) 5-HT excites globus pallidus neurons by multiple receptor mechanisms. *Neuroscience*, 151, no. 2, 439-451.

Chinaglia, G., Landwehrmeyer, B., Probst, A. and Palacios, J.M. (1993) Serotoninergic terminal transporters are differentially affected in Parkinson's disease and progressive supranuclear palsy: an autoradiographic study with [3H]citalopram. *Neuroscience*, 54, no. 3, 691-699.

Chu, Y.X., Liu, J., Feng, J., Wang, Y., Zhang, Q.J. and Li, Q. (2004) [Changes of discharge rate and pattern of 5-hydroxytrypamine neurons of dorsal raphe nucleus in a rat model of Parkinson's disease]. *Sheng Li Xue Bao*, 56, no. 5, 597-602.

Cicin-Sain, L. and Jenner, P. (1993) Reduction in cortical 5-HT3 binding sites following a unilateral 6-hydroxydopamine lesion of the medial forebrain bundle in rats. *J. Neurol. Sci.*, 115, no. 1, 105-110.

Clayton, A.H. (1995) Antidepressant-induced tardive dyskinesia: review and case report. *Psychopharmacol. Bull.*, 31, no. 2, 259-264.

Collingridge, G.L. and Davies, J. (1981) The influence of striatal stimulation and putative neurotransmitters on identified neurones in the rat substantia nigra. *Brain Res.*, 212, no. 2, 345-359.

Commins, D.L., Shaughnessy, R.A., Axt, K.J., Vosmer, G. and Seiden, L.S. (1989) Variability among brain regions in the specificity of 6-hydroxydopamine (6-OHDA)-induced lesions. *J. Neural Transm.*, 77, no. 2-3, 197-210.

Compan, V., Daszuta, A., Salin, P., Sebben, M., Bockaert, J. and Dumuis, A. (1996) Lesion study of the distribution of serotonin 5-HT4 receptors in rat basal ganglia and hippocampus. *Eur. J. Neurosci.*, 8, no. 12, 2591-2598.

Compan, V., Segu, L., Buhot, M.C. and Daszuta, A. (1998) Selective increases in serotonin 5-HT1B/1D and 5-HT2A/2C binding sites in adult rat basal ganglia following lesions of serotonergic neurons. *Brain Res.*, 793, no. 1-2, 103-111.

Cornea-Hébert, V., Riad, M., Wu, C., Singh, S.K. and Descarries, L. (1999) Cellular and subcellular distribution of the serotonin 5-HT2A receptor in the central nervous system of adult rat. *J. Comp. Neurol.*, 409, no. 2, 187-209.

Corvaja, N., Doucet, G. and Bolam, J.P. (1993) Ultrastructure and synaptic targets of the raphe-nigral projection in the rat. *Neuroscience*, 55, no. 2, 417-427.

D'Addario, C., Di Benedetto, M., Izenwasser, S., Candeletti, S. and Romualdi, P. (2007) Role of serotonin in the regulation of the dynorphinergic system by a kappa-opioid agonist and cocaine treatment in rat CNS. *Neuroscience*, 144, no. 1, 157-164.

Dahlström, A. and Fuxe, K. (1964) Evidence for the Existence of Monoamine-Containing Neurons in the Central Nervous System. I. Demonstration of Monoamines in the Cell Bodies of Brain Stem Neurons. *Acta Physiol. Scand.*, 62, no. 232, 1-55.

Darmani, N.A., Shaddy, J. and Gerdes, C.F. (1996) Differential ontogenesis of three DOI-induced behaviors in mice. *Physiol. Behav.*, 60, no. 6, 1495-1500.

Davies, J. and Tongroach, P. (1978) Neuropharmacological studies on the nigro-striatal and raphe-striatal system in the rat. *Eur. J. Pharmacol.*, 51, no. 2, 91-100.

De Deurwaerdere, P. and Chesselet, M.F. (2000) Nigrostriatal lesions alter oral dyskinesia and c-Fos expression induced by the serotonin agonist 1-(m-chlorophenyl)piperazine in adult rats. *J. Neurosci.*, 20, no. 13, 5170-5178.

del Arco, C., Galende, I. and Pazos, A. (1993) Autoradiographic mapping of 5-HT1 receptors in the guinea-pig brain with particular reference to the 5-HT1D receptor sites. *Naunyn Schmiedebergs Arch. Pharmacol.*, 347, no. 3, 248-256.

DeLong, M.R. (1990) Primate models of movement disorders of basal ganglia origin. *Trends Neurosci.*, 13, no. 7, 281-285.

Deniau, J.M. and Chevalier, G. (1985) Disinhibition as a basic process in the expression of striatal functions. II. The striato-nigral influence on thalamocortical cells of the ventromedial thalamic nucleus. *Brain Res.*, 334, no. 2, 227-233.

Di Giovanni, G. (2008) Will it Ever Become Possible to Prevent Dopaminergic Neuronal Degeneration? *CNS and neurological disorders drug targets*, 7, no. 1, 28-44.

Di Giovanni, G., Di Matteo, V., La Grutta, V. and Esposito, E. (2001) m-Chlorophenylpiperazine excites non-dopaminergic neurons in the rat substantia nigra and ventral tegmental area by activating serotonin-2C receptors. *Neuroscience*, 103, no. 1, 111-116.

Di Giovanni, G., Di Matteo, V., Pierucci, M., Benigno, A. and Esposito, E. (2006a) Central serotonin2C receptor: from physiology to pathology. *Current topics in medicinal chemistry*, 6, no. 18, 1909-1925.

Di Giovanni, G., Di Matteo, V., Pierucci, M., Benigno, A. and Esposito, E. (2006b) Serotonin involvement in the basal ganglia pathophysiology: could the 5-HT2C receptor be a new target for therapeutic strategies? *Curr. Med. Chem.*, 13, no. 25, 3069-3081.

Di Matteo, V., Cacchio, M., Di Giulio, C., Di Giovanni, G. and Esposito, E. (2002) Biochemical evidence that the atypical antipsychotic drugs clozapine and risperidone block 5-HT(2C) receptors in vivo. *Pharmacol. Biochem. Behav.*, 71, no. 4, 607-613.

Dijk, S.N., Francis, P.T., Stratmann, G.C. and Bowen, D.M. (1995) NMDA-induced glutamate and aspartate release from rat cortical pyramidal neurones: evidence for modulation by a 5-HT1A antagonist. *Br. J. Pharmacol.*, 115, no. 7, 1169-1174.

Doder, M., Rabiner, E.A., Turjanski, N., Lees, A.J. and Brooks, D.J. (2003) Tremor in Parkinson's disease and serotonergic dysfunction: an 11C-WAY 100635 PET study. *Neurology*, 60, no. 4, 601-605.

Doucet, E., Miquel, M.C., Nosjean, A., Verge, D., Hamon, M. and Emerit, M.B. (1999) Immunolabeling of the rat central nervous system with antibodies partially selective of the short form of the 5-HT3 receptor. *Neuroscience*, 95, no. 3, 881-892.

Dray, A., Gonye, T.J. and Oakley, N.R. (1976) Effects of alpha-flupenthixol on dopamine and 5-hydroxytryptamine responses of substantia nigra neurones. *Neuropharmacology*, 15, no. 12, 793-796.

Duncan, G.E., Knapp, D.J., Breese, G.R., Crews, F.T. and Little, K.Y. (1998) Species Differences in Regional Patterns of 3H-8-OH-DPAT and 3H-Zolpidem Binding in the Rat and Human Brain. *Pharmacol. Biochem. Behav.*, 60, no. 2, 439-448.

Durif, F., Debilly, B., Galitzky, M., Morand, D., Viallet, F., Borg, M., Thobois, S., Broussolle, E. and Rascol, O. (2004) Clozapine improves dyskinesias in Parkinson disease: a double-blind, placebo-controlled study. *Neurology*, 62, no. 3, 381-388.

Duvoisin, R.C. (1967) Cholinergic-anticholinergic antagonism in parkinsonism. *Arch. Neurol.*, 17, no. 2, 124-136.

Eberle-Wang, K., Lucki, I. and Chesselet, M.F. (1996) A role for the subthalamic nucleus in 5-HT2C-induced oral dyskinesia. *Neuroscience*, 72, no. 1, 117-128.

Eberle-Wang, K., Mikeladze, Z., Uryu, K. and Chesselet, M.F. (1997) Pattern of expression of the serotonin2C receptor messenger RNA in the basal ganglia of adult rats. *J. Comp. Neurol.*, 384, no. 2, 233-247.

Eisensamer, B., Uhr, M., Meyr, S., Gimpl, G., Deiml, T., Rammes, G., Lambert, J.J., Zieglgansberger, W., Holsboer, F. and Rupprecht, R. (2005) Antidepressants and antipsychotic drugs colocalize with 5-HT3 receptors in raft-like domains. *J. Neurosci.*, 25, no. 44, 10198-10206.

el Mansari, M. and Blier, P. (1997) In vivo electrophysiological characterization of 5-HT receptors in the guinea pig head of caudate nucleus and orbitofrontal cortex. *Neuropharmacology*, 36, no. 4-5, 577-588.

el Mansari, M., Radja, F., Ferron, A., Reader, T.A., Molina-Holgado, E. and Descarries, L. (1994) Hypersensitivity to serotonin and its agonists in serotonin-hyperinnervated neostriatum after neonatal dopamine denervation. *Eur. J. Pharmacol.*, 261, no. 1-2, 171-178.

Ellison, G. (1991) Spontaneous orofacial movements in rodents induced by long-term neuroleptic administration: a second opinion. *Psychopharmacology (Berl).* 104, no. 3, 404-408.

Ellison, G. and See, R.E. (1989) Rats administered chronic neuroleptics develop oral movements which are similar in form to those in humans with tardive dyskinesia. *Psychopharmacology (Berl).* 98, no. 4, 564-566.

Esposito, E., Di Matteo, V., Benigno, A., Pierucci, M., Crescimanno, G. and Di Giovanni, G. (2007a) Non-steroidal anti-inflammatory drugs in Parkinson's disease. *Exp. Neurol.*, 205, no. 2, 295-312.

Esposito, E., Di Matteo, V. and Di Giovanni, G. (2007b) Death in the substantia nigra: a motor tragedy. *Expert review of neurotherapeutics*, 7, no. 6, 677-697.

Esposito, E., Di Matteo, V., Pierucci, M., Benigno, A. and Di Giovanni, G. (2007c). Role of central 5-HT_{2C} receptor in the control of basal ganglia functions. In G. Di Giovanni (Ed.), *The Basal Ganglia Pathophysiology: Recent Advances.* Transworld research network, Trivandrum, 97-127.

Fibiger, H.C., Miller, J.J. (1977) An Anatomical and electrophysiological investigation of the serotoninergic projection from the dorsal raphe nucleus to the substantia nigra in the rat. *Neuroscience*, 2, 975-987.

Filip, M., Bubar, M.J. and Cunningham, K.A. (2004) Contribution of serotonin (5-hydroxytryptamine; 5-HT) 5-HT2 receptor subtypes to the hyperlocomotor effects of cocaine: acute and chronic pharmacological analyses. *J. Pharmacol. Exp. Ther.*, 310, no. 3, 1246-1254.

Filip, M. and Cunningham, K.A. (2002) Serotonin 5-HT(2C) receptors in nucleus accumbens regulate expression of the hyperlocomotive and discriminative stimulus effects of cocaine. *Pharmacol. Biochem. Behav.*, 71, no. 4, 745-756.

Fletcher, S. and Barnes, N.M. (1999) Autoradiographic localization of the [3H]-(S)-zacopride labelled 5-HT3 receptor in porcine brain. *Neurosci. Lett.*, 269, no. 2, 91-94.

Fletcher, P.J., Grottick, A.J. and Higgins, G.A. (2002) Differential effects of the 5-HT(2A) receptor antagonist M100907 and the 5-HT(2C) receptor antagonist SB242084 on cocaine-induced locomotor activity, cocaine self-administration and cocaine-induced reinstatement of responding. *Neuropsychopharmacology*, 27, no. 4, 576-586.

Flores, G., Rosales, M.G., Hernandez, S., Sierra, A. and Aceves, J. (1995) 5-Hydroxytryptamine increases spontaneous activity of subthalamic neurons in the rat. *Neurosci. Lett.*, 192, no. 1, 17-20.

Fox, S.H. and Brotchie, J.M. (2000a) 5-HT(2C) receptor antagonists enhance the behavioural response to dopamine D(1) receptor agonists in the 6-hydroxydopamine-lesioned rat. *Eur. J. Pharmacol.*, 398, no. 1, 59-64.

Fox, S.H. and Brotchie, J.M. (2000b) 5-HT2C receptor binding is increased in the substantia nigra pars reticulata in Parkinson's disease. *Mov. Disord.*, 15, no. 6, 1064-1069.

Fox, S.H., Moser, B. and Brotchie, J.M. (1998) Behavioral effects of 5-HT2C receptor antagonism in the substantia nigra zona reticulata of the 6-hydroxydopamine-lesioned rat model of Parkinson's disease. *Exp. Neurol.*, 151, no. 1, 35-49.

Frechilla, D., Cobreros, A., Saldise, L., Moratalla, R., Insausti, R., Luquin, M. and Del Río, J. (2001) Serotonin 5-HT_{1A} receptor expression is selectively enhanced in the striosomal compartment of chronic parkinsonian monkeys. *Synapse*, 39, no. 4, 288-296.

Garcia, L., D'Alessandro, G., Bioulac, B. and Hammond, C. (2005) High-frequency stimulation in Parkinson's disease: more or less? *Trends Neurosci.*, 28, no. 4, 209-216.

Gardell, L.R., Vanover, K.E., Pounds, L., Johnson, R.W., Barido, R., Anderson, G.T., Veinbergs, I., Dyssegaard, A., Brunmark, P., Tabatabaei, A., Davis, R.E., Brann, M.R., Hacksell, U. and Bonhaus, D.W. (2007) ACP-103, a 5-hydroxytryptamine 2A receptor inverse agonist, improves the antipsychotic efficacy and side-effect profile of haloperidol and risperidone in experimental models. *J. Pharmacol. Exp. Ther.*, 322, no. 2, 862-870.

Gehlert, D.R., Gackenheimer, S.L., Wong, D.T. and Robertson, D.W. (1991) Localization of 5-HT3 receptors in the rat brain using [3H]LY278584. *Brain Res.*, 553, no. 1, 149-154.

Gehlert, D.R., Schober, D.A., Gackenheimer, S.L., Mais, D.E., Ladouceur, G. and Robertson, D.W. (1993) Synthesis and evaluation of [125I]-(S)-iodozacopride, a high affinity radioligand for 5HT3 receptors. *Neurochem. Int.*, 23, no. 4, 373-383.

Gerard, C., el Mestikawy, S., Lebrand, C., Adrien, J., Ruat, M., Traiffort, E., Hamon, M. and Martres, M.P. (1996) Quantitative RT-PCR distribution of serotonin 5-HT_6 receptor mRNA in the central nervous system of control or 5,7-dihydroxytryptamine-treated rats. *Synapse*, 23, no. 3, 164-173.

Gerard, C., Martres, M.P., Lefevre, K., Miquel, M.C., Verge, D., Lanfumey, L., Doucet, E., Hamon, M. and el Mestikawy, S. (1997) Immuno-localization of serotonin 5-HT_6 receptor-like material in the rat central nervous system. *Brain Res.*, 746, no. 1-2, 207-219.

Gerber, R., Altar, C.A. and Liebman, J.M. (1988) Rotational behavior induced by 8-hydroxy-DPAT, a putative 5HT-1A agonist, in 6-hydroxydopamine-lesioned rats. *Psychopharmacology (Berl).* 94, no. 2, 178-182.

Gerfen, C.R. (1984) The neostriatal mosaic: compartmentalization of corticostriatal input and striatonigral output systems. *Nature*, 311, no. 5985, 461-464.

Gerfen, C.R. (1985) The neostriatal mosaic. I. Compartmental organization of projections from the striatum to the substantia nigra in the rat. *J. Comp. Neurol.*, 236, no. 4, 454-476.

Goldstein, M., Anagnoste, B., Battista, A.F., Owen, W.S. and Nakatani, S. (1969) Studies of amines in the striatum in monkeys with nigral lesions. The disposition, biosynthesis and metabolites of [3H]dopamine and [14C]serotonin in the striatum. *J. Neurochem.*, 16, no. 4, 645-653.

Gong, L. and Kostrzewa, R.M. (1992) Supersensitized oral responses to a serotonin agonist in neonatal 6-OHDA-treated rats. *Pharmacol. Biochem. Behav.*, 41, no. 3, 621-623.

Gongora-Alfaro, J.L., Hernandez-Lopez, S., Flores-Hernandez, J. and Galarraga, E. (1997) Firing frequency modulation of substantia nigra reticulata neurons by 5-hydroxytryptamine. *Neurosci. Res.*, 29, no. 3, 225-231.

Granoff, M.I. and Ashby, C.R., Jr. (1998) The effect of the repeated administration of the compound 3,4-methylenedioxymethamphetamine on the response of rats to the 5-HT2A,C receptor agonist (+/-)-1-(2,5-dimethoxy-4-iodophenyl)-2-aminopropane (DOI). *Neuropsychobiology*, 37, no. 1, 36-40.

Grottick, A.J., Fletcher, P.J. and Higgins, G.A. (2000) Studies to investigate the role of 5-$HT_{(2C)}$ receptors on cocaine- and food-maintained behavior. *J. Pharmacol. Exp. Ther.*, 295, no. 3, 1183-1191.

Guerra, M.J., Liste, I. and Labandeira-Garcia, J.L. (1997) Effects of lesions of the nigrostriatal pathway and of nigral grafts on striatal serotonergic innervation in adult rats. *Neuroreport*, 8, no. 16, 3485-3488.

Guiard, B.P., El Mansari, M., Merali, Z. and Blier, P. (2008) Functional interactions between dopamine, serotonin and norepinephrine neurons: an in-vivo electrophysiological study in rats with monoaminergic lesions. *Int. J. Neuropsychopharmacol.*, 21, 1-15.

Gunes, A., Scordo, M., Jaanson, P. and Dahl, M.-L. (2007) Serotonin and dopamine receptor gene polymorphisms and the risk of extrapyramidal side effects in perphenazine-treated schizophrenic patients. *Psychopharmacology (Berl).* 190, no. 4, 479-484.

Gunes, A., Dahl, M.-L., Spina, E. and Scordo, M. (2008) Further evidence for the association between 5-HT2C receptor gene polymorphisms and extrapyramidal side effects in male schizophrenic patients. *Eur. J. Clin. Pharmacol.*, 64, no. 5, 477-482.

Haapaniemi, T.H., Ahonen, A., Torniainen, P., Sotaniemi, K.A. and Myllyla, V.V. (2001) [123I]beta-CIT SPECT demonstrates decreased brain dopamine and serotonin transporter levels in untreated parkinsonian patients. *Mov. Disord.*, 16, no. 1, 124-130.

Haleem, D.J. and Khan, N.H. (2003) Enhancement of serotonin-1A receptor dependent responses following withdrawal of haloperidol in rats. *Prog. Neuropsychopharmacol. Biol. Psychiatry*, 27, no. 4, 645-651.

Haleem, D.J., Samad, N. and Haleem, M.A. (2007a) Reversal of haloperidol-induced extrapyramidal symptoms by buspirone: a time-related study. *Behav. Pharmacol.*, 18, no. 2, 147-153.

Haleem, D.J., Samad, N. and Haleem, M.A. (2007b) Reversal of haloperidol-induced tardive vacuous chewing movements and supersensitive somatodendritic serotonergic response by buspirone in rats. *Pharmacol. Biochem. Behav.*, 87, no. 1, 115-121.

Haleem, D.J., Shireen, E. and Haleem, M.A. (2004) Somatodendritic and postsynaptic serotonin-1A receptors in the attenuation of haloperidol-induced catalepsy. *Prog. Neuropsychopharmacol. Biol. Psychiatry*, 28, no. 8, 1323-1329.

Hall, H., Lundkvist, C., Halldin, C., Farde, L., Pike, V.W., McCarron, J.A., Fletcher, A., Cliffe, I.A., Barf, T., Wikstrom, H. and Sedvall, G. (1997) Autoradiographic localization of 5-HT1A receptors in the post-mortem human brain using [3H]WAY-100635 and [11C]WAY-100635. *Brain Res.*, 745, no. 1-2, 96-108.

Halliday, G.M., Blumbergs, P.C., Cotton, R.G.H., Blessing, W.W. and Geffen, L.B. (1990) Loss of brainstem serotonin- and substance P-containing neurons in Parkinson's disease. *Brain Res.*, 510, no. 1, 104-107.

Hameleers, R., Blokland, A., Steinbusch, H.W.M., Visser-Vandewalle, V. and Temel, Y. (2007) Hypomobility after DOI administration can be reversed by subthalamic nucleus deep brain stimulation. *Behav. Brain Res.*, 185, no. 1, 65-67.

Hamon, M., Doucet, E., Lefevre, K., Miquel, M.C., Lanfumey, L., Insausti, R., Frechilla, D., Del Rio, J. and Verge, D. (1999) Antibodies and antisense oligonucleotide for probing the distribution and putative functions of central 5-HT_6 receptors. *Neuropsychopharmacology*, 21, no. 2 Suppl, 68S-76S.

Hashimoto, K. and Kita, H. (2008) Serotonin Activates Presynaptic and Postsynaptic Receptors in Rat Globus Pallidus. *J. Neurophysiol.*, 99, no. 4, 1723-1732.

Hawkins, M.F., Uzelac, S.M., Baumeister, A.A., Hearn, J.K., Broussard, J.I. and Guillot, T.S. (2002) Behavioral responses to stress following central and peripheral injection of the 5-HT2 agonist DOI. *Pharmacol. Biochem. Behav.*, 73, no. 3, 537-544.

Heidenreich, B.A. and Napier, T.C. (2000) Effects of serotonergic 5-HT_{1A} and 5-HT_{1B} ligands on ventral pallidal neuronal activity. *Neuroreport*, 11, no. 13, 2849-2853.

Herrick-Davis, K., Grinde, E. and Teitler, M. (2000) Inverse Agonist Activity of Atypical Antipsychotic Drugs at Human 5-$Hydroxytryptamine_{2C}$ Receptors. *J. Pharmacol. Exp. Ther.*, 295, no. 1, 226-232.

Hervé, D., Pickel, V.M., Joh, T.H. and Beaudet, A. (1987) Serotonin axon terminals in the ventral tegmental area of the rat: fine structure and synaptic input to dopaminergic neurons. *Brain Res.*, 435, no. 1-2, 71-83.

Hicks, P.B. (1990) The effect of serotonergic agents on haloperidol-induced catalepsy. *Life Sci.*, 47, no. 18, 1609-1615.

Higgins, G.A., Jordan, C.C. and Skingle, M. (1991) Evidence that the unilateral activation of 5-HT_{1D} receptors in the substantia nigra of the guinea-pig elicits contralateral rotation. *Br. J. Pharmacol.*, 102, no. 2, 305-310.

Hirst, W.D., Abrahamsen, B., Blaney, F.E., Calver, A.R., Aloj, L., Price, G.W. and Medhurst, A.D. (2003) Differences in the Central Nervous System Distribution and Pharmacology of the Mouse 5-Hydroxytryptamine-6 Receptor Compared with Rat and Human Receptors Investigated by Radioligand Binding, Site-Directed Mutagenesis, and Molecular Modeling. 1295-1308.

Hirst, W.D., Minton, J.A., Bromidge, S.M., Moss, S.F., Latter, A.J., Riley, G., Routledge, C., Middlemiss, D.N. and Price, G.W. (2000) Characterization of [(125)I]-SB-258585 binding to human recombinant and native 5-HT(6) receptors in rat, pig and human brain tissue. *Br. J. Pharmacol.*, 130, no. 7, 1597-1605.

Hoffman, B.J. and Mezey, E. (1989) Distribution of serotonin 5-HT1C receptor mRNA in adult rat brain. *FEBS Lett.*, 247, no. 2, 453-462.

Horner, K.A., Adams, D.H., Hanson, G.R. and Keefe, K.A. (2005) Blockade of stimulant-induced preprodynorphin mRNA expression in the striatal matrix by serotonin depletion. *Neuroscience*, 131, no. 1, 67-77.

Hornykiewicz, O. (1973) Dopamine in the Basal Ganglia: Its Role and Therapeutic Implications (Including the Clinical Use of L-DOPA). *Br. Med. Bull.*, 29, no. 2, 172-178.

Hornykiewicz, O. (1998) Biochemical aspects of Parkinson's disease. *Neurology*, 51, no. 2, S2-9.

Hoyer, D., Hannon, J.P. and Martin, G.R. (2002) Molecular, pharmacological and functional diversity of 5-HT receptors. *Pharmacol. Biochem. Behav.*, 71, no. 4, 533-554.

Hoyer, D., Pazos, A., Probst, A. and Palacios, J.M. (1986) Serotonin receptors in the human brain. I. Characterization and autoradiographic localization of 5-HT1A recognition sites. Apparent absence of 5-HT1B recognition sites. *Brain Res.*, 376, no. 1, 85-96.

Ikeguchi, K. and Kuroda, A. (1995) Mianserin treatment of patients with psychosis induced by antiparkinsonian drugs. *Eur. Arch. Psychiatry Clin. Neurosci.*, 244, no. 6, 320-324.

Ikram, H., Samad, N. and Haleem, D.J. (2007) Neurochemical and behavioral effects of m-CPP in a rat model of tardive dyskinesia. *Pakistan journal of pharmaceutical sciences*, 20, no. 3, 188-195.

Invernizzi, R.W., Cervo, L. and Samanin, R. (1988) 8-Hydroxy-2-(di-n-propylamino) tetralin, a selective serotonin1A receptor agonist, blocks haloperidol-induced catalepsy by an action on raphe nuclei medianus and dorsalis. *Neuropharmacology*, 27, no. 5, 515-518.

Invernizzi, R.W., Pierucci, M., Calcagno, E., Di Giovanni, G., Di Matteo, V., Benigno, A. and Esposito, E. (2007) Selective activation of 5-HT2C receptors stimulates GABA-ergic function in the rat substantia nigra pars reticulata: A combined in vivo electro-physiological and neurochemical study. *Neuroscience*, 144, no. 4, 1523-1535.

Ito, H., Halldin, C. and Farde, L. (1999) Localization of 5-HT1A Receptors in the Living Human Brain Using [Carbonyl-11C]WAY-100635: PET with Anatomic Standardization Technique. *J. Nucl. Med.*, 40, no. 1, 102-109.

Jackson, M.J., Al-Barghouthy, G., Pearce, R.K.B., Smith, L., Hagan, J.J. and Jenner, P. (2004) Effect of 5-HT1B/D receptor agonist and antagonist administration on motor function in haloperidol and MPTP-treated common marmosets. *Pharmacol. Biochem. Behav.*, 79, no. 3, 391-400.

Jacobs, B.L. and Azmitia, E.C. (1992) Structure and function of the brain serotonin system. *Physiol. Rev.*, 72, no. 1, 165-229.

James, T.A. and Starr, M.S. (1980) Rotational behaviour elicited by 5-HT in the rat: evidence for an inhibitory role of 5-HT in the substantia nigra and corpus striatum. *J. Pharm. Pharmacol.*, 32, no. 3, 196-200.

Jellinger, K. (1987) Overview of morphological changes in Parkinson's disease. *Adv. Neurol.*, 45, no., 1-18.

Johnson, S.W., Mercuri, N.B. and North, R.A. (1992) 5-hydroxytryptamine$_{1B}$ receptors block the GABA$_B$ synaptic potential in rat dopamine neurons. *J. Neurosci.*, 12, no. 5, 2000-2006.

Johnston, T.H. and Brotchie, J.M. (2006) Drugs in development for Parkinson's disease: an update. *Curr Opin Investig Drugs*, 7, no. 1, 25-32.

Kalkman, H.O., Neumann, V. and Tricklebank, M.D. (1997) Clozapine inhibits catalepsy induced by olanzapine and loxapine, but prolongs catalepsy induced by SCH 23390 in rats. *Naunyn Schmiedebergs Arch. Pharmacol.*, 355, no. 3, 361-364.

Kehne, J.H., Ketteler, H.J., McCloskey, T.C., Sullivan, C.K., Dudley, M.W. and Schmidt, C.J. (1996) Effects of the selective 5-HT2A receptor antagonist MDL 100,907 on MDMA-induced locomotor stimulation in rats. *Neuropsychopharmacology*, 15, no. 2, 116-124.

Kennett, G.A., Lightowler, S., de Biasi, V., Stevens, N.C., Wood, M.D., Tulloch, I.F. and Blackburn, T.P. (1994) Effect of chronic administration of selective 5-hydroxytryptamine and noradrenaline uptake inhibitors on a putative index of 5-HT2C/2B receptor function. *Neuropharmacology*, 33, no. 12, 1581-1588.

Kennett, G.A., Wood, M.D., Bright, F., Cilia, J., Piper, D.C., Gager, T., Thomas, D., Baxter, G.S., Forbes, I.T., Ham, P. and Blackburn, T.P. (1996) In vitro and in vivo profile of SB 206553, a potent 5-HT2C/5-HT2B receptor antagonist with anxiolytic-like properties. *Br. J. Pharmacol.*, 117, no. 3, 427-434.

Kennett, G.A., Wood, M.D., Bright, F., Trail, B., Riley, G., Holland, V., Avenell, K.Y., Stean, T., Upton, N., Bromidge, S., Forbes, I.T., Brown, A.M., Middlemiss, D.N. and Blackburn, T.P. (1997) SB 242084, a selective and brain penetrant 5-HT2C receptor antagonist. *Neuropharmacology*, 36, no. 4-5, 609-620.

Kerenyi, L., Ricaurte, G.A., Schretlen, D.J., McCann, U., Varga, J., Mathews, W.B., Ravert, H.T., Dannals, R.F., Hilton, J., Wong, D.F. and Szabo, Z. (2003) Positron Emission Tomography of Striatal Serotonin Transporters in Parkinson Disease. *Arch. Neurol.*, 60, no. 9, 1223-1229.

Khawaja, X. (1995) Quantitative autoradiographic characterisation of the binding of [3H]WAY-100635, a selective 5-HT1A receptor antagonist. *Brain Res.*, 673, no. 2, 217-225.

Kienzl E, Riederer P, Jellinger K, Wesemann W. (1981) Transitional states of central serotonin receptors in Parkinson's disease. *J. Neural. Transm.*, 51, no. 1-2, 113-122.

Kilpatrick, G.J., Jones, B.J. and Tyers, M.B. (1987) Identification and distribution of 5-HT3 receptors in rat brain using radioligand binding. *Nature*, 330, no. 6150, 746-748.

Kim, S.E., Choi, J.Y., Choe, Y.S., Choi, Y. and Lee, W.Y. (2003) Serotonin Transporters in the Midbrain of Parkinson's Disease Patients: A Study with 123I-{beta}-CIT SPECT. *J. Nucl. Med.*, 44, no. 6, 870-876.

Kish, S.J., Tong, J., Hornykiewicz, O., Rajput, A., Chang, L.-J., Guttman, M. and Furukawa, Y. (2008) Preferential loss of serotonin markers in caudate versus putamen in Parkinson's disease. *Brain*, 131, no. 1, 120-131.

Kita, H., Chiken, S., Tachibana, Y. and Nambu, A. (2007) Serotonin Modulates Pallidal Neuronal Activity in the Awake Monkey. *J. Neurosci.*, 27, no. 1, 75-83.

Kita, H. and Kitai, S.T. (1987) Efferent projections of the subthalamic nucleus in the rat: light and electron microscopic analysis with the PHA-L method. *J. Comp. Neurol.*, 260, no. 3, 435-452.

Kleven, M.S., Barret-Grevoz, C., Slot, L.B. and Newman-Tancredi, A. (2005) Novel antipsychotic agents with 5-HT1A agonist properties: Role of 5-HT1A receptor activation in attenuation of catalepsy induction in rats. *Neuropharmacology*, 49, no. 2, 135-143.

Knobelman, D.A., Kung, H.F. and Lucki, I. (2000) Regulation of Extracellular Concentrations of 5-Hydroxytryptamine (5-HT) in Mouse Striatum by 5-HT1A and 5-HT1B Receptors. 1111-1117.

Kohen, R., Metcalf, M.A., Khan, N., Druck, T., Huebner, K., Lachowicz, J.E., Meltzer, H.Y., Sibley, D.R., Roth, B.L. and Hamblin, M.W. (1996) Cloning, characterization, and chromosomal localization of a human 5-HT6 serotonin receptor. *J. Neurochem.*, 66, no. 1, 47-56.

Krack, P., Benazzouz, A., Pollak, P., Limousin, P., Piallat, B., Hoffmann, D., Xie, J. and Benabid, A.L. (1998) Treatment of tremor in Parkinson's disease by subthalamic nucleus stimulation. *Mov. Disord.*, 13, no. 6, 907-914.

Krack, P., Batir, A., Van Blercom, N., Chabardes, S., Fraix, V., Ardouin, C., Koudsie, A., Limousin, P.D., Benazzouz, A., LeBas, J.F., Benabid, A.-L. and Pollak, P. (2003) Five-Year Follow-up of Bilateral Stimulation of the Subthalamic Nucleus in Advanced Parkinson's Disease. *N. Engl. J. Med.*, 349, no. 20, 1925-1934.

Krebs-Thomson, K. and Geyer, M.A. (1996) The role of 5-HT(1A) receptors in the locomotor-suppressant effects of LSD: WAY-100635 studies of 8-OH-DPAT, DOI and LSD in rats. *Behav. Pharmacol.*, 7, no. 6, 551-559.

Kung, M.P., Frederick, D., Mu, M., Zhuang, Z.P. and Kung, H.F. (1995) 4-(2'-Methoxy-phenyl)-1-[2'-(n-2"-pyridinyl)-p-iodobenzamido]-ethyl- piperazine ([125I]p-MPPI) as a new selective radioligand of serotonin-1A sites in rat brain: in vitro binding and autoradiographic studies. *J. Pharmacol. Exp. Ther.*, 272, no. 1, 429-437.

Kuoppamaki, M., Palvimaki, E.P., Hietala, J. and Syvalahti, E. (1995) Differential regulation of rat 5-HT2A and 5-HT2C receptors after chronic treatment with clozapine, chlorpromazine and three putative atypical antipsychotic drugs. *Neuropsychopharmacology*, 13, no. 2, 139-150.

Kuoppamaki, M., Syvalahti, E. and Hietala, J. (1993) Clozapine and N-desmethylclozapine are potent 5-HT1C receptor antagonists. *Eur. J. Pharmacol.*, 245, no. 2, 179-182.

Laporte, A.M., Koscielniak, T.M., Ponchant, D., Vergé, M., Hamon, H. and Gozlan, H. (1992) Quantitative autoradiographic mapping of 5-HT$_3$ receptors in the rat CNS using [^{125}I]iodo-zacopride and [^{1}H]zacopride as radioligands. *Synapse*, 10, no. 4, 271-281.

Laprade, N., Radja, F., Reader, T.A. and Soghomonian, J.-J. (1996) Dopamine Receptor Agonists Regulate Levels of the Serotonin 5-HT2A Receptor and its mRNA in a Subpopulation of Rat Striatal Neurons. *J. Neurosci.*, 16, no. 11, 3727-3736.

Lavoie, B. and Parent, A. (1990) Immunohistochemical study of the serotoninergic innervation of the basal ganglia in the squirrel monkey. *J. Comp. Neurol.*, 299, no. 1, 1-16.

Lee, M.S., Rinne, J.O. and Marsden, C.D. (2000) The pedunculopontine nucleus: its role in the genesis of movement disorders. *Yonsei Med. J.*, 41, no. 2, 167-184.

Leentjens, A.F.G. (2004) Depression in Parkinson's Disease: Conceptual Issues and Clinical Challenges. *J Geriat Psychiatr Neurol*, 17, no. 3, 120-126.

Leentjens, A.F.G., Scholtissen, B., Vreeling, F.W. and Verhey, F.R.J. (2006) The Serotonergic Hypothesis for Depression in Parkinson's Disease: an Experimental Approach. *Neuropsychopharmacology*, 31, no. 5, 1009-1015.

Leysen, J.E., Gommeren, W., Van Gompel, P., Wynants, J., Janssen, P.F. and Laduron, P.M. (1985) Receptor-binding properties in vitro and in vivo of ritanserin: A very potent and long acting serotonin-S2 antagonist. *Mol. Pharmacol.*, 27, no. 6, 600-611.

Limousin, P., Pollak, P., Benazzouz, A., Hoffmann, D., Le Bas, J.F., Broussolle, E., Perret, J.E. and Benabid, A.L. (1995) Effect of parkinsonian signs and symptoms of bilateral subthalamic nucleus stimulation. *Lancet*, 345, no. 8942, 91-95.

Lopez-Gimenez, J.F., Mengod, G., Palacios, J.M. and Vilaro, M.T. (1997) Selective visualization of rat brain 5-HT2A receptors by autoradiography with [3H]MDL 100,907. *Naunyn Schmiedebergs Arch. Pharmacol.*, 356, no. 4, 446-454.

Lopez-Gimenez, J.F., Mengod, G., Palacios, J.M. and Vilaro, M.T. (1999) Human striosomes are enriched in 5-HT2A receptors: autoradiographical visualization with [3H]MDL100,907, [125I](andplusmn;)DOI and [3H]ketanserin. *Eur. J. Neurosci.*, 11, no. 10, 3761-3765.

Lucas, G., Bonhomme, N., Deurwaerdère, P.D., Moal, M.L. and Spampinato, U. (1997) 8-OH-DPAT, a 5-HT1A agonist and ritanserin, a 5-HT2A/C antagonist, reverse haloperidol-induced catalepsy in rats independently of striatal dopamine release. *Psychopharmacology (Berl).* 131, no. 1, 57-63.

Lucas, G., De Deurwaerdère, P., Caccia, S. and Umberto, S. (2000) The effect of serotonergic agents on haloperidol-induced striatal dopamine release in vivo: opposite role of 5-HT2A and 5-HT2C receptor subtypes and significance of the haloperidol dose used. *Neuropharmacology*, 39, no. 6, 1053-1063.

Maeda, T., Kannari, K., Shen, H., Arai, A., Tomiyama, M., Matsunaga, M. and Suda, T. (2003) Rapid induction of serotonergic hyperinnervation in the adult rat striatum with extensive dopaminergic denervation. *Neurosci. Lett.*, 343, no. 1, 17-20.

Mailly, P., Charpier, S., Menetrey, A. and Deniau, J.-M. (2003) Three-Dimensional Organization of the Recurrent Axon Collateral Network of the Substantia Nigra Pars Reticulata Neurons in the Rat. 5247-5257.

Mander, A., McCausland, M., Workman, B., Flamer, H. and Christophidis, N. (1994) Fluoxetine induced dyskinesia. *Aust. N. Z. J. Psychiatry*, 28, no. 2, 328-330.

Marazziti, D., Betti, L., Giannaccini, G., Rossi, A., Masala, I., Baroni, S., Cassano, G. and Lucacchini, A. (2001) Distribution of [3H]GR65630 Binding in Human Brain Postmortem. *Neurochem. Res.*, 26, no. 3, 187-190.

Martin-Cora, F.J. and Pazos, A. (2004) Autoradiographic distribution of 5-HT7 receptors in the human brain using [3H]mesulergine: comparison to other mammalian species. *Br. J. Pharmacol.*, 141, no. 1, 92-104.

Martinez-Price, D.L. and Geyer, M.A. (2002) Subthalamic 5-HT1A and 5-HT1B receptor modulation of RU 24969-induced behavioral profile in rats. *Pharmacology Biochemistry and Behavior*, 71, no. 4, 569-580.

Matsubara, K., Shimizu, K., Suno, M., Ogawa, K., Awaya, T., Yamada, T., Noda, T., Satomi, M., Ohtaki, K.-i., Chiba, K., Tasaki, Y. and Shiono, H. (2006) Tandospirone, a 5-HT1A agonist, ameliorates movement disorder via non-dopaminergic systems in rats with unilateral 6-hydroxydopamine-generated lesions. *Brain Res.*, 1112, no. 1, 126-133.

Mayeux, R. (1990) The "serotonin hypothesis" for depression in Parkinson's disease. *Adv. Neurol.*, 53, no., 163-166.

McQuade, R. and Sharp, T. (1995) Release of cerebral 5-hydroxytryptamine evoked by electrical stimulation of the dorsal and median raphe nuclei: effect of a neurotoxic amphetamine. *Neuroscience*, 68, no. 4, 1079-1088.

Mehta, A., Eberle-Wang, K. and Chesselet, M.-F. (2001) Increased m-CPP-induced oral dyskinesia after lesion of serotonergic neurons. *Pharmacol. Biochem. Behav.*, 68, no. 2, 347-353.

Mendlin, A., Martín, F.J., Jacobs, B.L. (1999) Dopaminergic input is required for increases in serotonin output produced by behavioral activation: an in vivo microdialysis study in rat forebrain. *Neuroscience*, 93, no. 3, 897-905.

Mengod, G., Pompeiano, M., Martinez-Mir, M.I. and Palacios, J.M. (1990) Localization of the mRNA for the 5-HT2 receptor by in situ hybridization histochemistry. Correlation with the distribution of receptor sites. *Brain Res.*, 524, no. 1, 139-143.

Mengod, G., Vilaro, M.T., Raurich, A., Lopez-Gimenez, J.F., Cortes, R. and Palacios, J.M. (1996) 5-HT receptors in mammalian brain: receptor autoradiography and in situ hybridization studies of new ligands and newly identified receptors. *Histochem. J.*, 28, no. 11, 747-758.

Middlemiss, D.N. and Hutson, P.H. (1990) The 5-HT1B receptors. *Ann. N. Y. Acad. Sci.*, 600, 132-147; discussion 347-348.

Mignon, L. and Wolf, W. (2002) Postsynaptic 5-HT1A receptors mediate an increase in locomotor activity in the monoamine-depleted rat. *Psychopharmacology (Berl).* 163, no. 1, 85-94.

Mignon, L. and Wolf, W. (2007) Postsynaptic 5-HT1A receptor stimulation increases motor activity in the 6-hydroxydopamine-lesioned rat: implications for treating Parkinson's disease. *Psychopharmacology (Berl).* 192, no. 1, 49-59.

Mignon, L.J. and Wolf, W.A. (2005) 8-hydroxy-2-(di-n-propylamino)tetralin reduces striatal glutamate in an animal model of Parkinson's disease. *Neuroreport*, 16, no. 7, 699-703.

Miller, C.H., Fleischhacker, W.W., Ehrmann, H. and Kane, J.M. (1990) Treatment of neuroleptic induced akathisia with the 5-HT2 antagonist ritanserin. *Psychopharmacol. Bull.*, 26, no. 3, 373-376.

Miller, K.M., Okun, M.S., Fernandez, H.F., Jacobson, C.E., Rodriguez, R.L. and Bowers, D. (2007) Depression symptoms in movement disorders: Comparing Parkinson's disease, dystonia, and essential tremor. *Mov. Disord.*, 22, no. 5, 666-672.

Miquel, M.C., Doucet, E., Boni, C., El Mestikawy, S., Matthiessen, L., Daval, G., Verge, D. and Hamon, M. (1991) Central serotonin1A receptors: Respective distributions of encoding mRNA, receptor protein and binding sites by in situ hybridization histochemistry, radioimmunohistochemistry and autoradiographic mapping in the rat brain. *Neurochem. Int.*, 19, no. 4, 453-465.

Mitchell, I.J., Sambrook, M.A. and Crossman, A.R. (1985) Subcortical changes in the regional uptake of [3H]-2-deoxyglucose in the brain of the monkey during experimental choreiform dyskinesia elicited by injection of a gamma-aminobutyric acid antagonist into the subthalamic nucleus. *Brain*, 108, no. 2, 405-422.

Miyawaki, E., Meah, Y. and Koller, W.C. (1997) Serotonin, dopamine, and motor effects in Parkinson's disease. *Clin. Neuropharmacol.*, 20, no. 4, 300-310.

Molina-Holgado, E., Dewar, K.M., Descarries, L. and Reader, T.A. (1994) Altered dopamine and serotonin metabolism in the dopamine-denervated and serotonin-hyperinnervated neostriatum of adult rat after neonatal 6- hydroxydopamine. *J. Pharmacol. Exp. Ther.*, 270, no. 2, 713-721.

Monsma, F.J., Jr., Shen, Y., Ward, R.P., Hamblin, M.W. and Sibley, D.R. (1993) Cloning and expression of a novel serotonin receptor with high affinity for tricyclic psychotropic drugs. *Mol. Pharmacol.*, 43, no. 3, 320-327.

Morales, M., Battenberg, E. and Bloom, F.E. (1998) Distribution of neurons expressing immunoreactivity for the $5HT_3$ receptor subtype in the rat brain and spinal cord. *J. Comp. Neurol.*, 402, no. 3, 385-401.

Moukhles, H., Bosler, O., Bolam, J.P., Vallée, A., Umbriaco, D., Geffard, M. and Doucet, G. (1997) Quantitative and morphometric data indicate precise cellular interactions between serotonin terminals and postsynaptic targets in rat substantia nigra. *Neuroscience*, 76, no. 4, 1159-1171.

Mrini, A., Soucy, J.-P., Lafaille, F., Lemoine, P. and Descarries, L. (1995) Quantification of the serotonin hyperinnervation in adult rat neostriatum after neonatal 6-hydroxydopamine lesion of nigral dopamine neurons. *Brain Res.*, 669, no. 2, 303-308.

Naidu, P.S. and Kulkarni, S.K. (2001a) Effect of 5-HT1A and 5-HT2A/2C receptor modulation on neuroleptic-induced vacuous chewing movements. *Eur. J. Pharmacol.*, 428, no. 1, 81-86.

Naidu, P.S. and Kulkarni, S.K. (2001b) Reversal of neuroleptic-induced orofacial dyskinesia by 5-HT3 receptor antagonists. *Eur. J. Pharmacol.*, 420, no. 2-3, 113-117.

Navailles, S., De Deurwaerdère, P. and Spampinato, U. (2006) Clozapine and Haloperidol Differentially Alter the Constitutive Activity of Central Serotonin2C Receptors In Vivo. *Biol. Psychiatry*, 59, no. 6, 568-575.

Nayak, S.V., Ronde, P., Spier, A.D., Lummis, S.C.R. and Nichols, R.A. (1999) Calcium changes induced by presynaptic 5-hydroxytryptamine-3 serotonin receptors on isolated terminals from various regions of the rat brain. *Neuroscience*, 91, no. 1, 107-117.

Neal-Beliveau, B.S., Joyce, J.N. and Lucki, I. (1993) Serotonergic involvement in haloperidol-induced catalepsy. *J. Pharmacol. Exp. Ther.*, 265, no. 1, 207-217.

Nichols, R.A. and Mollard, P. (1996) Direct observation of serotonin 5-HT3 receptor-induced increases in calcium levels in individual brain nerve terminals. *J. Neurochem.*, 67, no. 2, 581-592.

Nicholson, S.L. and Brotchie, J.M. (2002) 5-hydroxytryptamine (5-HT, serotonin) and Parkinson's disease - opportunities for novel therapeutics to reduce the problems of levodopa therapy. *Eur. J. Neurol.*, 9 Suppl 3, no., 1-6.

Nishio, H., Kohno, Y., Fujii, A., Negishi, Y., Inoue, A. and Nakata, Y. (1996) 5-HT3 receptor blocking properties of the antiparkinsonian agent, talipexole. *Gen. Pharmacol.*, 27, no. 5, 779-785.

Numan, S., Lundgren, K.H., Wright, D.E., Herman, J.P. and Seroogy, K.B. (1995) Increased expression of 5HT2 receptor mRNA in rat striatum following 6-OHDA lesions of the adult nigrostriatal pathway. *Brain Res. Mol. Brain Res.*, 29, no. 2, 391-396.

O'Neill, M.F., Heron-Maxwell, C.L. and Shaw, G. (1999) 5-HT2 receptor antagonism reduces hyperactivity induced by amphetamine, cocaine, and MK-801 but not D1 agonist C-APB. *Pharmacol. Biochem. Behav.*, 63, no. 2, 237-243.

Oberlander, C., Hunt, P.F., Dumont, C. and Boissier, J.R. (1981) Dopamine independent rotational response to unilateral intranigral injection of serotonin. *Life Sci.*, 28, no. 23, 2595-2601.

Oberlander, C., Demassey, Y., Verdu, A., Van de Velde, D. and Bardelay, C. (1987) Tolerance to the serotonin 5-HT1 agonist RU 24969 and effects on dopaminergic behaviour. *Eur. J. Pharmacol.*, 139, no. 2, 205-214.

Okazawa, H., Yamane, F., Blier, P. and Diksic, M. (1999) Effects of acute and chronic administration of the serotonin1A agonist buspirone on serotonin synthesis in the rat brain. *J. Neurochem.*, 72, no. 5, 2022-2031.

Oliver, K.R., Kinsey, A.M., Wainwright, A. and Sirinathsinghji, D.J. (2000) Localization of 5-ht(5A) receptor-like immunoreactivity in the rat brain. *Brain Res.*, 867, no. 1-2, 131-142.

Olpe, H.R. and Koella, W.P. (1977) The response of striatal cells upon stimulation of the dorsal and median raphe nuclei. *Brain Res.*, 122, no. 2, 357-360.

Pakhotin, P. and Bracci, E. (2007) Cholinergic interneurons control the excitatory input to the striatum. *J. Neurosci.*, 27, no. 2, 391-400.

Park, M.R., Gonzales-Vegas, J.A. and Kitai, S.T. (1982) Serotonergic excitation from dorsal raphe stimulation recorded intracellularly from rat caudate-putamen. *Brain Res.*, 243, no. 1, 49-58.

Parker, R.M.C., Barnes, J.M., Ge, J., Barber, P.C. and Barnes, N.M. (1996) Autoradiographic distribution of [3H]-(S)-zacopride-labelled 5-HT3 receptors in human brain. *J. Neurol. Sci.*, 144, no. 1-2, 119-127.

Pasqualetti, M., Nardi, I., Ladinsky, H., Marazziti, D. and Cassano, G.B. (1996) Comparative anatomical distribution of serotonin 1A, 1D[alpha] and 2A receptor mRNAs in human brain postmorten. *Brain Res. Mol. Brain Res.*, 39, no. 1-2, 223-233.

Paulus, W. and Jellinger, K. (1991) The neuropathologic basis of different clinical subgroups of Parkinson's disease. *J. Neuropathol. Exp. Neurol.*, 50, no. 6, 743-755.

Pazos, A., Cortes, R. and Palacios, J.M. (1985) Quantitative autoradiographic mapping of serotonin receptors in the rat brain. II. Serotonin-2 receptors. *Brain Res.*, 346, no. 2, 231-249.

Pazos, A. and Palacios, J.M. (1985) Quantitative autoradiographic mapping of serotonin receptors in the rat brain. I. Serotonin-1 receptors. *Brain Res.*, 346, no. 2, 205-230.

Pazos, A., Probst, A. and Palacios, J.M. (1987a) Serotonin receptors in the human brain--III. Autoradiographic mapping of serotonin-1 receptors. *Neuroscience*, 21, no. 1, 97-122.

Pazos, A., Probst, A. and Palacios, J.M. (1987b) Serotonin receptors in the human brain--IV. Autoradiographic mapping of serotonin-2 receptors. *Neuroscience*, 21, no. 1, 123-139.

Perkins, M.N. and Stone, T.W. (1983) Neuronal responses to 5-hydroxytryptamine and dorsal raphe stimulation within the globus pallidus of the rat. *Exp. Neurol.*, 79, no. 1, 118-129.

Phelps, P.E., Houser, C.R. and Vaughn, J.E. (1985) Immunocytochemical localization of choline acetyltransferase within the rat neostriatum: a correlated light and electron microscopic study of cholinergic neurons and synapses. *J. Comp. Neurol.*, 238, no. 3, 286-307.

Pike, V.W., McCarron, J.A., Lammerstma, A.A., Hume, S.P., Poole, K., Grasby, P.M., Malizia, A., Cliffe, I.A., Fletcher, A. and Bench, C.J. (1995) First delineation of 5-HT1A receptors in human brain with PET and [11C]WAY-100635. *Eur. J. Pharmacol.*, 283, no. 1-3, R1-3.

Pineyro, G. and Blier, P. (1999) Autoregulation of serotonin neurons: role in antidepressant drug action. *Pharmacol. Rev.*, 51, no. 3, 533-591.

Pires, J.G., Bonikovski, V. and Futuro-Neto, H.A. (2005) Acute effects of selective serotonin reuptake inhibitors on neuroleptic-induced catalepsy in mice. *Braz. J. Med. Biol. Res.*, 38, no. 12, 1867-1872.

Pompeiano, M., Palacios, J.M. and Mengod, G. (1992) Distribution and cellular localization of mRNA coding for 5-HT1A receptor in the rat brain: correlation with receptor binding. *J. Neurosci.*, 12, no. 2, 440-453.

Pompeiano, M., Palacios, J.M. and Mengod, G. (1994) Distribution of the serotonin 5-HT2 receptor family mRNAs: comparison between 5-HT2A and 5-HT2C receptors. *Brain Res. Mol. Brain Res.*, 23, no. 1-2, 163-178.

Porras, G., Di Matteo, V., Fracasso, C., Lucas, G., De Deurwaerdere, P., Caccia, S., Esposito, E. and Spampinato, U. (2002) 5-HT2A and 5-HT2C/2B receptor subtypes modulate dopamine release induced in vivo by amphetamine and morphine in both the rat nucleus accumbens and striatum. *Neuropsychopharmacology*, 26, no. 3, 311-324.

Prinssen, E.P., Koek, W. and Kleven, M.S. (2000) The effects of antipsychotics with 5-HT(2C) receptor affinity in behavioral assays selective for 5-HT(2C) receptor antagonist properties of compounds. *Eur. J. Pharmacol.*, 388, no. 1, 57-67.

Queiroz, C.M. and Frussa-Filho, R. (1999) Effects of buspirone on an animal model of tardive dyskinesia. *Prog. Neuropsychopharmacol. Biol. Psychiatry*, 23, no. 8, 1405-1418.

Querejeta, E., Oviedo-Chavez, A., Araujo-Alvarez, J.M., Quinones-Cardenas, A.R. and Delgado, A. (2005) In vivo effects of local activation and blockade of 5-HT1B receptors on globus pallidus neuronal spiking. *Brain Res.*, 1043, no. 1-2, 186-194.

Quirion, R. and Richard, J. (1987) Differential effects of selective lesions of cholinergic and dopaminergic neurons on serotonin-type 1 receptors in rat brain. *Synapse*, 1, no. 1, 124-130.

Radja, F., Descarries, L., Dewar, K.M. and Reader, T.A. (1993) Serotonin 5-HT1 and 5-HT2 receptors in adult rat brain after neonatal destruction of nigrostriatal dopamine neurons: a quantitative autoradiographic study. *Brain Res.*, 606, no. 2, 273-285.

Rammes, G., Eisensamer, B., Ferrari, U., Shapa, M., Gimpl, G., Gilling, K., Parsons, C., Riering, K., Hapfelmeier, G., Bondy, B., Zieglgansberger, W., Holsboer, F. and Rupprecht, R. (2004) Antipsychotic drugs antagonize human serotonin type 3 receptor currents in a noncompetitive manner. *Mol. Psychiatry*, 9, no. 9, 846-858.

Rauser, L., Savage, J.E., Meltzer, H.Y. and Roth, B.L. (2001) Inverse agonist actions of typical and atypical antipsychotic drugs at the human 5-hydroxytryptamine(2C) receptor. *J. Pharmacol. Exp. Ther.*, 299, no. 1, 83-89.

Reavill, C., Kettle, A., Holland, V., Riley, G. and Blackburn, T.P. (1999) Attenuation of haloperidol-induced catalepsy by a 5-HT2C receptor antagonist. *Br. J. Pharmacol.*, 126, no. 3, 572-574.

Rees, S., den Daas, I., Foord, S., Goodson, S., Bull, D., Kilpatrick, G. and Lee, M. (1994) Cloning and characterisation of the human 5-HT5A serotonin receptor. *FEBS Lett.*, 355, no. 3, 242-246.

Rempel, N.L., Callaway, C.W. and Geyer, M.A. (1993) Serotonin1B receptor activation mimics behavioral effects of presynaptic serotonin release. *Neuropsychopharmacology*, 8, no. 3, 201-211.

Reynolds, G.P. (2004) Receptor mechanisms in the treatment of schizophrenia. *Journal of psychopharmacology (Oxford, England)*, 18, no. 3, 340-345.

Reynolds, G.P., Mason, S.L., Meldrum, A., De Keczer, S., Parnes, H., Eglen, R.M. and Wong, E.H. (1995) 5-Hydroxytryptamine (5-HT)4 receptors in post mortem human brain tissue: distribution, pharmacology and effects of neurodegenerative diseases. *Br. J. Pharmacol.*, 114, no. 5, 993-998.

Riad, M., Mestikawy, S.E., Verge, D., Gozlan, H. and Hamon, M. (1991) Visualization and quantification of central 5-HT1A receptors with specific antibodies. *Neurochem. Int.*, 19, no. 4, 413-423.

Rick, C.E., Stanford, I.M. and Lacey, M.G. (1995) Excitation of rat substantia nigra pars reticulata neurons by 5-hydroxytryptamine in vitro: evidence for a direct action mediated by 5-hydroxytryptamine2C receptors. *Neuroscience*, 69, no. 3, 903-913.

Ring, H.A. and Serra-Mestre, J. (2002) Neuropsychiatry of the basal ganglia. *J. Neurol. Neurosurg. Psychiatry.*, 72, 12-21.

Roberts, J.C., Reavill, C., East, S.Z., Harrison, P.J., Patel, S., Routledge, C. and Leslie, R.A. (2002) The distribution of 5-HT(6) receptors in rat brain: an autoradiographic binding study using the radiolabelled 5-HT(6) receptor antagonist [(125)I]SB-258585. *Brain Res.*, 934, no. 1, 49-57.

Rodríguez, J.J., Garcia, D.R. and Pickel, V.M. (1999) Subcellular distribution of 5-hydroxytryptamine$_{2A}$ and N-methyl-D-aspartate receptors within single neurons in rat motor and limbic striatum. *J. Comp. Neurol.*, 413, no. 2, 219-231.

Ronde, P. and Nichols, R.A. (1998) High calcium permeability of serotonin 5-HT3 receptors on presynaptic nerve terminals from rat striatum. *J. Neurochem.*, 70, no. 3, 1094-1103.

Rosengarten, H., Bartoszyk, G.D., Quartermain, D. and Lin, Y. (2006) The effect of chronic administration of sarizotan, 5-HT1A agonist/D3/D4 ligand, on haloperidol-induced repetitive jaw movements in rat model of tardive dyskinesia. *Prog. Neuropsychopharmacol. Biol. Psychiatry*, 30, no. 2, 273-279.

Roth, B.L., Ciaranello, R.D. and Meltzer, H.Y. (1992) Binding of typical and atypical antipsychotic agents to transiently expressed 5-HT1C receptors. *J. Pharmacol. Exp. Ther.*, 260, no. 3, 1361-1365.

Roth, B.L., Meltzer, H.Y. and Khan, N. (1998) Binding of typical and atypical antipsychotic drugs to multiple neurotransmitter receptors. *Adv. Pharmacol.*, 42, no., 482-485.

Ruat, M., Traiffort, E., Arrang, J.M., Tardivel-Lacombe, J., Diaz, J., Leurs, R. and Schwartz, J.C. (1993a) A novel rat serotonin (5-HT6) receptor: molecular cloning, localization and stimulation of cAMP accumulation. *Biochem. Biophys. Res. Commun.*, 193, no. 1, 268-276.

Ruat, M., Traiffort, E., Leurs, R., Tardivel-Lacombe, J., Diaz, J., Arrang, J.M. and Schwartz, J.C. (1993b) Molecular cloning, characterization, and localization of a high-affinity serotonin receptor (5-HT7) activating cAMP formation. *Proc. Natl. Acad. Sci. U. S. A.*, 90, no. 18, 8547-8551.

Rueter, L.E., Tecott, L.H. and Blier, P. (2000) In vivo electrophysiological examination of 5-HT2 responses in 5-HT2C receptor mutant mice. *Naunyn Schmiedebergs Arch. Pharmacol.*, 361, no. 5, 484-491.

Samad, N., Khan, A., Perveen, T., Haider, S., Abdul Haleem, M. and Haleem, D.J. (2007) Increase in the effectiveness of somatodendritic 5-HT-1A receptors in a rat model of tardive dyskinesia. *Acta Neurobiol Exp*, 67, no. 4, 389-397.

Sari, Y., Miquel, M.C., Brisorgueil, M.J., Ruiz, G., Doucet, E., Hamon, M. and Verge, D. (1999) Cellular and subcellular localization of 5-hydroxytryptamine1B receptors in the rat central nervous system: immunocytochemical, autoradiographic and lesion studies. *Neuroscience*, 88, no. 3, 899-915.

Sawada, M., Nagatsu, T., Nagatsu, I., Ito, K., Iizuka, R., Kondo, T. and Narabayashi, H. (1985) Tryptophan hydroxylase activity in the brains of controls and parkinsonian patients. *J. Neural Transm.*, 62, no. 1-2, 107-115.

Scatton, B., Javoy-Agid, F., Rouquier, L., Dubois, B. and Agid, Y. (1983) Reduction of cortical dopamine, noradrenaline, serotonin and their metabolites in Parkinson's disease. *Brain Res.*, 275, no. 2, 321-328.

Schiller, L., Jahkel, M., Kretzschmar, M., Brust, P. and Oehler, J. (2003) Autoradiographic analyses of 5-HT1A and 5-HT2A receptors after social isolation in mice. *Brain Res.*, 980, no. 2, 169-178.

Scholtissen, B., Verhey, F.R., Steinbusch, H.W. and Leentjens, A.F. (2006) Serotonergic mechanisms in Parkinson's disease: opposing results from preclinical and clinical data. *J. Neural Transm.*, 113, no. 1, 59-73.

Schotte, A., Janssen, P.F., Megens, A.A. and Leysen, J.E. (1993) Occupancy of central neurotransmitter receptors by risperidone, clozapine and haloperidol, measured ex vivo by quantitative autoradiography. *Brain Res.*, 631, no. 2, 191-202.

Sethi, K.D. (2003) Tremor. *Curr. Opin. Neurol.*, 16, no. 4, 481-485.

Shen, K.Z. and Johnson, S.W. (2008) 5-HT inhibits synaptic transmission in rat subthalamic nucleus neurons in vitro. *Neuroscience*, 151, no. 4, 1029-1033.

Shen, K.Z., Kozell, L.B. and Johnson, S.W. (2007) Multiple conductances are modulated by 5-HT receptor subtypes in rat subthalamic nucleus neurons. *Neuroscience*, 148, no. 4, 996-1003.

Shilliam, C.S. and Dawson, L.A. (2005) The effect of clozapine on extracellular dopamine levels in the shell subregion of the rat nucleus accumbens is reversed following chronic administration: comparison with a selective 5-HT(2C) receptor antagonist. *Neuropsychopharmacology*, 30, no. 2, 372-380.

Shink, E., Bevan, M.D., Bolam, J.P. and Smith, Y. (1996) The subthalamic nucleus and the external pallidum: two tightly interconnected structures that control the output of the basal ganglia in the monkey. *Neuroscience*, 73, no. 2, 335-357.

Sian, J., Gerlach, M., Youdim, M.B. and Riederer, P. (1999) Parkinson's disease: a major hypokinetic basal ganglia disorder. *J. Neural Transm.*, 106, no. 5-6, 443-476.

Simola, N., Morelli, M. and Carta, A.R. (2007) The 6-hydroxydopamine model of Parkinson's disease. *Neurotoxicity research*, 11, no. 3-4, 151-167.

Sivam, S.P., Breese, G.R., Krause, J.E., Napier, T.C., Mueller, R.A. and Hong, J.S. (1987) Neonatal and adult 6-hydroxydopamine-induced lesions differentially alter tachykinin and enkephalin gene expression. *J. Neurochem.*, 49, no. 5, 1623-1633.

Smith, I.D. and Grace, A.A. (1992) Role of the subthalamic nucleus in the regulation of nigral dopamine neuron activity. *Synapse*, 12, no. 4, 287-303.

Stachowiak, M.K., Bruno, J.P., Snyder, A.M., Stricker, E.M. and Zigmond, M.J. (1984) Apparent sprouting of striatal serotonergic terminals after dopamine-depleting brain lesions in neonatal rats. *Brain Res.*, 291, no. 1, 164-167.

Stanford, I.M., Kantaria, M.A., Chahal, H.S., Loucif, K.C. and Wilson, C.L. (2005) 5-Hydroxytryptamine induced excitation and inhibition in the subthalamic nucleus: action at 5-HT(2C), 5-HT(4) and 5-HT(1A) receptors. *Neuropharmacology*, 49, no. 8, 1228-1234.

Stanford, I.M. and Lacey, M.G. (1996) Differential actions of serotonin, mediated by 5-HT1B and 5-HT2C receptors, on GABA-mediated synaptic input to rat substantia nigra pars reticulata neurons in vitro. *J. Neurosci.*, 16, no. 23, 7566-7573.

Stefani, A., Surmeier, D.J. and Kitai, S.T. (1990) Serotonin enhances excitability in neostriatal neurons by reducing voltage-dependent potassium currents. *Brain Res.*, 529, no. 1-2, 354-357.

Stefani A, Fedele E, Mazzone P, Galati S, Tropepi P, Stanzione P. (2006) In vivo microdialysis in parkinsonian patients undergoing stereotactic neurosurgery: key insights on DBS mechanisms of actions. *Proceedings of the 11th International Conference of In Vivo Methods* 74–76. (Valentini V, Di Chiara G, eds) Sardinia, Italy: University of Cagliari.

Steffensen, S.C., Svingos, A.L., Pickel, V.M. and Henriksen, S.J. (1998) Electrophysiological Characterization of GABAergic Neurons in the Ventral Tegmental Area. 8003-8015.

Steinbusch, H.W. (1981) Distribution of serotonin-immunoreactivity in the central nervous system of the rat-cell bodies and terminals. *Neuroscience*, 6, no. 4, 557-618.

Steward, L.J., Bufton, K.E., Hopkins, P.C., Davies, W.E. and Barnes, N.M. (1993) Reduced levels of 5-HT3 receptor recognition sites in the putamen of patients with Huntington's disease. *Eur. J. Pharmacol.*, 242, no. 2, 137-143.

Sturman, M.M., Vaillancourt, D.E., Metman, L.V., Bakay, R.A. and Corcos, D.M. (2004) Effects of subthalamic nucleus stimulation and medication on resting and postural tremor in Parkinson's disease. *Brain*, 127, no. Pt 9, 2131-2143.

Tarsy, D. and Baldessarini, R.J. (1984) Tardive dyskinesia. *Annu. Rev. Med.*, 35, no., 605-623.

Tauscher, J., Kapur, S., Verhoeff, N.P., Hussey, D.F., Daskalakis, Z.J., Tauscher-Wisniewski, S., Wilson, A.A., Houle, S., Kasper, S. and Zipursky, R.B. (2002) Brain serotonin 5-HT(1A) receptor binding in schizophrenia measured by positron emission tomography and [11C]WAY-100635. *Arch. Gen. Psychiatry*, 59, no. 6, 514-520.

Tepper, J.M. and Bolam, J.P. (2004) Functional diversity and specificity of neostriatal interneurons. *Curr. Opin. Neurobiol.*, 14, no. 6, 685-692.

Trevitt, J.T., Lyons, M., Aberman, J., Carriero, D., Finn, M. and Salamone, J.D. (1997) Effects of clozapine, thioridazine, risperidone and haloperidol on behavioral tests related to extrapyramidal motor function. *Psychopharmacology (Berl).* 132, no. 1, 74-81.

Trevitt, J., Atherton, A., Aberman, J. and Salamone, J.D. (1998) Effects of subchronic administration of clozapine, thioridazine and haloperidol on tests related to extrapyramidal motor function in the rat. *Psychopharmacology (Berl).* 137, no. 1, 61-66.

Twarog, B.M. and Page, I.H. (1953) Serotonin content of some mammalian tissues and urine and a method for its determination. *Am. J. Physiol.*, 175, no. 1, 157-161.

Ullmer, C., Engels, P., Abdel'Al, S. and Lubbert, H. (1996) Distribution of 5-HT4 receptor mRNA in the rat brain. *Naunyn Schmiedebergs Arch. Pharmacol.*, 354, no. 2, 210-212.

Utter, A.A. and Basso, M.A. (2008) The basal ganglia: an overview of circuits and function. *Neurosci. Biobehav. Rev.*, 32, no. 3, 333-342.

Van Bockstaele, E.J., Biswas, A. and Pickel, V.M. (1993) Topography of serotonin neurons in the dorsal raphe nucleus that send axon collaterals to the rat prefrontal cortex and nucleus accumbens. *Brain Res.*, 624, no. 1-2, 188-198.

Van Bockstaele, E.J., Cestari, D.M. and Pickel, V.M. (1994) Synaptic structure and connectivity of serotonin terminals in the ventral tegmental area: potential sites for modul-ation of mesolimbic dopamine neurons. *Brain Res.*, 647, no. 2, 307-322.

Van Bockstaele, E.J. and Pickel, V.M. (1995) GABA-containing neurons in the ventral tegmental area project to the nucleus accumbens in rat brain. *Brain Res.*, 682, no. 1-2, 215-221.

Vandermaelen, C.P., Bonduki, A.C. and Kitai, S.T. (1979) Excitation of caudate-putamen neurons following stimulation of the dorsal raphe nucleus in the rat. *Brain Res.*, 175, no. 2, 356-361.

Varnas, K., Hall, H., Bonaventure, P. and Sedvall, G. (2001) Autoradiographic mapping of 5-HT(1B) and 5-HT(1D) receptors in the post mortem human brain using [(3)H]GR 125743. *Brain Res.*, 915, no. 1, 47-57.

Varnas, K., Hurd, Y.L. and Hall, H. (2005) Regional expression of 5-HT1B receptor mRNA in the human brain. *Synapse*, 56, no. 1, 21-28.

Varnas, K., Thomas, D.R., Tupala, E., Tiihonen, J. and Hall, H. (2004) Distribution of 5-HT7 receptors in the human brain: a preliminary autoradiographic study using [3H]SB-269970. *Neurosci. Lett.*, 367, no. 3, 313-316.

Veazey, C., Aki, S.O., Cook, K.F., Lai, E.C. and Kunik, M.E. (2005) Prevalence and treatment of depression in Parkinson's disease. *J. Neuropsychiatry Clin. Neurosci.*, 17, no. 3, 310-323.

Verge, D., Daval, G., Marcinkiewicz, M., Patey, A., el Mestikawy, S., Gozlan, H. and Hamon, M. (1986) Quantitative autoradiography of multiple 5-HT1 receptor subtypes in the brain of control or 5,7-dihydroxytryptamine-treated rats. *J. Neurosci.*, 6, no. 12, 3474-3482.

Vilaro, M.T., Cortes, R., Gerald, C., Branchek, T.A., Palacios, J.M. and Mengod, G. (1996) Localization of 5-HT4 receptor mRNA in rat brain by in situ hybridization histochemistry. *Brain Res. Mol. Brain Res.*, 43, no. 1-2, 356-360.

Vilaro, M.T., Cortes, R. and Mengod, G. (2005) Serotonin 5-HT4 receptors and their mRNAs in rat and guinea pig brain: distribution and effects of neurotoxic lesions. *J. Comp. Neurol.*, 484, no. 4, 418-439.

Waddington, J.L., Molloy, A.G., O'Boyle, K.M. and Mashurano, M. (1986) Motor consequences of D-1 dopamine receptor stimulation and blockade. *Clin. Neuropharmacol.*, 9, no. 4, 20-22.

Wadenberg, M.L. (1996) Serotonergic mechanisms in neuroleptic-induced catalepsy in the rat. *Neurosci. Biobehav. Rev.*, 20, no. 2, 325-339.

Waeber, C., Dietl, M.M., Hoyer, D. and Palacios, J.M. (1989) 5.HT1 receptors in the vertebrate brain. Regional distribution examined by autoradiography. *Naunyn Schmiedebergs Arch. Pharmacol.*, 340, no. 5, 486-494.

Waeber, C., Schoeffter, P., Hoyer, D. and Palacios, J.M. (1990a) The serotonin 5-HT1D receptor: a progress review. *Neurochem. Res.*, 15, no. 6, 567-582.

Waeber, C., Zhang, L.A. and Palacios, J.M. (1990b) 5-HT1D receptors in the guinea pig brain: pre- and postsynaptic localizations in the striatonigral pathway. *Brain Res.*, 528, no. 2, 197-206.

Waeber, C., Sebben, M., Nieoullon, A., Bockaert, J. and Dumuis, A. (1994) Regional distribution and ontogeny of 5-HT4 binding sites in rodent brain. *Neuropharmacology*, 33, no. 3-4, 527-541.

Ward, R.P. and Dorsa, D.M. (1996) Colocalization of serotonin receptor subtypes 5-HT2A, 5-HT2C, and 5-HT6 with neuropeptides in rat striatum. *J. Comp. Neurol.*, 370, no. 3, 405-414.

Ward, R.P., Hamblin, M.W., Lachowicz, J.E., Hoffman, B.J., Sibley, D.R. and Dorsa, D.M. (1995) Localization of serotonin subtype 6 receptor messenger RNA in the rat brain by in situ hybridization histochemistry. *Neuroscience*, 64, no. 4, 1105-1111.

Weiner, D.M., Vanover, K.E., Brann, M.R., Meltzer, H.Y. and Davis, R.E. (2003) Psychosis of Parkinson's disease: serotonin 2A receptor inverse agonists as potential therapeutics. *Curr Opin Investig Drugs*, 4, no. 7, 815-819.

Wesolowska, A. (2002) In the search for selective ligands of 5-HT5, 5-HT6 and 5-HT7 serotonin receptors. *Pol. J. Pharmacol.*, 54, no. 4, 327-341.

Wilms, K., Vierig, G. and Davidowa, H. (2001) Interactive effects of cholecystokinin-8S and various serotonin receptor agonists on the firing activity of neostriatal neuronesin rats. *Neuropeptides*, 35, no. 5-6, 257-270.

Wolf, W.A., Bieganski, G.J., Guillen, V. and Mignon, L. (2005) Enhanced 5-HT2C receptor signaling is associated with haloperidol-induced "early onset" vacuous chewing in rats: implications for antipsychotic drug therapy. *Psychopharmacology (Berl).* 182, no. 1, 84-94.

Wright, D.E., Seroogy, K.B., Lundgren, K.H., Davis, B.M. and Jennes, L. (1995) Comparative localization of serotonin1A, 1C, and 2 receptor subtype mRNAs in rat brain. *J. Comp. Neurol.*, 351, no. 3, 357-373.

Xiang, Z., Wang, L. and Kitai, S.T. (2005) Modulation of Spontaneous Firing in Rat Subthalamic Neurons by 5-HT Receptor Subtypes. *J. Neurophysiol.*, 93, no. 3, 1145-1157.

Yakel, J.L., Trussell, L.O. and Jackson, M.B. (1988) Three serotonin responses in cultured mouse hippocampal and striatal neurons. *J. Neurosci.*, 8, no. 4, 1273-1285.

Yoshioka, M., Matsumoto, M., Togashi, H. and Mori, K. (1998) Central Distribution and Function of 5-ht6 Receptor Subtype in the Rat Brain. *Ann. N. Y. Acad. Sci.*, 861, no. 1, 244.

Zhang, Q.J., Gao, R., Liu, J., Liu, Y.P. and Wang, S. (2007) Changes in the firing activity of serotonergic neurons in the dorsal raphe nucleus in a rat model of Parkinsonos disease. *Sheng Li Xue Bao*, 59, no. 2, 183-189.

Zhang, X., Andren, P.E. and Svenningsson, P. (2007) Changes on 5-HT2 receptor mRNAs in striatum and subthalamic nucleus in Parkinson's disease model. *Physiol. Behav.*, 92, no. 1-2, 29-33.

Zhang, X., Andren, P.E., Greengard, P. and Svenningsson, P. (2008) Evidence for a role of the 5-HT1B receptor and its adaptor protein, p11, in L-DOPA treatment of an animal model of Parkinsonism. *Proc. Natl. Acad. Sci. U. S. A.*, 105, no. 6, 2163-2168.

Zhou, F.C., Bledsoe, S. and Murphy, J. (1991) Serotonergic sprouting is induced by dopamine-lesion in substantia nigra of adult rat brain. *Brain Res.*, 556, no. 1, 108-116.

Zhou, F.M., Wilson, C.J. and Dani, J.A. (2002) Cholinergic interneuron characteristics and nicotinic properties in the striatum. *J. Neurobiol.*, 53, no. 4, 590-605.

In: Movement Disorders: Causes, Diagnoses and Treatments ISBN 978-1-61209-200-3
Editor: Barbara J. Larsen

Chapter II

Peripheral and Central Changes Combined Induce Movement Disorders on the Basis of Disuse or Overuse

Jacques-Olivier Coq[1,*] and Mary F. Barbe[†,2]
[1]UMR 6149 Neurobiologie Intégrative et Adaptative, CNRS/Aix-Marseille Université, Marseille, France
[2]Department of Anatomy and Cell Biology, Temple University, Philadelphia, USA

Abstract

To gain new insights into the underpinning mechanisms of movement disorders observed with both cerebral palsy and repetitive motion disorders, we have investigated the long-term effects of movement disuse or overuse on musculoskeletal tissues and topographical organization of the primary somatosensory and primary motor cortices, using two different rat models. We provide strong evidence that experience-dependent movements play a crucial role in shaping normal as well as aberrant movement abilities. Cerebral palsy is a developmental neurological disorder characterized by spasticity of some muscles, but also disuse in other muscles, and motor abnormalities. Our data from a rat model of cerebral palsy shows that aberrant sensorimotor inputs during development resulting from prolonged disuse (i.e. hind limb immobilization during the first month of life) induces peripheral tissue changes, such as muscle atrophy and extracellular matrix changes, joint degeneration, and drastic topographical disorganization of primary somatosensory and motor cortical hind limb representations. These peripheral and central tissue changes were associated with increased muscular tone at rest and with active flexion and extension around movement-restricted joints that resulted in abnormal walking patterns. Observed tissue changes and movement disorders were worsened when

* Email: jacques-olivier.coq@univ-provence.fr, UMR6149 Neurobiologie Intégrative et Adaptative, CNRS/Aix-Marseille Université, Pôle 3C, Case B, 3 Place Victor Hugo, 13331, Marseille Cedex 03, France. Tel: +33 413 55 08 63, Fax: +33 413 55 08 69.
† Email: mary.barbe@temple.edu. Department of Anatomy and Cell Biology, Temple University, 3500 North Broad Street, Philadelphia, PA 19140, USA,Tel: +1 215/707-6422 fax: +1 215/738-2966.

developmental disuse was combined with neonatal asphyxia. In contrast, repetitive motion disorders, such as carpal tunnel syndrome and focal hand dystonia, are a type of overuse associated with tasks that require prolonged, repetitive behaviors. Our data from a rat model of repetitive reaching and grasping shows that peripheral tissue changes are induced with cumulative task exposure, including myofiber fray, fibrotic nerve compression, and increased macrophages and inflammatory cytokines. These tissue changes were associated with declines in reach performance, grip strength and agility. The motor declines also correlated with disorganization of the forepaw representation in the primary somatosensory cortex, including the emergence of large receptive fields, and a drastic enlargement of the overall forepaw map area of the primary motor cortex, in which emerged the representation of joint movements specifically involved in the repetitive task. Peripheral inflammation correlated with signs of central sensitization (mechanical allodynia, myalgia, and increased neurochemicals and cytokines in the spinal cord), and with the reduced amount of current needed in the motor cortex to evoke forelimb movements. Our data from a rat model of repetitive motion injuries show that peripheral inflammation, spinal cord neuroplasticity and cortical neuroplasticity jointly contribute to the development of chronic repetitive motion disorders. In conclusion, both prolonged disuse and overuse lead to both peripheral and central changes that are interdependent to drive cerebral plasticity and altered motor output function.

Introduction

The changes in skeletal muscle physiology, gait, posture and brain adaptation to microgravity exposure has been a medical and physiological concern since the early 1960 and the human flight in space (more than 500 human beings have flown into space since 1961; Narici and De Boer, 2010). Many studies in animals and humans have been devoted to investigate peripheral and central changes in presumed models of disuse, such as spaceflight, bed rest, hind limb immobilization or suspension, tetrodotoxin (TTX), spinal cord transection or denervation, which are actually models of normal or decreased use, but appear to be interesting models of abnormal inputs to the brain. For instance, early sensory input deprivation has been shown to impact the development of brain cortical function and structure.

An other line of work on disuse have been dedicated to study the impact of spontaneous movements on the development of gait, posture and adaptive motor behavior in both normal infants and children with cerebral palsy (Hadders-Algra, 2001, 2004, 2007, 2008; Heineman et al., 2010). Cerebral palsy (CP) describes a group of permanent disorders of the development of movement and posture, causing activity limitation, that are attributed to non-progressive disturbances occurring in the developing fetal or infant brain. The motor disorders of CP are often accompanied by disturbances of sensation, perception, cognition, communication, behavior, by epilepsy and secondary musculoskeletal problems (Rosenbaum et al., 2007; Pakula et al., 2009). Normal infants produce a large and rich repertoire of spontaneous movements from early fetal life until the end of the first half of a year of life. In contrast, children with CP display scarce, monotonous and stereotypical patterns of cramped-synchronized spontaneous movements that lack complexity, variation, and fluency (Prechtl, 1997; Hadders-Algra, 2004; Einspieler and Prechtl, 2005; Hadders-Algra et al., 2010). Deficits in these spontaneous movements could account for musculoskeletal tissue changes found in these children. Indeed, varying degrees of atrophy and hypertrophy of muscle fibers

(Lindboe and Platou, 1982; Romanini et al., 1989; Rose et al., 1994; Marbini et al., 2002) and increased fat and connective tissue within muscles (Castle et al., 1979; Järvinen et al., 2002) have been reported in children with spastic CP. These muscle changes could be responsible for abnormal forces on bones and joints resulting in secondary bone malformations (Banks, 1972; Gormley, 2001) and/or articular cartilage degenerative changes (Banks, 1972; Lundy et al., 1998). In previous studies, we hypothesized that peripheral changes have a deleterious impact on brain structure, physiology and function following abnormal inputs during development (Strata et al., 2004; Coq et al., 2008). Indeed, recent studies in humans have provided evidence of maladaptive somatosensory and cortex reorganization and of impairments in tactile and kinesthesic discrimination abilities in patients with CP (Clayton et al., 2003; Gordon et al., 2006; Hadders-Algra and Gramsbergen, 2007; Hadders-Algra, 2008; Burton et al., 2008, 2009; Wingert et al., 2008, 2009, 2010; Andiman et al., 2010).

In contrast to the above disuse model, several types of overuse injuries are associated with performance of tasks that require prolonged, repetitive behaviors. These disorders are also known as repetitive motion injuries (RMIs) and musculoskeletal disorders (MSDs), and include peripheral neuropathies (e.g. carpal tunnel syndrome), tendinitis, tendinopathies, myalgias, myopathies and stress fractures (Forwood and Parker, 1991; Fredericson et al., 1995; Ljung et al., 1999; Larsson et al., 2000; Freeland et al., 2002; Luime et al., 2004; Keir and Rempel, 2005; Szabo et al., 2006; see Barr et al., 2004 for further review). Focal hand dystonias can also develop in patients with performance of repetitive tasks, although they are thought to be the consequence of central nervous system changes rather than peripheral tissue changes (Byl et al., 2000; Byl, 2009).

Overuse injuries of the upper extremity are painful, potentially disabling and costly. Work-related overuse injuries accounted for 30% of lost workday injuries and illnesses in US industry in 2006 (Bureau of Labor Statistics, 2007). Upper extremity overuse injuries have a high impact on lost workdays and cause substantial worker discomfort, disability and loss of productivity. For example, carpal tunnel syndrome and repetitive motion tasks (e.g. grasping tools) resulted in the longest work absences, with a median of 27 and 19 lost workdays, respectively. The most common musculoskeletal disorder in a study by Gerr et al. (2002) was somatic pain syndrome. Patients with upper extremity overuse injuries have increased frequency of local pain and tenderness, peripheral nerve irritation, weakness and increased frequency of symptoms such as pain and tenderness at multiple anatomical sites (Carp et al., 2007). In this last study, patient symptoms interestingly correlated with increased serum inflammatory cytokines (Carp et al, 2007).

However, in spite of numerous epidemiological studies demonstrating a positive relationship between exposure to repetitive and/or forceful motion and the prevalence of overuse injuries (Bernard, 1997), the mechanisms of pathophysiology are incompletely understood. In part, this is due to ethical constraints in obtaining tissue biopsies from healthy working populations in order to study the natural history of these disorders. Also, if there is a surgical intervention, the initiating injury stimulus is often long since past. It is thus hard to conclude which biochemical changes cause or follow the physiological mechanisms leading to a patient's clinical presentation. Animal models provide an opportunity to examine such tissue effects at a much earlier time point and under experimental conditions in which exposure can be controlled.

To gain new insights into the underlying mechanisms of movement disorders, we have investigated the long-term effects of movement disuse or overuse on musculoskeletal tissues and topographical organization of the primary somatosensory and motor cortices. We provide evidence that experience-dependent movements, through physiological mechanisms of plasticity, play a crucial role in building normal or abnormal motor capabilities during development and in adulthood.

I. Disuse During Development

1. Our Animal Model of Sensorimotor Disuse

We utilized hind limb immobilization during development as a means to produce limited and abnormal patterns of movements during maturation. We hypothesized that repetitive, reduced and abnormal movement would provide abnormal sensorimotor feedback to the primary somatosensory (S1) and motor (M1) cortices that would lead to S1 and M1 deleterious reorganization. We also hypothesized that prolonged limb disuse would also induce deleterious changes in musculoskeletal tissues, which in turn would contribute to aberrant sensory inputs to the immature brain. The S1 and M1 deleterious reorganization in combination with hind limb tissue degradation should then result in degraded motor function.

Sprague-Dawley rat pups from different litters were pseudo-randomly assigned to several experimental groups, one of which was hind limb immobilization from P1 to P28. A detailed description of the restriction procedures has been previously published (Strata et al., 2004; Coq et al., 2007, 2008; Delcour et al., 2009). Pups were restrained for 16 hours per day from P1 or P2 to P28. The feet of the pups were first gently bound together with medical tape. The feet were not taped so tight as to cause anoxia (changes in color) in peripheral tissues. The hind limbs were then immobilized in an extended position by firmly taping them to a cast (Figure 1), which allowed only limited movements around the hip joint. The cast made of hand-moldable epoxy putty stick was well tolerated by pups and mothers, and allowed the pups to urinate, defecate and to receive maternal cares necessary for good health conditions. After casting, pups were returned to their mother and unrestrained littermates. The restrained rats were allowed to move freely for 8 hours per day as the epoxy casts were removed for that period of time per day. The size of the casts was adapted to the growth of the rats from P1 to P28. We observed that body growth of restrained pups was significantly lower than that of unrestricted littermates (see Strata et al. 2004 for details). However, the differences in body growth between restricted and unrestrained rats decreased over time after the cessation of sensorimotor restriction (Strata et al., 2004).

2. Motor Outputs Affected by Disuse: Open-Field Exploration, Locomotion and Motor Skills

A. Open-Field Activity

To our knowledge, no studies dealing with hind limb unloading have been devoted to open-field measurements.

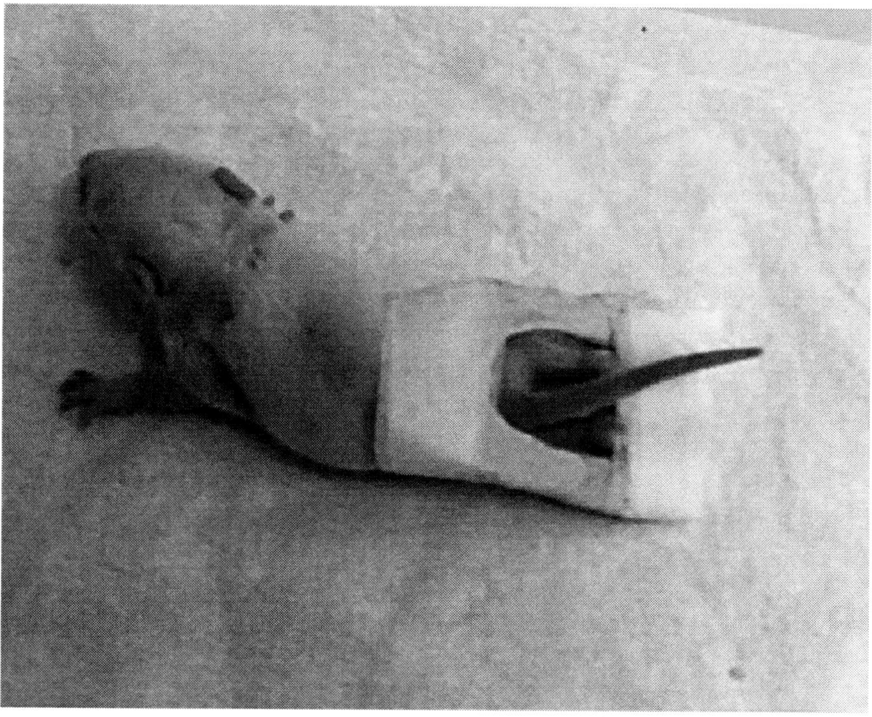

Figure 1. Young rat experiencing sensorimotor restriction (SMR). The feet of the pup were first tied together with medical tape and then were firmly attached to a cast made of epoxy stick. The proximal part of the hind limbs was also taped to the cast. The sensorimotor restriction lasted for 16 hours a day every day from P1 to P28. The casting was well tolerated by pups and mothers.

We examined spontaneous exploratory and locomotor activity of the rats by counting the number of square (10 x 10 cm) crossings, rearings, defecations and cleanings during 10 min in an empty arena. Sensorimotor-restrained (SMR) rats displayed fewer square crossings, rearings and cleanings than control rats (Coq et al., 2007).

B. Posture and Gait

We also explored posture and gait changes in order to assess gross motor function. Qualitative observation revealed that SMR rats exhibited irregular step cycles, difficulty in coordination between homolateral (fore vs. hind) limbs, elevated hindquarters, externally rotated feet, widened support base and some rats dragged their feet and/or toes behind, so the forelimbs propelled them (Strata et al., 2004).

Gait was also assessed via treadmill walking. Using a treadmill speed of 0.23 $m.s^{-1}$, preliminary data (Coq et al., 2007) on SMR rats at P30 showed that they displayed hind limb hyperextension, which was characterized by larger knee and ankle angles at the beginning of the stance (toe-contact on the belt) and swing (toe-off), and at the maximal height of the swing than control rats, while the angle of hip was comparable in each phase. While gait was degraded in restrained rats, with multiple drifting on the treadmill and little hopping capacity, the number of steps per second performed by SMR was similar to that performed by controls. The length of the swing was also shorter in SMR rats while duration was greater and the height of the swing was shorter (Coq et al., 2007). In a study from a different laboratory using the same procedure and duration of hind limb immobilization as ours, Marcuzzo et al. (2008) also found an elevation of the hindquarters during posture and walking, which was caused by abnormal extension of both ankle and knee joints. They also showed a decrease in the stride length and wider foot angle at toe-contact, suggesting greater foot rigidity. In addition, their SMR rats underwent treadmill training once a day for 3 weeks, an intervention that improved stride length, but not the foot angle (Marcuzzo et al., 2008).

Hind limb unloading (HU) in adulthood has provided interesting data on the effects of disuse on gait and posture. Canu et al. (2005) showed that HU rats exhibited increased stride length during treadmill locomotion, hyperextensions at the end of the stance, and a decrease in ankle angle during the remaining part of the stride compared to controls. The ankle remained overflexed from paw contact to the end of midstance, whereas ankle extension increased during push-off. During this overextension, rats appeared to walk on their toes although soleus muscle (ankle extensor) activity was not altered in HU rats (Canu et al., 2005). In addition, HU slightly altered the patterns of neuromuscular activation during treadmill locomotion, suggesting alterations of peripheral afferent information that regulates gait (Canu and Falempin, 1997, 1998). In fictive rhythmic motor episodes elicited by electrical stimulation of the mesencephalic locomotor area, the overall motor pattern was not affected by HU, but extensor muscle nerves were frequently activated and their burst duration were increased relative to control rats (Canu et al., 2001). Consistent with SMR and HU, a 9-day space flight induced overextension of the knee and ankle in rats during both stance and swing phases(Walton, 1998). In addition, it appears that a postnatal critical period (from P14 to P30) exists for the development and maturation of some movement patterns, such as surface righting (Walton et al., 2005).

C. Motor Skill Development

More challenging situations than treadmill locomotion, such as walking on a narrow suspended bar (beam), ladder or rotarod, may allow one to detect additional deficits and to differentiate the involvement of spinal and supraspinal structures in locomotion (Beloozerova et al., 2003; Drew et al., 2008; Garnier et al., 2008). Our SMR rats were barely able to stay on the beam at P17, they often hung on the bar before falling off, and then gradually but slowly improved over time relative to controls (Strata et al., 2004). Using the same SMR methods, Marcuzzo et al. (2008) found comparable results with beam walking.

Our SMR rats spent much less time than controls on the rotarod, and propelled their body using the forelimb rather than the hind limbs, along with their belly in contact with the rotarod (Strata et al., 2004).

Using the ladder walking, Marcuzzo et al. (2008) showed that SMR rats made more stepping errors than controls with increasing numbers of errors over time. These authors also found that SMR delayed stability on an inclined plane (negative geotaxis) but accelerated the appearance of the proprioceptive placing reflex. During ladder walking, HU rats exhibited enhanced duration of step, stance and swing phases, increased ankle flexion during stance, hyperextension at the beginning of the swing (toe-off), and lower protraction during swing, with increased flexor and extensor burst duration in this challenging gait situation (Canu and Garnier, 2009).

3. Peripheral Musculoskeletal Changes Induced by Disuse

Limb disuse can alter physiology and function of muscles and joints as well as bone structure mainly through degenerative processes, as explained further below.

A. Muscle Changes

Disuse resulted in decreased individual myofiber diameters of the triceps surae muscle, a knee and ankle plantar flexor, whereas the myofiber diameters of the quadriceps muscle and the hamstrings, a knee extensor and a knee flexor, respectively, were unchanged (Coq et al., 2008). We used bin frequency counts of myofiber diameters and found that the triceps surae of SMR rats exhibited greater numbers of myofibers with diameters $\leq$ 10 μm than controls and a loss of all myofibers with diameters over 60 μm. According to (Johnson and Kucukyalcin, 1978), myofiber diameters smaller than 10 μm represent an index of myofiber atrophy. These results are similar to those of Marcuzzo et al.'s (2008), in which they observed smaller myofiber areas in the soleus muscle, a foot plantar flexor, in SMR rats than in controls. They also observed a higher percentage of atrophied fibers (0-500 μm), with more rounded profile, and thus increased fiber density, as a consequence of the reduction in the mean fiber area. In their study, treadmill training for 3 weeks after restriction increased the myofiber area and decreased the percentage of atrophied fibers of the soleus (Marcuzzo et al., 2008).

It is now well admitted that hind limb unloading (HU), used as a chronic weightless bearing and movement disuse, have long lasting effects on muscle physiology and function, as well as denervation, tenotomy, spaceflight in both rats and humans or bed rest in the latter (see Booth, 1982; Talmadge et al., 1995; Ohira et al., 2002a; Narici and de Boer, 2010). Briefly, HU induces i) myofiber atrophy (i.e. a reduction in cross-sectional area), especially in predominant slow extensor muscles while fast muscles are almost unaffected (Booth, 1982; Stevens et al., 1990; Ohira et al., 2002b; Kawano et al., 2002; Deschenes et al., 2003; Vermaelen et al., 2005, Wang et al., 2006, Fujita et al., 2009; Schuenke et al., 2009; Narici and de Boer, 2010), ii) changes in fiber phenotypes, such as increases in the expression of fast myosin heavy chains in normally slow muscles (Talmadge et al., 1995; De-Doncker et al., 2002; Kawano et al., 2002; Ohira et al., 2002a; Stevens et al., 2004; Giger et al., 2005, 2009; Yu et al., 2007; Narici and de Boer, 2010; see however Schuenke et al., 2009), iii) drastic reductions of EMG activity of muscles in immobilized limbs and neural drive (Booth, 1982; Ohira et al., 2002a; Westerga and Gramsbergen, 1993; Leterme and Falempin, 1998; Narici and de Boer, 2010), and iv) decreases in muscle glucose consumption and contraction dynamic performance, such as muscle strength, force and power (Booth, 1982; Shenkman et al., 2002; Stein et al., 2002; Stevenson et al., 2003; Kourtidou-Papadeli et al., 2004; Narici and de Boer, 2010).

In our study on disuse, muscle atrophy was accompanied by intramuscular connective tissue changes in all hind limb muscles (Coq et al., 2008). Collagen type I showed a small increase in SMR rats, but connective tissue growth factor (CTGF) increased significantly after restriction compared to controls. CTGF is a cytokine and growth factor that induces fibroblast proliferation and matrix production, and it correlates with fibrotic tissue disorders (Hayashi et al., 2002). Many of the CTGF immunoreactive cells were small cells surrounding the myofibers in the perimysium and endomysium (Coq et al., 2008; Figure 2A,B).

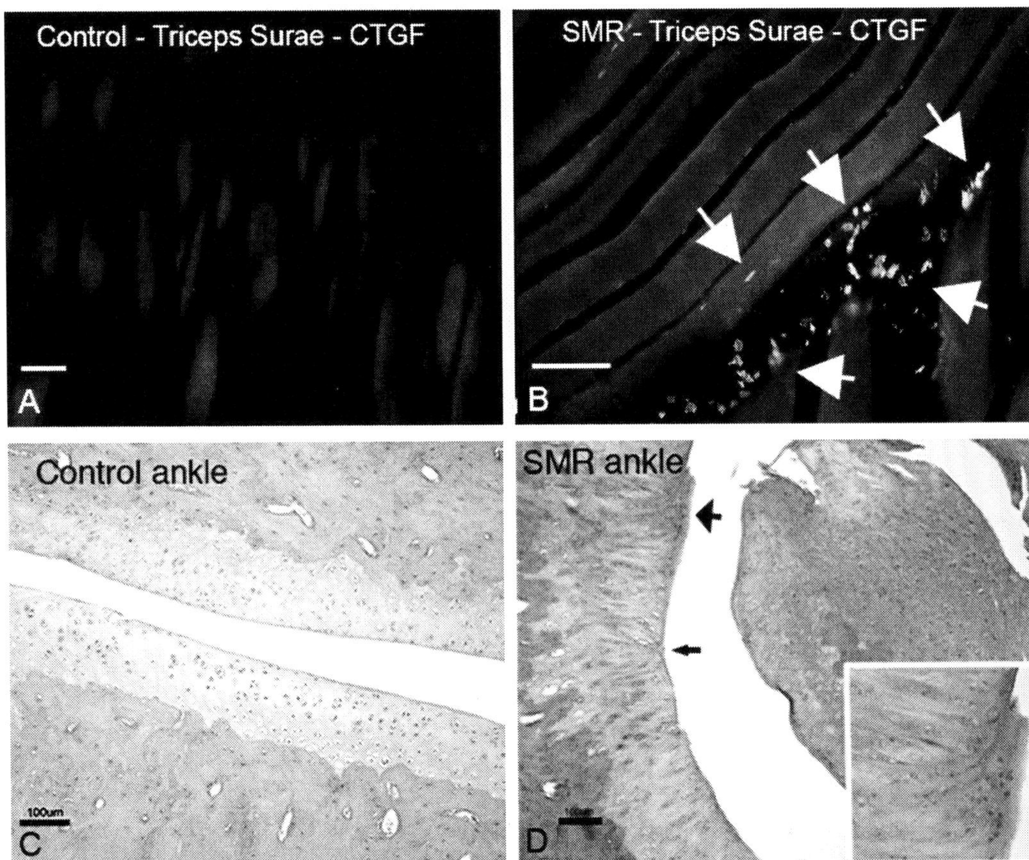

Figure 2. Muscle and ankle histopathlogy in control and sensorimotor restricted (SMR) rats. A-B) Photomicrographs showing connective tissue growth factor (CTGF) immunoreactivity in hind limb muscles from a control rat and a SMR rat. Specifically, longitudinal sections of the triceps surae muscle, also known as gastrocnemius and soleus, are shown. A) Control muscle shows no CTGF immunostaining. B) SMR muscle shows increased CTGF-positive cells that appear to be fibroblasts by location (between muscle fibers primarily), size, and CTGF production. The myofibers themselves also have a low level increase of CTGF within their cytoplasm. Scale bars are 50 μm. C-D) Photos of ankle joints from control and SMR rats. C) Control joint showing healthy articular cartilage. D) SMR joint showing eburnations (small arrow) in the superficial cartilage layers, tidemark changes between the bone and cartilage, and fibrotic cartilage (large arrow). Inset shows a higher power of fibrotic area. Hematoxylin and eosin staining. Scale bars correspond to 100 μm. Figure modified with permission from Coq et al. (2008).

Marcuzzo et al. (2008) also found significant increases in interstitial connective tissue, in their case in the soleus muscle of SMR rats. In that study, treadmill training attenuated the increase in connective tissue and also led to increased polygonal myofibers, instead of rounded fibers. As in SMR, HU also increased connective tissue and satellite cells in muscles (Wang et al., 2006; Kawano et al., 2008; Heinemeier et al., 2009). In regard to disuse-induced changes in muscle force and tension, HU decreased tendon stiffness, especially Achilles tendon, so that the extensibility of tendons increased to compensate some muscle changes (Heinemeier et al., 2009; Narici and de Boer, 2010). Proprioceptive information from muscle afferent fibers is crucial in contraction force regulation and HU has been showed to decrease the dynamic peak but to increase the static sensitivity of Ib afferent fibers (Treffort et al., 2005).

B. Alterations of Joints and Bones

Lastly, we observed articular cartilage degradation in the hind limbs as a result of disuse (Figure 2C,D). For example, medial menisci in the knee joints of SMR rats were undergoing the initial stages of calcification, changes not observed in control rats. The knee articular cartilage was only mildly affected after SMR, with increased condensations in upper cartilage layers in 50% of the rats, but no signs of eburnation or thinning. In contrast, articular cartilages of ankle joints of 62% of the SMR rats showed eburnations, tidemark changes, and fibrocartilage degenerative changes. These degenerative cartilage thickenings were immunoreactive for CTGF, indicative of fibrotic cartilage formation, a type of cartilage degeneration (Coq et al., 2008). The hip joint was not studied in these animals, although in several of the SMR rats, femoral internal rotation was observed (unpublished data), a finding reminiscent of femoral anteversion in children with cerebral palsy. In the same line, HU appears to weaken bone and cartilage structures, in relation to enhanced apoptosis of osteocytes and chondrocytes (Basso and Heersche, 2006; David et al., 2006; Pan et al., 2008; Shimano and Volpon, 2009). As a general physiological adaptation, HU increases sympathetic but reduces parasympathetic cardiac tone, and also induces anhedonia (Moffitt et al., 2008).

4. Central Changes Related to Disuse

To our knowledge, there are no studies dealing with the effects of disuse, such as SMR or HU, on spinal central pattern generators and other subcortical structures, whereas many studies have been devoted to cortical areas.

A. Map Reorganization in the Primary Somatosensory Cortex (S1)

Electrophysiological S1 maps of the hind limb skin representation were recorded in layer IIIb-IV and were located between -1 and +3 mm from bregma in the rostrocaudal axis and between 1 and 4 mm in the mediolateral direction and often overlapped with the M1 layer V representation of hind limb movements (see also Donoghue, 1995). Despite idiosyncratic differences, the S1 hind limb representation in controls presented common somatotopic features (Coq et al., 2008). The hind paw representation was usually located medial to the forepaw map and rostral to the tail and back/ventrum representations. From rostral to caudal, cortical sites progressed from the toes, plantar pads of the sole to the heel and leg. From lateral to medial in the rostral portion of the hind paw map, the toes were topographically represented from toe 1 (t1) to toe 5 (t5) (Figure 3A). The hairy representation of the toes was generally located medially (t1 to t3, innervated by the saphenous nerve) and laterally (t3 to t5, innervated by the sciatic nerve) to the glabrous representation of the toes (innervated by the sciatic nerve).

The overall somatotopy of the foot maps was preserved in our SMR rats in which the representation of contiguous skin surfaces of the foot was partially disrupted (Figure 3B).

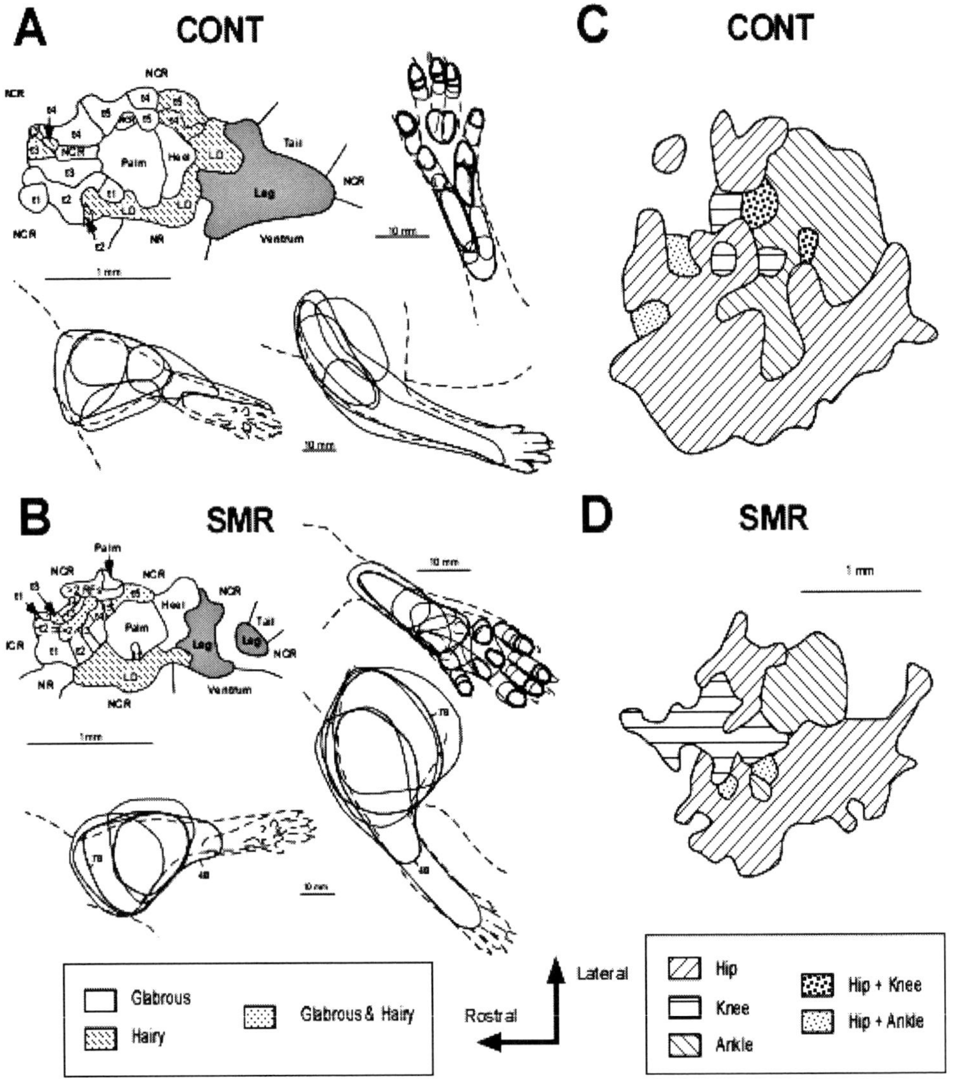

Figure 3. Effects of sensorimotor restriction (SMR) during development on the topographical organization of the hind limb maps in the primary somatosensory (S1) and motor (M1) cortices. A-B) Illustration of the S1 representation of the hind paw and receptive fields (RFs) located on the glabrous foot skin and leg. A) Example of the S1 hind limb map and RFs in a representative control rat (CONT). B) Representative S1 map and RFs of the hind limb in a rat that experienced developmental SMR. Relative to controls the organization of the S1 foot map was degraded in SMR rats and RFs were enlarged. More multiple RFs were recorded in SMR rats. In addition, we found the emergence of RFs that encompassed the two sides of the leg in SMR rats (RFs # 48 and #78), while none in CONT animals. C-D) Illustration of the movement representation of the hind limb joints in M1. C) Representative M1 hind limb map in a control rat (CONT). Note the absence of precise topographical organization of the movements of the joints. D) Developmental SMR induced a reduction in the overall size of the M1 hind limb maps while the relative areas devoted to the different joint representations were not significantly altered. Abbreviations: LD, large dorsum of hind paw; NCR, non cutaneous responses; NR, no response; t1-t5, toe1 to toe 5; >2 and >2 RFs, cortical zones whose RFs encompassed more than 2 distinct hind paw subdivision, i.e. toe or plantar pad. Figure modified with permission from Coq et al. (2007, 2008).

The total S1 area devoted to the foot representation was not statistically different from controls, but the proportions of cortical sites responding to both hind paw cutaneous stimulation and nail movements were about twice in SMR than in control rats (Coq et al., 2008). These results show a change in neuronal selectivity between cutaneous and nail movement inputs and emphasize the sensorimotor restriction-induced alterations of the S1 neuronal properties. Using the same SMR procedures, (Marcuzzo et al., 2010) found a reduction in neuronal counts in the layer V of S1 while the number of glial cells increased, suggesting gliosis and pathological conditions often related to stroke.

The proportions of cortical sites with at least three disjunctive, multiple receptive fields (RFs) were more than 10 times greater in SMR rats than in controls, while the percentages of disjunctive, double RFs did not differ between both groups. As the numbers of multiple RFs increased with disuse the RF size also increased (Figure 3B). The sizes of all RFs were about twice as large in SMR as in controls. This enlargement led to a greater overlap between glabrous RFs, a coarser-grained representation of these surfaces and patchy representations of glabrous and hairy foot surfaces after SMR. To better understand the topographic disruption of the S1 foot maps, the proportions of RFs that encompass both glabrous and hairy foot surfaces were greater in SMR. As a consequence of larger and overlapping RFs, and numerous multiple RFs located on both sides of the foot, the delineation of toe and pad representation borders was difficult in our SMR rats, so that penetrations with at least three multiple RFs were pooled together in specific cortical sectors of the foot maps (Figure 3B).

The proportions of RFs covering both sides of the leg were also greater after SMR since no such double-sided RFs were present in the control rats. The presence of abnormally large RFs covering both sides of either the foot or leg in restrained rats (Coq et al. 2007, 2008) seems in accordance with the level of spasticity reported in our previous studies. Indeed, Strata et al. (2004) reported that restrained rats displayed hind limb rigidity and hypertonicity, as well as increased velocity-dependent resistance to passive motion in all joints of the hind limbs, sign of disabling levels of spasticity, as defined by (Lance and McLeod, 1981). Co-contractions of antagonist muscles of the leg may have induced synchronous activations of cutaneous mechanoreceptors, thus leading to very large RFs covering the entire leg by physiological mechanisms of plasticity (e.g. Wang et al., 1995; Byl et al., 1996, 1997). In the same line, hypertonicity and rigidity of toes and other joints found in SMR rats (Strata et al., 2004) may have contributed to the increase in S1 nail movement representation and to the decrease in neuronal selectivity to afferent inputs in S1 (Coq et al., 2008).

Thus, disuse induced the emergence of RFs located on both sides of the leg, as well as RFs on both glabrous and hairy sides of the foot. In addition, SMR also increased the cortical responsiveness to tactile stimulation. And disuse during development induced a topographical degradation of the S1 foot maps and alterations of the neuronal properties (Coq et al., 2008). Interestingly, Canu et al. recently found changes in cortical neuron properties, such as decreased intrinsic excitability (reduction in input membrane resistance and slow after hyperpolarization, increased rheobase, but unchanged resting membrane potential) of cortical cells in layer II to VI of the sensorimotor cortex in adult rats that experienced 2 weeks of HU (Canu et al., 2010).

Previous studies based on disuse during adulthood partially confirm our results. Forepaw immobilization with a plaster cast for one or two weeks degraded the S1 topographic organization and drastically reduced the contralateral S1 map area, while the size of the corresponding RFs was unchanged (Coq and Xerri, 1999). Two weeks of HU also reduced the

S1 map but increased the proportion of large foot RFs (Langlet et al., 1999a, 1999b) and induced abnormal locomotor patterns, such as hind limb hyperextension (Canu and Falempin, 1996). However, we cannot rule out possible effects of restraint-induced stress on S1 map reorganization (Canu et al., 2007), but we previously reported no increase in stress induced by forepaw immobilization in young adult rats and no significant impact of possible stress on the S1 map plasticity (Coq and Xerri, 1999).

In a nice series of studies on the central effects of HU, Canu, Falempin and colleagues showed that the HU-induced S1 map reorganization was related to changes in reduced nerve velocity, and spinal and cortical responsiveness (Canu et al., 2003), neurotrophin expression such as NGF and BDNF (Dupont et al., 2005), cholinergic transmission (Dupont et al., 2002) and the balance between excitation and inhibition (Dupont et al., 2003; Canu et al., 2006; Treffort et al., 2006). More precisely, these authors reported that HU in adulthood increased the *in vivo* levels of both excitatory (glutamate and aspartate) and inhibitory (GABA and taurine) transmission in the L5 spinal cord (Treffort et al., 2006), while excitation levels did not change but GABA inhibition was reduced in the S1 cortex (Dupont et al., 2003; Canu et al., 2006). Thus, they showed the cortical S1 maps changes related to disuse in adulthood was mainly induced by reduced GABA inhibition but not by increased excitation. Likewise, whisker trimming, nerve transection or partial hind limb deafferentation led to a marked, but reversible reduction of GAD (gamma amino decarboxylase) immunostaining within layer IV of the cortical zone representing the deprived body part (Warren et al., 1989; Land et al., 1995; Fuchs and Salazar, 1998). Relevant to our studies is the observation that reduction in GABAergic inhibition tends also to induce cutaneous RF enlargement, as found after SMR and HU. Such a RF enlargement has been found with micro-iontophoretic injections of bicuculline methiodide to antagonize GABA-mediated inhibition in the cat S1 cortex (Dykes et al., 1984; Alloway et al., 1989).

B. Maps in the Primary Motor Cortex (M1)

The movement representations of the hind limbs in rat are located in the primary motor cortex at the rostrocaudal level of bregma, and slightly lateral (+1 to +5) to it (Strata et al., 2004; Coq et al., 2007). The representation of the hind limb joints is not topographically organized but distributed throughout the hind limb map. In control rats, the hip representation occupied in average 73.5 % of the M1 total hind limb area (3.92 ± 0.40 mm^2 in average), while 3.5 % was knee, 16 % the ankle, 1.5% the toes and 1.6 % was devoted to complex movements involving several joints (Coq et al., 2007; Figure 3C).

After developmental SMR, we found no change in the size of the overall M1 hind limb maps, although the proportion of hip movements increased while that of the knee decreased (Strata et al., 2004). More recently, we found slightly different results after developmental SMR. It decreased the overall size of M1 hind limb maps, although the relative areas devoted to the different joint representations were not significantly altered, except for a decrease in hip movement representations (Coq et al., 2007; Figure 3D). To our knowledge, there are no data on the effects of HU or other comparable types of disuse on M1 maps. However, neonatal amputation of the forearm induced a loss of the motor representation of this limb in the adult rat. The deafferented cortical territory was then devoted to represent movements of the trunk, shoulder and whiskers, whose cortical representation increased (Donoghue and Sanes, 1988; Donoghue et al., 1990). In contrast, whisker sensory denervation did not alter the motor representation of these whiskers, but increased the stimulation threshold (Franchi,

2000, 2001). In our study, disuse during development induced a partial deafferentation of sensory inputs, which reduces the motor representation but did not alter the muscular activation threshold. Recently, we showed that unilateral cervical spinal hemisection in adult rat drastically reduced the size of M1 forepaw movement representations and that the absence or drastic reduction of afferent inputs from S1 did not seem to be the main cause of such a large M1 forelimb map remodeling in adulthood (Martinez et al., 2010), as found after sensory facial nerve section in adult rats (Franchi, 2001; Franchi and Veronesi, 2006; see however, Liepert et al., 2003). In contrast, small and large scale changes in the M1 maps have been shown to depend mainly upon intracortical horizontal connections, synaptogenesis, and alterations of LTP/LTD and excitation-inhibition balance, all of which may lead to masking or unmasking of connections in relation to the neuronal activity within M1 cortex (Rioult-Pedotti et al., 2000; Kleim et al., 2002; see Sanes and Donoghue, 2000; Raineteau and Schwab, 2001; Teskey et al., 2008 for reviews).

In developmental disuse, although the overall M1 maps of the hind limb either decreased (Coq et al., 2007) or were not altered (Strata et al., 2004), the average thresholds (i.e. minimal amount current to evoke movements) did not differ from controls. These results differ from those of studies in which neonatal motor nerve section or limb amputation led to enlarged M1 representation of intact muscles concomitant with decreased stimulation thresholds in the newly occupied cortical territories (Donoghue and Sanes, 1987, 1988). Along the same line, sensory vibrissal pad denervation in adult rats has been found to increase the thresholds required to evoke movements of the whiskers, whereas those to produce other types of movements were similar between control and input-deprived rats (Franchi, 2001; Franchi and Veronesi, 2006). Decreased or similar thresholds seem to correspond to unmasking of pre-existing horizontal connections, whereas increased stimulation thresholds suggest high-threshold representation may be unmasked (Donoghue and Sanes, 1987; 1988; Franchi, 2001; see Sanes and Donoghue, 2000 for review).

5. Conclusion for the Disuse Model

Our studies on developmental disuse confirm and emphasize the preponderant role of individual experience in shaping the body and brain during maturation. Indeed, we have shown that abnormal inputs, through disuse, during development induced some of the motor dysfunctions (Strata et al., 2004) and hind limb histopathologies (Coq et al., 2008) which recapitulate those observed in patients with cerebral palsy (CP; Booth et al., 2001; Liptak and Accardo, 2004; Foran et al., 2005). In addition, the presence of abnormal sensorimotor experience has been shown in infants with CP (Prechtl, 1997; Hadders-Algra, 2004; Einspieler and Prechtl, 2005; Hadders-Algra et al., 2010), with its possible deleterious impact on musculoskeletal tissues (Lieber, 1986; Foran et al., 2005) and cortical reorganization in humans (Clayton et al., 2003; Hadders-Algra and Gramsbergen, 2007; Hadders-Algra, 2008; Burton et al., 2008, 2009; Wingert et al., 2008, 2009; Andiman et al., 2010). In other studies, we also showed that the combination of disuse during development with either neonatal asphyxia or prenatal ischemia increased the deleterious impact of disuse on peripheral histopathology as well as on cortical M1 and S1 reorganization (Strata et al., 2004; Coq et al., 2007, 2008; Delcour et al., 2009). It is possible that perinatal asphyxia or ischemia impinges physiological mechanisms of plasticity (see Vannucci et al., 1999; Vannucci and Vannucci,

2005 for reviews), which could even worsen the already deleterious effects of disuse during development. Thus, abnormal and limited movements, through hind limb immobilization, may account for the musculoskeletal tissue changes, which in turn contribute to provide repetitive, aberrant sensory inputs to the immature brain. These aberrant inputs induce abnormal sensory feedback leading to degradation of the topographic maps in S1 and M1 and consequently to degraded motor function.

II. Overuse Model

1. Our Animal Model of Overuse Injury

In an effort to understand the underlying mechanisms of these disorders, Barbe and Barr and a number of other labs have developed animal models of overuse injuries (Topp and Byl, 1999; Remple et al., 2001; Barbe et al., 2003; Diao et al., 2005; Sommerich et al., 2007; ; Dourte et al., 2010; Hollander et al., 2010; Willems et al., 2010). Our model is a unique rat model of voluntary repetitive reaching in which rats can be trained to perform an upper limb repetitive hand and wrist-intensive task at ranges of reach rates and force levels derived from clinical and epidemiological evidence for risk exposure in humans (See Barr and Barbe, 2002 for a review). Investigations of industrial workers by Silverstein and colleagues (Silverstein et al., 1986, 1998) defined risk levels for repetitiveness to be high when reaching and grasping motions are performed faster than 30 sec/cycle. Force is considered negligible to low if less than 15% of maximum voluntary contraction (MVC) is required and high if it is above 50% MVC. In our model, rats are trained to perform one of several levels of paced reaching and grasping tasks, as shown in Table 1. Whishaw has quantified the similarities between rats and humans in targeted reach submovements of the upper extremity (Whishaw et al., 1992). In our model, the repetition and force parameters in the rat were scaled to resemble occupational tasks in humans, as explained further in Barr and Barbe (2002). Viikari-Juntura and colleagues state that laboratory studies of animals examining the effect of repetitive loading on tissue function may be extrapolated to human exposures and responses (Viikari-Juntura, 1997; Viikari-Juntura and Silverstein, 1999). Therefore, our rat model of a paced reaching and grasping task may be generalized to humans in terms of both behavioral and tissue responses for some types of physically constrained and paced occupational tasks. An example of such a paced task would be packing, in which a worker repeatedly places small objects presented on a conveyor belt into a package crate.

In this model, rats are placed into operant test chambers for rodents with a portal located in one wall, as described previously (Barbe et al., 2003; Clark et al., 2004; Rani et al., 2009a, 2009b; Elliott et al., 2009, 2009). They are trained to perform a repetitive reaching task in which they reach through the portal to grasp and retrieve a food pellet, or to grasp and isometrically pull a force handle, which is attached to force transducer, until a predetermined force threshold is reached and held for at least 50 ms. Upon successful achievement of reach force and time criteria, the rat releases the handle and retrieves a food pellet reward by mouth from a food trough. Using this apparatus, the short-term effects (3-12 weeks) of a voluntary low force task performed at low, moderate or high reach rates, with force requirements of low or high (see details in Table 1), on sensorimotor behavior, forelimb musculoskeletal and nerve tissues, spinal cord and brain have been determined.

Table 1. Repetitive task group parameters of the Barbe and Barr rat model of overuse

Group	Target Reach Rate (reaches/min)	Actual Reach Rate (reaches/min)	Reach Force (% of Maximum Pull Force)
HRHF	8	12	60 ± 5
MRHF	4	9.4	60 ± 5
HRLF	8	12	15 ± 5
HRNF = MRNF	4	8	<5[a]
LRNF	2	3.3	<5[a]

HRHF = high repetition high force; MRHF = moderate repetition high force; HRLF = high repetition low force; HRNF = high repetition negligible force, redefined as MRNF based on the repetition rate; LRNF = Low repetition negligible force. [a] The negligible force rats retrieved a 45 mg food pellet, which was estimated to be < 5% maximum pulling force.

Specifically, the short-term effects of repetitive and/or forceful tasks on tissue pathophysiology have been characterized, focusing on injury, inflammation, inflammation-induced catabolic changes, and fibrotic changes, that might contribute to peripheral tissue degeneration or sensorimotor behavior declines. Inflammation-induced central nervous system changes that might contribute to sensorimotor behavior changes, such as the development of pain behaviors, have also been investigated.

2. Sensorimotor Behavioral Changes with Overuse

Only a few investigative teams are studying degradation of movement and associated tissue changes in animal models of overuse injuries. The Barbe and Barr's, Sommerich's and Byl's models are the only models of repetitive motion induced overuse injuries at this time that utilize voluntary tasks in which pathophysiological tissue responses and behavioral responses, indicative of sensorimotor function, can be determined simultaneously. Voluntary movement paradigms allow the linking of tissue pathology with outward physical signs of dysfunction. The behavioral changes are discussed in this section, while possible links to peripheral and central tissue changes are discussed in a subsequent section.

A. Gross Motor Function

In the Barbe and Barr rat model, several indicators offer insight into the behavioral consequences of repetitive task performance and induced tissue changes. Reach rate (reaches/minute) is an indicator of the animals' ability to maintain task pace, and undergoes exposure-dependent declines in this model. Across weeks of task performance, rats performing a low repetition negligible force (LRNF) task showed no decrease in reach rate (Elliott et al., 2008). Rats performing a high repetition negligible force (HRNF) task had significant but transient declines in reach rate (Barbe et al., 2003; Clark et al., 2003; Coq et al., 2009), while rats performing a high repetition high force (HRHF) task demonstrate a fluctuating and continual decline in reach rate over weeks of task performance (Barr et al., 2004; Clark et al., 2004). Grip strength is a sign of muscle integrity and mass, and declines in grip strength can result from muscle injury, neuropathic injury or muscle inflammation (described further later). In rats performing a LRNF food retrieval task, grip strength had a small but transient decline in week 6, while rats performing a HRNF food retrieval task had progressive declines in grip strength, with a 35% decline by week 6 and a 60% decline by week 8 (Barbe et al., 2008). Rats performing a MRHF handle-pulling task showed no decline in until week 12 (a 35% decline; Elliott et al., 2009a), suggesting that the handle-pulling task was easier to perform than the food retrieval task. New studies in our lab confirm that the food retrieval task required more fine motor skills to manipulate the food out of a pellet dispenser than performing an isometric pull on a fixed lever (unpublished data). In contrast, rats performing a HRHF task had progressive declines in grip strength to 53% in week 12 (Fedorczyk et al., 2010; Rani et al., 2010). Thus, gross motor function is preserved with lower demand tasks, but is more compromised with higher demand tasks, such as high repetition with high force, or tasks requiring very fine motor skills.

Task duration (number of hours/day the rats participated in this voluntary task) is an indicator of overall animal comfort. Similar to reach rate, animals exhibited exposure-dependent task avoidance with continued task performance. This was exhibited as decreased duration of performance of this voluntary task, and was likely due to discomfort from tissue inflammation, as discussed further below. LRNF rats showed no declines in task duration, HRNF/MRNF (moderate repetition negligible force task; see Table 1) rats declined transiently in week 3, MRHF rats declined only in week 12, while task duration declined progressively in HRHF rats from week 3 through 12 weeks (Barbe et al., 2003; Coq et al., 2009; Clark et al., 2004; Elliott et al., 2008; 2009a).

B. Fine Motor Skills

Movement pattern changes that are associated with chronic repetitive paw closing tasks, with or without force, have been demonstrated in both non-human primate and rodent models of repetitive motion disorder (Byl et al., 1996, 1997; Topp and Byl, 1999; Barbe et al., 2003; Sommerich et al., 2007; Elliott et al., 2008). In the Barbe and Barr model, a gradual increase in two distinct alternative reach movement patterns for food pellet retrieval was observed (Barbe et al., 2003; Coq et al., 2009). Scooping is a pattern in which the semi-open forepaw is placed over the food pellet and the pellet is dragged along the bottom or side surface of the tube and scooped into the mouth. Scooping peaked in week 5 in 47% of animals and then declined. Raking is an inefficient extreme of scooping in which repeated unsuccessful attempts to contact the food pellet with the semi-open forepaw result in repeated back and forth movements that resemble a raking motion. The raking pattern continued to increase beyond week 5 and was observed in 100% of animals by weeks 7 and 8. The "raking" reach pattern also included poor forepaw and digit closure and, thus, poor grasp control changes that are reminiscent of focal dystonia from somatosensory cortical map changes, as described by Byl et al. (1996, 1997) in an owl monkey model.

Another movement pattern degradation was increased extraneous movement reversals during the grasp phase of reach (Figure 4). All MRNF animals developed progressively increased extraneous movement reversals during the grasp phase of reach (Coq et al., 2009), while only 60% of LRNF animals developed increased extraneous movement reversals, although only transiently (Elliott et al., 2008).

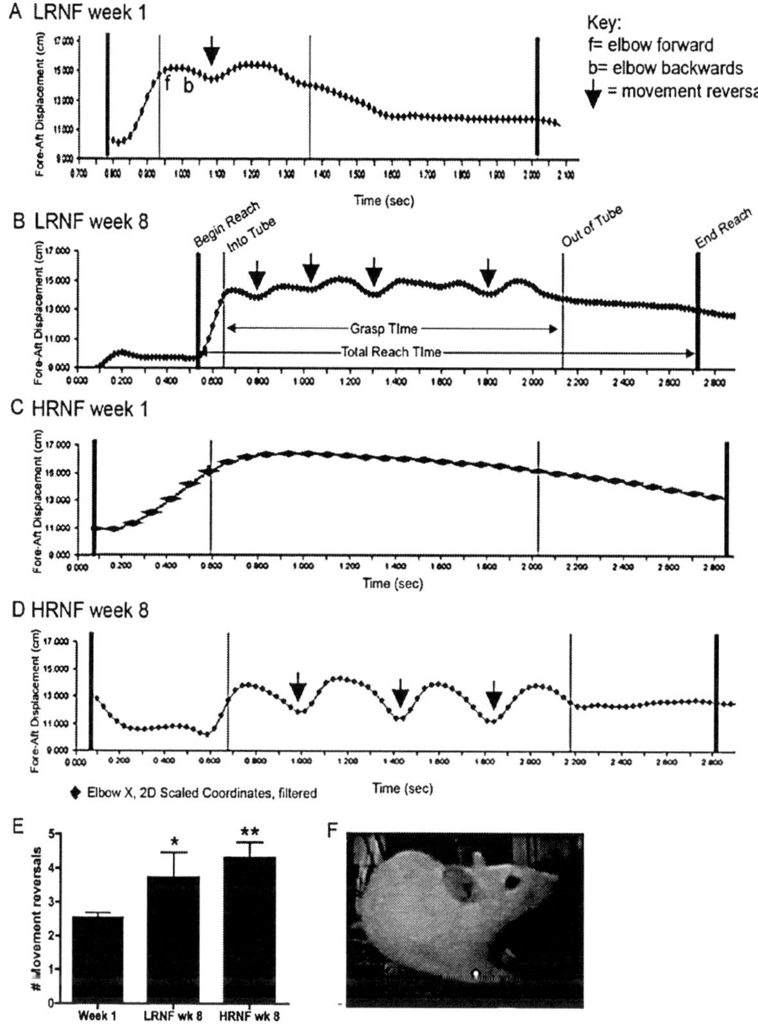

Figure. 4. Motor performance data in rats performing either a low repetition negligible force task (LRNF) or a high repetition negligible force task (HRNF) from baseline (week 1) to week 8. This task consisted of a reaching, grasping and food pellet retrieval. A-D) Representative reach sequences of LRNF and HRNF rats analyzed from video tape segments collected in weeks 1 or 8. Thick black lines indicate beginning and end time points of one entire reach, as indicated in panel B as Begin Reach and End Reach, respectively. This also defines the Total Reach Time. The thin grey lines indicate the point when the elbow enters the tube (Into Tube) and when it is withdrawn (Out of Tube). A food pellet is grasped and retrieved during this period (Grasp Time). X-axis indicates time required to perform these movements (in sec). Y-axis indicates fore-aft movement (in cm) of elbow from floor of behavior chamber, through the portal to retrieve the food, and back. Dashed lines indicate movement of elbow tracked using this 2D system. Key: f, forward movement of elbow; b, backward movement of elbow; arrows, extra movement reversals during grasp time. A-D) Not only do both LRNF and HRNF rats have more movement reversals (fore-aft displacements of elbow) in weeks 8 than weeks 1, but graph times are longer in weeks 8 than 1. (E) Mean number of extra movement reversals per reach is significantly increased in week 8 of both tasks compared to week 1, indicating more errors and thus a decline in fine motor abilities. *: $p < 0.05$, **: $p < 0.01$ compared to week 1. Mean per week ± SEM is shown. Number of animals per group: Week 1 (n = 15), LRNF 8 week (n = 7), HRNF week 8 (n = 8). F) Photo of rat showing placement of marker on elbow during analysis of video tape segments. Figure modified with permission from Elliott et al. (2008).

This latter movement pattern change was interpreted as decreased fine motor dexterity associated with declines in sensorimotor abilities, because these extra movement reversals occurring during a reach sequence are corrections for missed food pellets. These increases in arm movement reversals may be due to discomfort, changes in afferent or efferent nerve function, or both. Thus, fine motor control, like gross motor control, is preserved with lower demand tasks, but is more compromised with higher demand tasks (Elliott et al., 2008; Coq et al., 2009).

Using a voluntary repetitive pinching task in a monkey model, Sommerich and colleagues (2007) reported decreased performance as force level and pinch hold time increased. In one monkey, there was also a substantial reduction from a previously high work rate, as well as complete task cessation that lasted for days. The authors suggest that the animal was self-limiting the work rate. This suggestion may also explain the declines in task duration in our rat model.

Byl's primate model (1996, 1997) also used a voluntary task in which nonhuman primates were trained to perform stressful repetitive hand tasks of either: a) opening and closing a hand piece, or b) trying to meticulously place the thumb and the index finger on two points. Five of seven primates were trained until they could no longer perform the task. They began to have difficulty either closing or opening the hand on the target task. In addition, their training rate declined, as did their accuracy. As mentioned above, their poor grasp control changes were reminiscent of focal dystonia seen in patients. While some clinicians consider focal hand dystonia (occupational hand cramps) to be idiopathic, individuals performing tasks requiring intensive repetitive movements (e.g. working at computer, playing an instrument, pitching a ball, screwing nails, playing golf) appear to be at high risk.

C. Forepaw Sensation

Responses to sensory stimulation have also been examined in the Barbe and Barr rat model, and also appear to be exposure dependent. For example, no changes in withdrawal responses to mechanical stimulation was observed in LRNF rats across 12 weeks of task performance (unpublished observation), while MRHF rats exhibited forepaw hypersensitivity to mechanical stimuli in weeks 6 and 12 (Elliott et al., 2009a), as did HRHF rats in weeks 2-4 prior to their development of hyposensitivity to mechanical stimuli (Clark et al., 2004; Barr et al., 2004; Rani et al., 2010). The development of forepaw hypersensitivity is suggestive of an irritative nerve lesion or increased presence of nociceptive sensitization chemicals in and around peripheral nerve terminals. In contrast, the development of forepaw hyposensitivity is suggestive of a destructive nerve lesion, such as that produced by nerve compression. The presence or absence of these underlying tissue mechanisms is further discussed below.

3. Peripheral Changes with Overuse

A. Human Findings

Human studies examining tissue biopsies in patients with long-term chronic overuse syndromes find evidence of nerve compression and musculoskeletal and nerve injury, inflammation, fibrosis, degeneration and even necrosis (Ljung et al., 1999; Larsson et al., 2000; Kuiper et al., 2004; Rempel et al., 1999; Rempel and Diao, 2004; Diao et al., 2005; for more review see Barr et al., 2004). Imaging studies of patients show cortical stress fractures

(Forwood and Parker, 1991; Fredericson et al., 1995), and histological studies of articular cartilage examined after joint replacement in patients with osteoarthritis, a disorder with overuse etiology, show thinning, erosions and osteophytes. Freeland and colleagues (2002) detected increased tenosynovium IL-6, an inflammatory cytokine, and increased serum malondialdehyde, a cell injury biomarker and a reactive oxygen species that initiates arachidonic acid metabolism into products (e.g. PGE2) in patients with carpal tunnel syndrome (CTS). As mentioned earlier, increased inflammatory cytokines have also been detected in serum of patients with early onset of moderate to severe symptoms of upper limb overuse injury (Carp et al., 2007), presumably as a result of increased cytokines in injured or inflamed tissues.

B. Findings in Animal Models of Overuse

Recent work in animal models suggests that performance of repetitive tasks with or without force, induces injury, persistent inflammation, and damage in several tissues, including nerve, muscle, tendon and bone (Diao et al., 2005; Perry et al., 2005; Sommerich et al., 2007; Dourte et al., 2010; Hollander et al., 2010; Willems et al., 2010; for more review see Barr et al., 2004). In the Barbe and Barr rat model, repetitive reaching and grasping tasks induced nerve and musculoskeletal injury as well as inflammatory and degenerative responses. Specifically, observed signs of tissue injury included myofiber fray, the presence of moth eaten myofibers in forelimb muscles, declines in median nerve conduction velocity, degraded myelin and axonal swelling in the median nerve, and pathological bone morphology (Barbe et al., 2003; Clark et al., 2003, 2004; Rani et al., 2009a, 2009b; Elliott et al., 2010). The declines in median nerve conduction were exposure-dependent, ranging in reductions of 9-17% depending on the level of task intensity (Clark et al., 2003, 2004; Elliott et al., 2009b). Chronic task induced inflammatory responses were also induced, such as persistently increased macrophages and inflammatory cytokines in musculoskeletal tissues, nerves and serum (Barbe et al., 2003, Barr et al., 2003, Clark et al., 2003, Clark et al., 2004, Al-Shatti et al., 2005, Elliott et al., 2009b, Fedorczyk et al., 2010, Rani et al., 2010; Figure 5A,B). Task-induced degenerative changes also developed, including increased collagen deposition in and around the median nerve and tendon sheaths within the carpal tunnel, tendon disorganization, pathological woven bone formation as well as bone resorption (Barr et al., 2003; Fedorczyk et al., 2010; Rani et al., 2009ab, 2010). The degenerative changes, such as tendon disorganization and bone resorption, appeared to be linked at least partially to the inflammatory responses. The declines in nerve conduction velocity, nerve fibrosis, myelin degradation, axonal swelling also indicate the presence of a chronic nerve compression injury mechanism in this model, especially when high repetition is combined with high force.

4. Central Nervous System Changes with Overuse

Previous studies using animal models of repetitive motion have correlated cortical neuroplastic changes or peripheral tissue inflammation with changes in either gross or fine motor performance. However, the possibility that both peripheral inflammatory and central cortical neuroplastic changes mechanisms coexist with altered motor performance has only recently been studied (Coq et al., 2009).

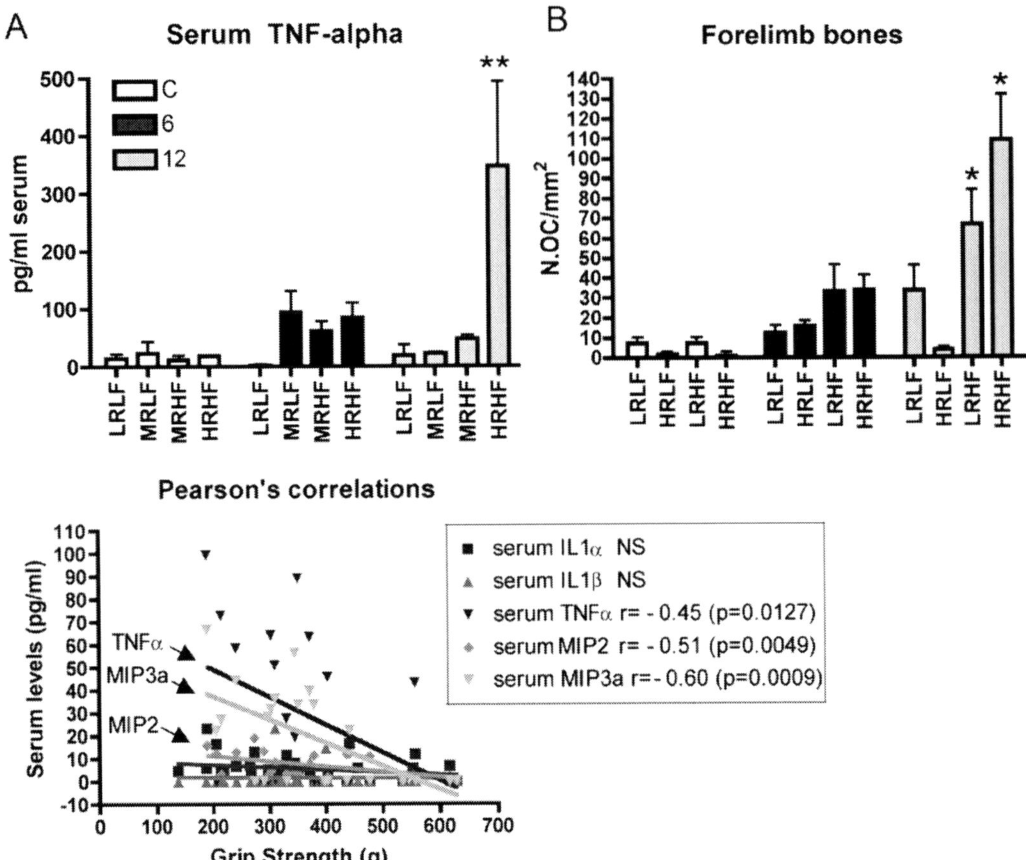

Figure 5. Task exposure dependent (i.e. dependent on weeks of task performance and demands of task) increases serum cytokines and bone osteoclasts, and correlation of grip with serum cytokines. A) Serum TNFα, a key pro-inflammatory cytokine, in all task groups at control (0), 6 or 12 weeks of task performance, tested via ELISA. Although serum TNFα was significant higher in MRLF and MRHF rats at 6 weeks compared to controls when 1 way ANOVAs were performed individually by task (see Barbe et al, 2008 and Elliott et al, 2009a), when HRHF serum data is included in a 2 way ANOVA (with factors weeks and tasks), highest serum TNFα is clearly in HRHF rats at 12 weeks. **: $p < 0.01$ compared to controls. B) Osteoclasts also increase in a dose dependent manner in distal radius and ulna with task performance, with greatest numbers (N.Oc/mm^2) in HRHF rats at 12 weeks. *: $p < 0.05$ compared to controls. Osteoclasts are known to increase bone resorptive activity in presence of increased TNFα. C) Graph showing Pearson's correlations of grip strength with 5 serum cytokines. Serum TNFα, MIP2 and MIP3 levels correlated negatively with grip strength. Reductions in grip strength also reduces loading on bone, contributing to decreased bone. Thus, increased serum cytokines can have detrimental effects on both motor function and bone integrity. See also Barr et al. (2004); Barbe et al. (2008); Elliott et al. (2008, 2009a) for more explanation.

We have also performed a series of studies examining peripheral inflammatory responses in combination with spinal cord neuroplastic changes (Elliott et al., 2008, 2009ab, 2010).

A. Spinal Cord Neuroplasticity

Several studies using chronic nerve compression injuries have found phenotypic changes in dorsal root ganglion neurons in which the expression of proteins, receptors, neurotransmitters, and neurotrophic factors were altered (Wallin and Schött, 2002; Hammond et al., 2004; Chao et al., 2008). For example, Substance P increases in spinal cord dorsal horns following chronic constriction injury from partial nerve ligation, peripheral nerve injury or inflammation (Abbadie et al., 1996; Delander et al., 1997; Allen et al., 1999; McCarson, 1999; Cruce et al., 2001; Rothman et al., 2005). This increase may be due to inflammation-induced increases in afferent synaptic input to the spinal cord through an increased rate of discharge, increased peptide production by the dorsal root ganglion, and/or afferent fiber phenotype alterations that favor Substance P expression (Pitcher and Henry, 2004). Schaible and colleagues described this type of afferent influx of excitatory transmitters into the spinal cord dorsal horn after injury as the presynaptic component of central sensitization (Schaible et al., 2002). An increase in neurokinin-1, a key receptor for Substance P, occur in the post-synaptic spinal cord neurons, and most likely occurs as a response to the increased release of Substance P from nociceptive afferent terminals (Pitcher and Henry, 2004).

Thus, it was not a surprise to us to see increased Substance P and neurokinin 1 in dorsal horns in cervical spinal cord regions with performance low and moderate repetitive tasks with or without high force (Elliott et al 2008, 2009ab, 2010). In each of these studies, the neurochemical response was associated temporally with a peripheral tissue macrophage or inflammatory cytokine response. This supports a hypothesis that task induced peripheral tissue injury and inflammation drives a spinal cord neurochemical response from nociceptive afferent terminals. Such increases in Substance P and neurokinin 1 are temporally associated with mechanical hypersensitivity (Sweitzer et al., 2001; Winkelstein et al., 2001; Rothman et al., 2005). These studies combined provide evidence that spinal cord plasticity under injury and inflammatory conditions may well be contributing to chronic pain conditions, such as mechanical hypersensitivity, in animal models and patients with overuse injury.

There are also an abundance of studies showing spinal cord inflammatory responses after unilateral peripheral nerve injury, e.g. increased activated microglia and increased pro-inflammatory cytokines production by spinal cord neuron and/or glia (DeLeo et al., 1997; Hunt et al., 2001; Shubayev and Myers, 2002; Schäfers et al., 2003a; Ohtori et al., 2004; Hubbard and Winkelstein, 2005; Hatashita et al., 2008). In a recent study, we observed increased IL-1β and TNFα immunoexpression in neurons within the dorsal horn superficial lamina in aged rats that had performed a moderate demand task (HRLF) for 12 weeks, compared to normal controls (Elliott et al., 2010). We have observed that the production of cytokines in the spinal cord in our rat model includes neurons. That said, the production of cytokines by glial cells is also plausible and still needs to be investigated in our model for understanding of the central changes induced by performance of repetitive tasks.

B. Overuse-Induced Remodeling of Somatosensory and Motor Cortical Maps

With regard to the cortical changes, we examined primary somatosensory cortical (S1) and primary motor cortical (M1) changes in rats performing a reaching and grasping task with moderate repetition and negligible force demands (MRNF task) for 2 hrs/day, 3 days/wk for 8 weeks (Coq et al., 2009).

In S1, the repetitive behavioral task did not alter the overall size of the S1 forepaw map, but that overall size was positively correlated with the ratio of grip strength in week 1 versus 8. The MRNF changed the neuronal selectivity between cutaneous and nail movement inputs, as the proportion of cortical sites responding to both forepaw cutaneous stimulation and nail movements was greater in MRNF rats than in control rats. We found other examples of MRNF-induced degradation of S1 neuronal properties, such as more RFs encompassing several forepaw subdivisions (i.e. several digits and/or palmar pads), more cortical sites exhibiting RFs located on both glabrous and hairy surfaces, and increased cortical responsiveness to light tactile stimulation. In addition, the RFs located on the glabrous forepaw were 1.5 times larger in MRNF rats than in controls and glabrous RFs overlapped much more (Figure 6A,B,D,E). The larger the glabrous RFs on the forepaw, the lower the mean percent of successful reaches. As a consequence, the forepaw representation appeared to be patchy and the S1 map topography was disrupted in MRNF rats relative to controls. For example, disruptions in the continuity of the S1 representation of contiguous skin surfaces of the forepaw and discontinuous representations of several single forepaw subdivisions into distinct cortical zones within the S1 forepaw map (see the patchy representation of digits 1 and 2 in Figure 6D), features not seen in untrained S1 maps. Another conspicuous feature in the S1 forepaw maps of trained rats was the higher proportion of RFs located on either palmer pads and digits or dorsal forepaw and wrist/forearm after the behavioral training (Figure 6E). These large RFs located on the forepaw and forearm correlated negatively with the percentage of successful reaches, positively correlated with percentage of rats using the inefficient food retrieval pattern of raking, and positively correlated with the reach phase time ratio of week 1 to week 8 (Coq et al. 2009). These data confirm and extend those found in primates in which repetitive, rewarded hand grasp led to a de-differentiation of the finger 3b maps, characterized by enlarged, overlapping RFs, the emergence of multidigit and hairy-glabrous RFs, as well as abnormal somatosensory maps in the thalamus (Byl et al., 1996, 1997; Blake et al., 2002). In previous studies, it has also been shown that abnormal sensorimotor experience (disuse) can result in a degradation of both the topographic organization of somatosensory maps and S1 neuronal properties (Coq and Xerri, 1999; Coq et al., 2008). A concordant degradation of the S1 forepaw map features has been correlated with poor tactile discrimination performance in rats (Xerri et al., 2005).

In the motor cortex, the MRNF reaching task drastically increased the total area of the forepaw movement representation (1.6 times larger) compared to controls. The areas occupied by the shoulder (6% of the total map area), elbow (41%), wrist (23%), digits (1%) and arm (3%) were not significantly affected by the behavioral training, but the cortical area devoted to multi-joint movements drastically increased in MRNF rats (Figure 6C,F). Indeed, the movement representation area of the elbow-wrist multi-joint responses tripled and the arm-digits multi-joint areal extent was 17 times larger than in untrained rats. Interestingly, the cortical increase in the multi-joint movement representation for elbow-wrist, arm and arm-digits correlated strongly with the increased prevalence of the raking strategy, as well as the elbow movement representation. The overall threshold (i.e. minimal current to evoke a movement) of neuronal M1 responses did not differ between groups nor did the threshold for most forelimb joints, except for digits (digits only and digit-arm), which were 2 times lower after behavioral training. Out of the motor forepaw map, the average thresholds required to evoke whisker and hind paw movements did not differ between both groups, so that the MRNF task specifically altered the M1 digit representation.

Thus, the MRNF task drastically increased the size of the M1 forepaw maps, especially the movement representation of the digits, digit-arm and elbow-wrist specifically involved in the behavioral task, and also decreased specifically the amount of current required to evoke movements of the digits. To a certain extent, the motor cortical reorganization induced by the prolonged performance of repetitive reaching in our model seems more adaptive than deleterious.

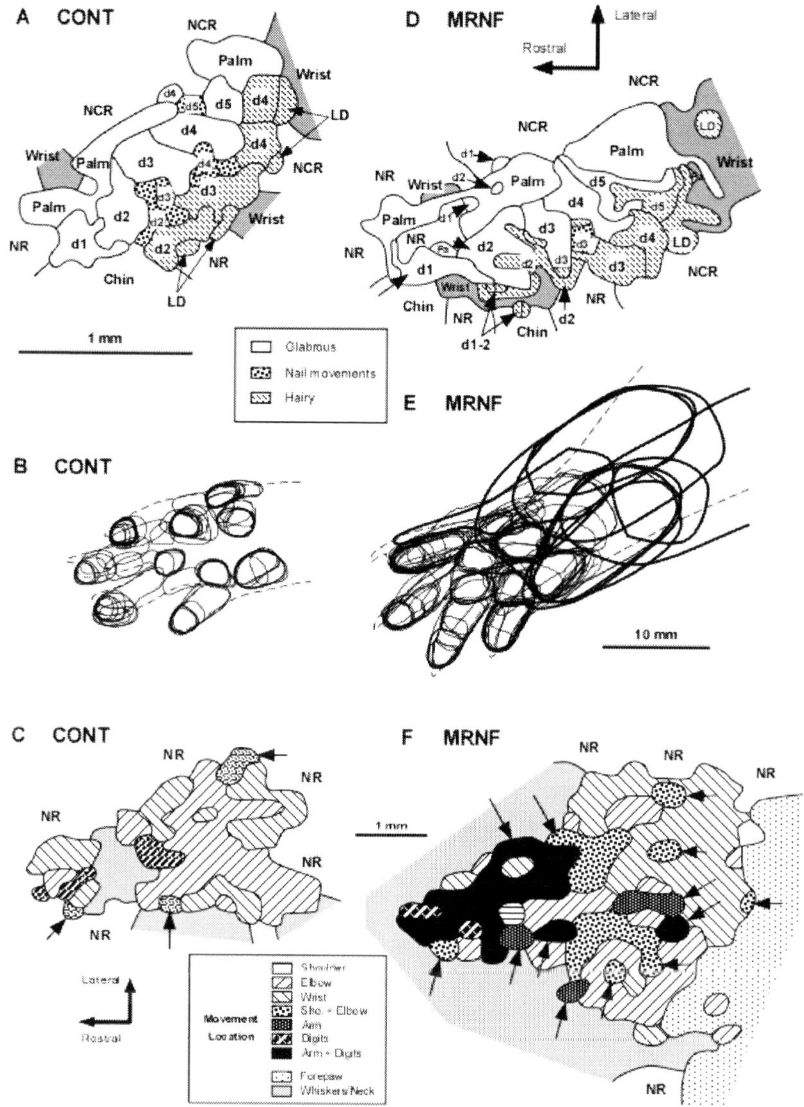

Figure 6. Primary somatosensory (S1) and motor (M1) cortical maps of the forepaw in control (CONT) and trained rats performing a moderate repetition, negligible force (MRNF) task. A) Representative S1 map devoted to the forepaw skin in a normal control rat. B) Typical glabrous receptive fields (RFs) in the same normal control rat showing single RFs encompassing mainly one or two forepaw subdivisions. C) Cortical map of the movement representation of the forepaw joints in a normal control rat. D) Representative map in an 8 week MRNF rat showing disruptions in the continuity of the S1 representation of contiguous forepaw skin surfaces and patchy representations of single forepaw subdivisions (e.g. digits 1 or 2; examples indicated by arrows) into distinct cortical zones. E) Glabrous RFs in the same MRNF rat showing many large RFs encompassing several forepaw subdivisions and even larger RFs located on both plantar pads or digits and wrist/forearm (examples indicated by thick RFs). Note the greater overlap of glabrous RFs in MRNF rats (E) than in CONT (B). F) Typical map in an 8 week MRNF rat showing a drastic enlargement of the M1 forelimb cortical map and the task-induced increase in the cortical area devoted to digit, arm-digit and multi-joint movements (multi-joint responses are highlighted by arrows). Abbreviations: d1-d5, digit 1 to digit 5; LD, large dorsum of forepaw; NCR, non cutaneous responses; NR, no response; Pa, palmar pads; Sho., shoulder. Figure modified with permission from Coq et al. (2009).

Several studies examined the effects of motor repetition related to any motor training experience on the M1 map organization. Extensive repetition of digit movements without motor learning in primate or unskilled pellet reaching in rats did not significantly alter the M1 forelimb map, while motor skill learning was associated with an expansion of the representation of distal forelimb movements (Kleim et al., 1998; Plautz et al., 2000). The M1 skill-related expansion has been shown to depend upon functional synaptogenesis (Kleim et al., 2002, 2004), long-term potentiation (Rioult-Pedotti et al., 2000), excitation-inhibition balance (see Teskey et al., 2008 for a review), synchronous firing (Schieber, 2002), tuning and signal-to-noise changes of M1 cells (Kargo and Nitz, 2003, 2004). In rats that reached for bundles of pasta strands, skilled reaching with targeting and grasping components requires coordinated forelimb joint movements (Remple et al., 2001). We also observed increases in elbow-wrist and in digit representations in our overuse model that are consistent with such increased skill. These findings support the learning hypothesis for the etiology of repetitive motion disorders (Byl and Melnick, 1997; Blake et al., 2005, 2006).

5. Links between Behavioral Changes and Peripheral and/Or Central Changes

A. Peripheral Sensitization

In our model, several peripheral tissue changes are associated temporally and correlate statistically with declines in reach performance, grip strength, agility and mechanical hypersensation. These changes include widespread musculoskeletal and peripheral nerve inflammation, nerve pathology, and perhaps musculoskeletal tissue injury. With regards to inflammation, we have observed that reach rate correlates negatively with changes in nerve and musculoskeletal inflammatory cytokines and macrophages (Barbe et al., 2003; Clark et al., 2003, 2004; Elliott et al., 2008, 2009a), as did grip strength (Barbe et al., 2008; Elliott et al., 2009ab; Fedorczyk et al., 2010; Rani et al., 2010). This latter finding is supportive of other work in which forelimb grip strength declines occurred after intramuscular injections of TNFα (Schäfers et al., 2003b; Beyreuther et al., 2007), suggesting that reduced grip strength can be a sign of muscle inflammation (also called muscle hyperalgesia). In a recent study from our lab, a two-week regimen of an anti-TNFα drug decreased repetitive task-induced increases of TNFα in flexor forelimb muscles and attenuated declines in grip strength (Rani et al., 2010). Grip strength was not entirely restored due to the presence of increased Substance P and neurokinin 1 in the spinal cord of these same rats (unpublished data), suggesting a central sensitization mechanism was also present that 2 week regimen of anti-TNFα could not ameliorate. Our observed degraded forelimb movement patterns, such as scooping and raking, was also concomitant with forelimb musculoskeletal and nerve inflammation (Barbe et al., 2003; Elliott et al., 2008; Coq et al., 2009).

Lastly, heightened pain sensitivity is a known consequence of increased inflammatory mediators, particularly TNFα. Pro-inflammatory cytokines activate and sensitize peripheral terminals of nociceptors both directly (such as within the nerve) and indirectly (such as in surrounding tissues) leading to hypersensitivity (Moalem and Tracey, 2006; Schäfers and Sorkin, 2008). We have recently reported a correlation between increased inflammatory cytokines in the median nerve and forepaw mechanical hypersensitivity (Elliott et al., 2010).

Alternatively, a task-induced systemic cytokine response may also be associated with the widespread mechanical hypersensitivity found in the present study; we have previously observed a significant correlation between reduced grip strength and task-induced increases in serum inflammatory cytokines (Barbe et al., 2008; Elliott et al., 2009; Figure 5C). These findings combined suggest that inflammation-driven peripheral sensitization contributes to sensorimotor changes with performance of repetitive tasks.

B. Peripheral Nerve Injury

A peripheral nerve injury mechanism has also been identified in our overuse model. We have observed nerve demyelination, axonal swelling, fibrosis, with subsequent decreased nerve conduction velocity, forepaw sensation and grip strength, each suggestive of a nerve compression injury (Clark et al., 2003; 2004; Elliott et al., 2010). Declines in grip strength can also be a sign of neuropathic injury (Schäfers et al., 2003a; Beyreuther et al., 2007). The contribution of nerve injury to grip strength changes in our model is supported by positive correlations grip strength declines and reductions of median nerve conduction velocity (Elliott et al., 2009, 2010). In conclusion, our findings suggest that several sensorimotor behavior outcomes are affected by peripheral muscle and nerve inflammation, nerve compression injury, or both, with performance of repetitive tasks.

C. Spinal Cord Central Sensitization

The phenomenon of central sensitization is characterized by adaptations in neurons and glia cells, such as changes in neuronal structure, protein production, function, and survival within the CNS, that then contribute to abnormal pain behaviors (Woolf and Salter, 2000). For example, it has been proposed that spinal cytokines released in the dorsal horn nerve terminal region ipsilateral to the affected peripheral nerve spread to nearby spinal nerve terminals that then effect uninvolved peripheral nerves and central sensory processing (Chacur et al., 2001). These changes may then promote remote and contralateral sensitization effects (Chacur et al., 2001). We have observed forepaw hypersensitivity bilaterally in our model (Barr et al., 2004, Elliott et al., 2010). However, we have also shown that the non-reach limb is used as a support limb in our model, as depicted in Fedorczyk et al. (2010). Thus, the bilateral hypersensitivity responses in our study are not a type of 'mirror allodynia', sometimes seen after unilateral nerve ligation, in which there is a contralateral spread of symptoms via spinal cord mechanisms (DeLeo et al., 1997; Chacur et al., 2001; Milligan et al., 2003; Kelly et al., 2007), but rather due to bilateral use of the forelimbs in performing the task, and then bilateral changes in the median nerves.

However, we have also reported the presence of hind paw mechanical hypersensitivity in our model (Barr et al., 2004; Elliott et al., 2010), limbs not involved in performing an upper extremity repetitive task. We observed hind paw mechanical hypersensitivity in aged rats performing a HRLF task for 12 weeks (Elliott et al., 2010), and an early increase in hind paw sensitivity at 3 weeks in young rats performing a HRHF task (prior to the development of hyposensation in these latter rats). These findings are suggestive of an extraterritorial spread of symptoms via central sensitization mechanisms that may contribute to pain behaviors with overuse injuries. Studies showing mirror allodynia (mechanical hypersensitivity) or extra-territorial hyperalgesia in cases of unilateral nerve injury provide evidence of nerve injury-induced mechanisms of central sensitization (Chacur et al., 2001; Gazda et al., 2001). We suggest that the hypersensitivity in the uninvolved hind paws in our model may be due to increased pro-inflammatory cytokines in cervical spinal cord affecting cells or processing in distal spinal cord segments. Unfortunately, we did not collect lumbar spinal cord segments in these studies, and therefore are limited in our interpretation of these results. Nevertheless, the finding of mechanical hypersensitivity in body regions not involved in performing a task is highly suggestive of central mechanisms of sensitivity and is of potential interest to clinicians considering appropriate therapies for patients with overuse injuries.

D. Does Sensitization Result from both Peripheral and Central Changes?

Signs of injury and inflammation occurring in the median nerve in addition to the spinal cord inflammatory response prevent us from separating peripheral versus central mechanisms contributing to observed cutaneous sensation changes in forepaws. Pro-inflammatory cytokines have been shown to sensitize peripheral terminals of nociceptors both directly and indirectly, leading to hypersensitivity (Moalem and Tracey, 2006; Schäfers and Sorkin, 2008). We have reported the presence of inflammatory cytokines in peripheral nerves, musculoskeletal tissues, and circulating widely in serum in our model (Al-Shatti et al., 2005; Barbe et al., 2008; Coq et al., 2009; Elliott et al., 2009, 2010). We have also reported statistical correlation between these cytokine increases, hypersensitivity and declines in grip strength in several studies, suggesting a link between increased peripheral cytokines and pain-related behaviors with overuse injuries.

Furthermore, nerve compression can be initially irritative to nerves, resulting in cutaneous hypersensitivity. Our findings of mechanical hypersensitivity in the presence of decreased nerve conduction velocity, and histological findings of increased extraneuronal connective tissue and axonal swelling in the median nerve, are suggestive of nerve compression with long-term repetitive task performance, particularly HRHF tasks. Hand and arm pain in the distribution of the median nerve is a common symptom in patients with electrophysiologically diagnosed carpal tunnel syndrome, particularly in those subjects involved in full time intensive manual work (Bonfiglioli et al., 2007).

With regard to central sensitivity, we can only point to an abundance of other studies showing spinal cord inflammatory responses after unilateral peripheral nerve injury, e.g. increased spinal cord neuron- and glia-produced cytokines, increases that are temporally associated with mechanical hypersensitivity (DeLeo et al., 1997, Hunt et al., 2001, Shubayev and Myers, 2002, Schäfers et al., 2003b, Ohtori et al., 2004, Hubbard and Winkelstein, 2005, Hatashita et al., 2008). The contribution of central sensitization to repetition-induced hypersensitivity is also suggested by studies from our lab showing increased Substance P and neurokinin-1 receptor in spinal cord dorsal horns, changes described earlier (Elliott et al., 2008, 2009ab). These increases in Substance P correlated statistically with declines in forelimb grip strength (Elliott et al., 2009b), and coincided with degraded forelimb movement patterns (Elliott et al., 2008). On the other hand, we have also observed increased Substance P in forelimb tendons with HRHF task performance, changes that correlated strongly with declines in grip strength (Fedorczyk et al., 2010), bringing us back to a potential peripheral sensitization mechanism. We hypothesize that both mechanisms are at work in our model and cases of overuse injury in which chronic pain is present.

E. Contribution of Cortical Map Changes to Sensorimotor Behavior Changes

It is now well established that S1 map organization and neuronal properties are correlated with sensorimotor and tactile performances (Xerri et al., 2005; Duncan and Boynton, 2007;

Bensmaia, 2008; Reed et al., 2008). The deterioration of the S1 map features and neuronal properties found in our model, described earlier, would likely result in ambiguous interpretation of tactile cues and undoubtedly contributed to a decline in grasp control, ultimately resulting in failed and repeated grasp attempts (i.e. the increased movement reversals observed in our model). Our observed "raking" reach pattern also includes poor forepaw and digit closure and, thus, poor grasp control changes that are reminiscent of focal dystonia as described by Byl et al. (1996, 1997) in an owl monkey model. In fact, in our Coq et al. (2009) study, the enlargement of S1 receptive fields and the emergence of large receptive fields that encompassed the whole forepaw (digits and palmar pads) or dorsal hand and wrist or forearm correlated statistically with a reduction in successful reaches, an increase in the inefficient raking food retrieval pattern, and an increase in reach time. These findings support our hypothesis that ambiguous interpretation of tactile cues result in reduced motor performance, particularly fine motor skills, as found in the monkey model of focal hand dystonia (Byl et al., 1996, 1997; Blake et al., 2002).

Similar movement pattern changes have been attributed to degradation of the S1 paw representation in owl monkey (Byl et al., 1996, 1997; Topp and Byl, 1999). Using somatosensory evoked potential measurements, Byl et al. (2000, 2002) detected somatosensory disorganization consistent with somatotopic dedifferentiation in human subjects with severe and moderate focal hand dystonia. These observations have led to a learning hypothesis for the origin of focal hand dystonia, and possibly other repetitive motion disorders, whereby the reversibility of the somatosensory cortical degradation is exploited in treatment interventions to restore normal cortical representations (Byl and Melnick, 1997; Byl and McKenzie, 2000; Byl, 2003, 2007; Byl et al., 2003; Candia et al., 2003; McKenzie et al., 2003).

The motor declines also correlated with a dramatic enlargement of the overall forepaw map area of the primary motor cortex, in which emerged the representation of joint movements specifically involved in the repetitive task. In fact, the movement representation areas leading to multi-joint movements, such as elbow-wrist, arm and mainly wrist-digits, increased in repetitive task rats. Interestingly, this increase in cortical multi-joint movement representations correlated strongly with the increased prevalence of the raking strategy.

Unexpectedly, but interesting to consider here, task-induced peripheral increases in inflammatory cytokines in muscles of repetitive task rats had a strong negative correlation with not only grip strength, but also with the amount of current required to evoke movements of the wrist, and elbow-wrist, and arm-digit multi-joints in the primary motor cortex. The higher the inflammation in flexor muscles specifically involved in the task, the lower the threshold required to elicit arm-digit movements, which was decreased in trained rats relative to controls.

6. Conclusions for Overuse Injury Model

Our data from a rat model of overuse injury show that peripheral nerve injury, peripheral inflammatory, spinal cord sensitization and central neuroplastic mechanisms co-exist. Each appear to contribute to motor behavior declines and the development of pain related behaviors. What was previously unknown was if peripheral inflammation was primarily responsible for the movement performance deficits that emerge in these rats over time (Barbe and Barr, 2006) or whether cortical degradation was responsible for the movement defects (Byl et al 1997). It is clear from our studies that *both* sensorimotor cortical reorganization and peripheral inflammation/injury mechanisms contribute to movement performance declines and movement pattern changes in the progression of the overuse injury.

Overall Conclusion

In conclusion, both prolonged disuse and overuse lead to both peripheral and central changes that are interdependent to drive cerebral plasticity and altered output function. From the findings of these two models combined, we postulate that abnormal movements, whether limited through hind limb immobilization, or excessive as in highly repetitive tasks, can lead to pathological musculoskeletal tissue changes, which in turn contribute to provide aberrant sensory inputs to the brain. These repetitive, aberrant inputs result in abnormal sensory feedback leading to S1 and M1 topographic reorganization, which can be either adaptive or deleterious. Indeed, sensorimotor disuse, rewarded-training and overuse drive long-term potentiation and depression (LTP and LTD), spike-timing dependent plasticity (STDP), homeostatic synaptic and structural plasticity in both S1 and M1 cortices (see Adkins et al., 2006; Moucha and Kilgard, 2006; Martin et al., 2007; Feldman, 2009; Wittenberg, 2010). Thus, disruptions in the S1 map topography and neuronal properties, as described in our models, suggest less ability to interpret inputs to selected parts of the body and the abnormal feedforward of somatosensory information to the motor cortex might be subsequently expressed in degraded motor functions, as found in patients with CP or focal hand dystonia (Byl, 2004; Gordon et al., 2006; Wingert et al., 2008, 2009, 2010; Burton et al., 2009; Hinkley et al., 2009).

Therefore, our studies emphasize the crucial role of early sensorimotor experience and suggest the critical importance for early interventions and sustained activity in children and infants with CP to hopefully restore sensorimotor functions or at least prevent further degradations (Damiano, 2006, 2009; Hadders-Algra and Gramsbergen, 2007). Our studies also emphasize the need for early intervention in repetitive/overuse injuries to reduce central phenotypic changes in dorsal root ganglia, spinal cord and cortical cells, in which the expression of proteins, receptors, neurotransmitters, and neurotrophic factors have been altered as a consequence of either chronic nerve compression injuries, chronic inflammation (local, widespread or systemic) and subsequent aberrant sensory inputs (Latremoliere and Woolf, 2009; Sorkin and Yaksh, 2009).

Acknowledgments

The work described in this review paper from the laboratory of Dr. J-Olivier Coq was supported by CNRS, Ministère de l'Enseignement Supérieur et de la Recherche, l'Agence Nationale de la Recherche, la Région Provence-Alpes-Côte-d'Azur, NIH grant NS-10414, the Cerebral Palsy Institute, la Fondation Motrice, Fondation NRJ – Institut de France and the Sandler Fundation. The work described in this review paper from the laboratory of Dr. Mary

Barbe was supported by a grant from NIOSH grants UO1 OH 03970 and RO1 OH 8599, and NIAMS grants R01 AR056019 and R01 AR051212.

References

Abbadie C, Brown JL, Mantyh PW, Basbaum AI (1996) Spinal cord substance P receptor immunoreactivity increases in both inflammatory and nerve injury models of persistent pain. *Neuroscience* 70:201-209

Adkins DL, Boychuk J, Remple MS, Kleim JA (2006) Motor training induces experience-specific patterns of plasticity across motor cortex and spinal cord. *J. Appl. Physiol.* 101:1776-1782

Allen BJ, Li J, Menning PM, Rogers SD, Ghilardi J, Mantyh PW, Simone DA (1999) Primary afferent fibers that contribute to increased substance P receptor internalization in the spinal cord after injury. *J. Neurophysiol.* 81:1379-1390

Alloway KD, Rosenthal P, Burton H (1989) Quantitative measurements of receptive field changes during antagonism of GABAergic transmission in primary somatosensory cortex of cats. *Exp. Brain Res.* 78:514-532

Al-Shatti T, Barr AE, Safadi FF, Amin M, Barbe MF (2005) Increase in inflammatory cytokines in median nerves in a rat model of repetitive motion injury. *J. Neuroimmunol.* 167:13-22

Andiman SE, Haynes RL, Trachtenberg FL, Billiards SS, Folkerth RD, Volpe JJ, Kinney HC (2010) The Cerebral Cortex Overlying Periventricular Leukomalacia: Analysis of Pyramidal Neurons. *Brain Pathol.* 20:803-14

Banks HH (1972) The knee and cerebral palsy. *Orthop. Clin. North Am..* 3:113-129

Barbe MF, Barr AE (2006) Inflammation and the pathophysiology of work-related musculoskeletal disorders. *Brain Behav. Immun.* .20:423-429

Barbe MF, Barr AE, Gorzelany I, Amin M, Gaughan JP, Safadi FF (2003) Chronic repetitive reaching and grasping results in decreased motor performance and widespread tissue responses in a rat model of MSD. *J. Orthop. Res.* 21:167-176

Barbe MF, Elliott MB, Abdelmagid SM, Amin M, Popoff SN, Safadi FF, Barr AE (2008) Serum and tissue cytokines and chemokines increase with repetitive upper extremity tasks. *J. Orthop. Res.* 26:1320-1326

Barr AE, Barbe MF (2002) Pathophysiological tissue changes associated with repetitive movement: a review of the evidence. *Phys .Ther.* 82:173-187

Barr AE, Barbe MF, Clark BD (2004) Work-related musculoskeletal disorders of the hand and wrist: epidemiology, pathophysiology, and sensorimotor changes. *J. Orthop. Sports Phys. Ther.* 34:610-627

Basso N, Heersche JNM (2006) Effects of hind limb unloading and reloading on nitric oxide synthase expression and apoptosis of osteocytes and chondrocytes. *Bone* 39:807-814

Beloozerova IN, Sirota MG, Swadlow HA (2003) Activity of different classes of neurons of the motor cortex during locomotion. *J. Neurosci.* 23:1087-1097

Bensmaia SJ (2008) Tactile intensity and population codes. *Behav. Brain Res* 190:165-173

Bernard B (1997) Musculoskeletal Disorders and Workplace Factors: A Critical Review of Epidemiologic Evidence for Work-Related Disorders of the Neck, Upper Extremities, and Low Back. National Institute of Occupational Safety and Health.

Beyreuther BK, Geis C, Stöhr T, Sommer C (2007) Antihyperalgesic efficacy of lacosamide in a rat model for muscle pain induced by TNF. Neuropharmacology 52:1312-1317

Blake DT, Byl NN, Merzenich MM (2002) Representation of the hand in the cerebral cortex. Behav. *Brain Res.* 135:179-184

Blake DT, Heiser MA, Caywood M, Merzenich MM (2006) Experience-dependent adult cortical plasticity requires cognitive association between sensation and reward. *Neuron* 52:371-381

Blake DT, Strata F, Kempter R, Merzenich MM (2005) Experience-dependent plasticity in S1 caused by noncoincident inputs. *J. Neurophysiol.* 94:2239-2250

Bonfiglioli R, Mattioli S, Fiorentini C, Graziosi F, Curti S, Violante FS (2007) Relationship between repetitive work and the prevalence of carpal tunnel syndrome in part-time and full-time female supermarket cashiers: a quasi-experimental study. *Int. Arch. Occup. Environ. Health* 80:248-253

Booth CM, Cortina-Borja MJ, Theologis TN (2001) Collagen accumulation in muscles of children with cerebral palsy and correlation with severity of spasticity. *Dev. Med. Child Neurol.* 43:314-320

Booth FW (1982) Effect of limb immobilization on skeletal muscle. *J. Appl .Physiol.* 52:1113-1118

Bureau of Labor Statistics (2007) Nonfatal occupational injuries and illnesses requiring days away from work, 2006. United States Department of Labor News.

Burton H, Dixit S, Litkowski P, Wingert JR (2009) Functional connectivity for somatosensory and motor cortex in spastic diplegia. *Somatosens. Mot. Res.* 26:90-104

Burton H, Sinclair RJ, Wingert JR, Dierker DL (2008) Multiple parietal operculum subdivisions in humans: tactile activation maps. *Somatosens Mot. Res.* 25:149-162

Byl NN (2003) What can we learn from animal models of focal hand dystonia? *Rev. Neurol.* (Paris) 159:857-873

Byl NN, McKenzie A (2000) Treatment effectiveness for patients with a history of repetitive hand use and focal hand dystonia: a planned, prospective follow-up study. *J. Hand Ther.* 13:289-301

Byl NN, McKenzie A, Nagarajan SS (2000) Differences in somatosensory hand organization in a healthy flutist and a flutist with focal hand dystonia: a case report. *J. Hand Ther.* 13:302-309

Byl NN, Melnick M (1997) The neural consequences of repetition: clinical implications of a learning hypothesis. *J. Hand Ther.* 10:160-174

Byl NN, Merzenich MM, Cheung S, Bedenbaugh P, Nagarajan SS, Jenkins WM (1997) A primate model for studying focal dystonia and repetitive strain injury: effects on the primary somatosensory cortex. *Phys. Ther.* 77:269-284

Byl NN, Merzenich MM, Jenkins WM (1996) A primate genesis model of focal dystonia and repetitive strain injury: I. Learning-induced dedifferentiation of the representation of the hand in the primary somatosensory cortex in adult monkeys. *Neurology* 47:508-520

Byl NN (2004) Focal hand dystonia may result from aberrant neuroplasticity. *Adv. Neurol.* 94:19-28

Byl NN (2007) Learning-based animal models: task-specific focal hand dystonia. *ILAR J.* 48:411-431

Byl NN (2009) Focal hand dystonia: a historical perspective from a clinician scholar. *J. Hand Ther.* 22:105-108

Byl NN, Nagajaran S, McKenzie AL (2003) Effect of sensory discrimination training on structure and function in patients with focal hand dystonia: a case series. *Arch. Phys. Med. Rehabil.* 84:1505-1514

Byl NN, Nagarajan SS, Merzenich MM, Roberts T, McKenzie A (2002) Correlation of clinical neuromusculoskeletal and central somatosensory performance: variability in controls and patients with severe and mild focal hand dystonia. *Neural Plast.* 9:177-203

Candia V, Wienbruch C, Elbert T, Rockstroh B, Ray W (2003) Effective behavioral treatment of focal hand dystonia in musicians alters somatosensory cortical organization. *Proc. Natl. Acad. Sci. U.S.A.* 100:7942-7946

Canu MH, Darnaudéry M, Falempin M, Maccari S, Viltart O (2007) Effect of hindlimb unloading on motor activity in adult rats: impact of prenatal stress. *Behav. Neurosci.* 121:177-185

Canu MH, Falempin M (1996) Effect of hindlimb unloading on locomotor strategy during treadmill locomotion in the rat. *Eur. J. Appl. Physiol. Occup. Physiol.* 74:297-304

Canu MH, Falempin M (1997) Effect of hindlimb unloading on two hindlimb muscles during treadmill locomotion in rats. *Eur J Appl Physiol Occup Physiol* 75:283-288

Canu MH, Falempin M (1998) Effect of hindlimb unloading on interlimb coordination during treadmill locomotion in the rat. *Eur. J. Appl. Physiol. Occup. Physiol.* 78:509-515

Canu MH, Falempin M, Orsal D (2001) Fictive motor activity in rat after 14 days of hindlimb unloading. *Exp. Brain Res.* 139:30-38

Canu MH, Langlet C, Dupont E, Falempin M (2003) Effects of hypodynamia-hypokinesia on somatosensory evoked potentials in the rat. *Brain Res.* 978:162-168

Canu M, Garnier C (2009) A 3D analysis of fore- and hindlimb motion during overground and ladder walking: comparison of control and unloaded rats. *Exp. Neurol.* 218:98-108

Canu M, Garnier C, Lepoutre F, Falempin M (2005) A 3D analysis of hindlimb motion during treadmill locomotion in rats after a 14-day episode of simulated microgravity. *Behav. Brain Res.* 157:309-321

Canu M, Picquet F, Bastide B, Falempin M (2010) Activity-dependent changes in the electrophysiological properties of regular spiking neurons in the sensorimotor cortex of the rat in vitro. *Behav. Brain Res.* 209:289-294

Canu M, Treffort N, Picquet F, Dubreucq G, Guerardel Y, Falempin M (2006) Concentration of amino acid neurotransmitters in the somatosensory cortex of the rat after surgical or functional deafferentation. *Exp. Brain Res.* 173:623-628

Carp SJ, Barbe MF, Winter KA, Amin M, Barr AE (2007) Inflammatory biomarkers increase with severity of upper-extremity overuse disorders. *Clin. Sci* 112:305-314

Castle ME, Reyman TA, Schneider M (1979) Pathology of spastic muscle in cerebral palsy. *Clin. Orthop. Relat. Res.* 142:223-232

Chacur M, Milligan ED, Gazda LS, Armstrong C, Wang H, Tracey KJ, Maier SF, Watkins LR (2001) A new model of sciatic inflammatory neuritis (SIN): induction of unilateral and bilateral mechanical allodynia following acute unilateral peri-sciatic immune activation in rats. *Pain* 94:231-244

Chao T, Pham K, Steward O, Gupta R (2008) Chronic nerve compression injury induces a phenotypic switch of neurons within the dorsal root ganglia. *J. Comp. Neurol.* 506:180-193

Clark BD, Al-Shatti TA, Barr AE, Amin M, Barbe MF (2004) Performance of a high-repetition, high-force task induces carpal tunnel syndrome in rats. *J. Orthop. Sports Phys. Ther.* 34:244-253

Clark BD, Barr AE, Safadi FF, Beitman L, Al-Shatti T, Amin M, Gaughan JP, Barbe MF (2003) Median nerve trauma in a rat model of work-related musculoskeletal disorder. *J. Neurotrauma* 20:681-695

Clayton K, Fleming JM, Copley J (2003) Behavioral responses to tactile stimuli in children with cerebral palsy. *Phys. Occup. Ther. Ped.* 23:43–62

Coq JO, Xerri C (1999) Tactile impoverishment and sensorimotor restriction deteriorate the forepaw cutaneous map in the primary somatosensory cortex of adult rats. *Exp. Brain Res.* 129:518-531

Coq JO, Barr AE, Strata F, Russier M, Kietrys DM, Merzenich MM, Byl NN, Barbe MF (2009) Peripheral and central changes combine to induce motor behavioral deficits in a moderate repetition task. *Exp. Neurol.* 220:234-245

Coq JO, Delcour M, Russier M, Olivier P, Fontaine R, Gestreau C, Baud O (2007) Prenatal ischemia and hind limb disuse induce locomotor deficits and S1 and M1 map degradation: what can we learn about cerebral palsy? In: From basic motor control to functional recovery – V, Sofia, Bulgaria: Gantchev N (Ed), pp 170-179

Coq JO, Strata F, Russier M, Safadi FF, Merzenich MM, Byl NN, Barbe MF (2008) Impact of neonatal asphyxia and hind limb immobilization on musculoskeletal tissues and S1 map organization: implications for cerebral palsy. *Exp. Neurol* .210:95-108

Cruce WL, Lovell JA, Crisp T, Stuesse SL (2001) Effect of aging on the substance P receptor, NK-1, in the spinal cord of rats with peripheral nerve injury. *Somatosens. Mot .Res.* 18:66-75

Damiano DL (2006) Activity, activity, activity: rethinking our physical therapy approach to cerebral palsy. *Phys. Ther.* 86:1534

Damiano DL (2009) Rehabilitative Therapies in Cerebral Palsy: The Good, the Not As Good, and the Possible. *J. Child Neurol.* 24:1200-1204

David V, Lafage-Proust M, Laroche N, Christian A, Ruegsegger P, Vico L (2006) Two-week longitudinal survey of bone architecture alteration in the hindlimb-unloaded rat model of bone loss: sex differences. *Am. J. Physiol. Endocrinol. Metab.* 290:E440-447

De-Doncker L, Picquet F, Browne GB, Falempin M (2002) Expression of myosin heavy chain isoforms along intrafusal fibers of rat soleus muscle spindles after 14 days of hindlimb unloading. *J. Histochem. Cytochem.* 50:1543-1554

Delander GE, Schött E, Brodin E, Fredholm BB (1997) Temporal changes in spinal cord expression of mRNA for substance P, dynorphin and enkephalin in a model of chronic pain. *Acta Physiol. Scand* 161:509-516

Delcour M, Olivier P, Chambon C, Russier M, Gestreau C, Alescio-Lautier B, Baud O, Coq JO (2009) Prenatal ischemia and sensorimotor disuse during development in rats: a promising new animal model of CP. *Dev. Med. Child Neur.* 51:S19

DeLeo JA, Colburn RW, Rickman AJ (1997) Cytokine and growth factor immunohistochemical spinal profiles in two animal models of mononeuropathy. *Brain Res.* 759:50-57

Deschenes MR, Will KM, Booth FW, Gordon SE (2003) Unlike myofibers, neuromuscular junctions remain stable during prolonged muscle unloading. *J. Neurol. Sci.* 210:5-10

Diao E, Shao F, Liebenberg E, Rempel D, Lotz JC (2005) Carpal tunnel pressure alters median nerve function in a dose-dependent manner: a rabbit model for carpal tunnel syndrome. *J. Orthop. Res.* 23:218-223

Donoghue JP (1995) Plasticity of adult sensorimotor representations. *Curr. Opin. Neurobiol.* 5:749-754

Donoghue JP, Sanes JN (1987) Peripheral nerve injury in developing rats reorganizes representation pattern in motor cortex. *Proc. Natl. Acad. Sci. U.S.A* 84:1123-1126

Donoghue JP, Sanes JN (1988) Organization of adult motor cortex representation patterns following neonatal forelimb nerve injury in rats. *J. Neurosci.* 8:3221-3232

Donoghue JP, Suner S, Sanes JN (1990) Dynamic organization of primary motor cortex output to target muscles in adult rats. II. Rapid reorganization following motor nerve lesions. *Exp. Brain Res.* 79:492-503

Dourte LM, Perry SM, Getz CL, Soslowsky LJ (2010) Tendon properties remain altered in a chronic rat rotator cuff model. *Clin. Orthop. Relat. Res.* 468:1485-1492

Drew T, Andujar J, Lajoie K, Yakovenko S (2008) Cortical mechanisms involved in visuomotor coordination during precision walking. *Brain Res. Rev.* 57:199-211

Duncan RO, Boynton GM (2007) Tactile hyperacuity thresholds correlate with finger maps in primary somatosensory cortex (S1). *Cereb. Cortex* 17:2878-2891

Dupont E, Canu M, Falempin M (2003) A 14-day period of hindpaw sensory deprivation enhances the responsiveness of rat cortical neurons. *Neuroscience* 121:433-439

Dupont E, Canu M, Falempin M (2002) Atropine prevents the changes in the hindlimb cortical area induced by hypodynamia-hypokinesia. *Brain Res.* 926:51-57

Dupont E, Canu M, Stevens L, Falempin M (2005) Effects of a 14-day period of hindpaw sensory restriction on mRNA and protein levels of NGF and BDNF in the hindpaw primary somatosensory cortex. *Brain Res. Mol.* 133:78-86

Dykes RW, Landry P, Metherate R, Hicks TP (1984) Functional role of GABA in cat primary somatosensory cortex: shaping receptive fields of cortical neurons. *J. Neurophysiol.* 52:1066-1093

Einspieler C, Prechtl HFR (2005) Prechtl's assessment of general movements: a diagnostic tool for the functional assessment of the young nervous system. *Ment. Retard Dev. Disabil. Res. Rev.* 11:61-67

Elliott MB, Barr AE, Clark BD, Amin M, Amin S, Barbe MF (2009) High force reaching task induces widespread inflammation, increased spinal cord neurochemicals and neuropathic pain. *Neuroscience* 158:922-931

Elliott MB, Barr AE, Clark BD, Wade CK, Barbe MF (2010) Performance of a repetitive task by aged rats leads to median neuropathy and spinal cord inflammation with associated sensorimotor declines. *Neuroscience* 170:929-941

Elliott MB, Barr AE, Barbe MF (2009) Spinal substance P and neurokinin-1 increase with high repetition reaching. *Neurosci. Lett.* 454:33-37

Elliott MB, Barr AE, Kietrys DM, Al-Shatti T, Amin M, Barbe MF (2008) Peripheral neuritis and increased spinal cord neurochemicals are induced in a model of repetitive motion injury with low force and repetition exposure. *Brain Res.* 1218:103-113

Fedorczyk JM, Barr AE, Rani S, Gao HG, Amin M, Amin S, Litvin J, Barbe MF (2010) Exposure-dependent increases in IL-1beta, substance P, CTGF, and tendinosis in flexor digitorum tendons with upper extremity repetitive strain injury. *J. Orthop. Res.* 28:298-307

Feldman DE (2009) Synaptic mechanisms for plasticity in neocortex. *Annu. Rev. Neurosci.* 32:33-55

Foran JR, Steinman S, Barash I, Chambers HG, Lieber RL (2005) Structural and mechanical alterations in spastic skeletal muscle. *Dev. Med. Child Neur.* 47:713–717

Forwood MR, Parker AW (1991) Repetitive loading, in vivo, of the tibiae and femora of rats: effects of repeated bouts of treadmill-running. *Bone Miner.* 13:35-46

Franchi G (2000) Changes in motor representation related to facial nerve damage and regeneration in adult rats. *Exp. Brain Res.* 135:53-65

Franchi G (2001) Persistence of vibrissal motor representation following vibrissal pad deafferentation in adult rats. *Exp. Brain Res.* 137:180-189

Franchi G, Veronesi C (2006) Short-term reorganization of input-deprived motor vibrissae representation following motor disconnection in adult rats. *J. Physiol.* (Lond.) 574:457-476

Fredericson M, Bergman AG, Hoffman KL, Dillingham MS (1995) Tibial stress reaction in runners. Correlation of clinical symptoms and scintigraphy with a new magnetic resonance imaging grading system. *Am. J. Sports Med.* 23:472-481

Freeland AE, Tucci MA, Barbieri RA, Angel MF, Nick TG (2002) Biochemical evaluation of serum and flexor tenosynovium in carpal tunnel syndrome. Microsurgery 22:378-385

Fuchs JL, Salazar E (1998) Effects of whisker trimming on GABA(A) receptor binding in the barrel cortex of developing and adult rats. *J. Comp. Neurol.* 395:209-216

Fujita N, Arakawa T, Matsubara T, Ando H, Miki A (2009) Influence of fixed muscle length and contractile properties on atrophy and subsequent recovery in the rat soleus and plantaris muscles. *Arch. Histol. Cytol.* 72:151-163

Garnier C, Falempin M, Canu M (2008) A 3D analysis of fore- and hindlimb motion during locomotion: comparison of overground and ladder walking in rats. *Behav. Brain Res.* 186:57-65

Gazda LS, Milligan ED, Hansen MK, Twining CM, Poulos NM, Chacur M, O'Connor KA, Armstrong C, Maier SF, Watkins LR, Myers RR (2001) Sciatic inflammatory neuritis (SIN): behavioral allodynia is paralleled by peri-sciatic proinflammatory cytokine and superoxide production. *J. Peripher. Nerv. Syst.* 6:111-129

Gerr F, Marcus M, Ensor C, Kleinbaum D, Cohen S, Edwards A, Gentry E, Ortiz DJ, Monteilh C (2002) A prospective study of computer users: I. Study design and incidence of musculoskeletal symptoms and disorders. *Am. J. Ind. Med.* 41:221-235

Giger JM, Bodell PW, Zeng M, Baldwin KM, Haddad F (2009) Rapid muscle atrophy response to unloading: pretranslational processes involving MHC and actin. J. *Appl. Physiol.* 107:1204-1212

Giger JM, Haddad F, Qin AX, Zeng M, Baldwin KM (2005) Effect of unloading on type I myosin heavy chain gene regulation in rat soleus muscle. *J. Appl. Physiol.* 98:1185-1194

Gordon AM, Charles J, Steenbergen B (2006) Fingertip Force Planning During Grasp Is Disrupted by Impaired Sensorimotor Integration in Children With Hemiplegic Cerebral Palsy. *Pediatric Research* 60:587-591

Gormley ME (2001) Treatment of neuromuscular and musculoskeletal problems in cerebral palsy. *Pediatr. Rehabil.* 4:5-16

Hadders-Algra M (2001) Early Brain Damage and the Development of Motor Behavior in Children: Clues Therapeutic Intel ention? Neural plasticity 8:31-49

Hadders-Algra M (2004) General movements: a window for early identification of children at high risk for developmental disorders. *J. Pediatrics* 145:12–18

Hadders-Algra M (2007) Putative neural substrate of normal and abnormal general movements. Neurosci Biobehav Rev 31:1181-1190

Hadders-Algra M (2008) Reduced variability in motor behaviour: an indicator of impaired cerebral connectivity? *Early Hum. Dev* 84:787-789

Hadders-Algra M, Gramsbergen A (2007) Discussion on the clinical relevance of activity-dependent plasticity after an insult to the developing brain. *Neurosci. Biobehav. Rev.* 31:1213-1219

Hadders-Algra M, Heineman KR, Bos AF, Middelburg KJ (2010) The assessment of minor neurological dysfunction in infancy using the Touwen Infant Neurological Examination: strengths and limitations. *Dev. Med. Child Neurol.* 52:87-92

Hammond DL, Ackerman L, Holdsworth R, Elzey B (2004) Effects of spinal nerve ligation on immunohistochemically identified neurons in the L4 and L5 dorsal root ganglia of the rat. *J. Comp. Neurol.* 475:575-589

Hatashita S, Sekiguchi M, Kobayashi H, Konno S, Kikuchi S (2008) Contralateral neuropathic pain and neuropathology in dorsal root ganglion and spinal cord following hemilateral nerve injury in rats. *Spine* 33:1344-1351

Hayashi N, Kakimuma T, Soma Y, Grotendorst GR, Tamaki K, Harada M, Igarashi A (2002) Connective tissue growth factor is directly related to liver fibrosis. *Hepatogastroenterology* 49:133-135

Heineman KR, Middelburg KJ, Hadders-Algra M (2010) Development of adaptive motor behaviour in typically developing infants. *Acta Paediatr.* 99:618-624

Heinemeier KM, Olesen JL, Haddad F, Schjerling P, Baldwin KM, Kjaer M (2009) Effect of unloading followed by reloading on expression of collagen and related growth factors in rat tendon and muscle. *J. Appl. Physiol.* 106:178-186

Hinkley LBN, Webster RL, Byl NN, Nagarajan SS (2009) Neuroimaging characteristics of patients with focal hand dystonia. *J. Hand Ther.* 22:125-134; quiz 135

Hollander MS, Baker BA, Ensey J, Kashon ML, Cutlip RG (2010) Effects of age and glutathione levels on oxidative stress in rats after chronic exposure to stretch-shortening contractions. *Eur. J. Appl. Physiol.* 108:589-597

Hubbard RD, Winkelstein BA (2005) Transient cervical nerve root compression in the rat induces bilateral forepaw allodynia and spinal glial activation: mechanical factors in painful neck injuries. *Spine* 30:1924-1932

Hunt JL, Winkelstein BA, Rutkowski MD, Weinstein JN, DeLeo JA (2001) Repeated injury to the lumbar nerve roots produces enhanced mechanical allodynia and persistent spinal neuroinflammation. *Spine* 26:2073-2079

Järvinen TAH, Józsa L, Kannus P, Järvinen TLN, Järvinen M (2002) Organization and distribution of intramuscular connective tissue in normal and immobilized skeletal muscles. An immunohistochemical, polarization and scanning electron microscopic study. *J. Muscle Res. Cell. Motil.* 23:245-254

Johnson MA, Kucukyalcin DK (1978) Patterns of abnormal histochemical fibre type differentitation in human muscle biopsies. *J. Neurol. Sci.* 37:159-178

Kargo WJ, Nitz DA (2003) Early skill learning is expressed through selection and tuning of cortically represented muscle synergies. *J. Neurosci.* 23:11255-11269

Kargo WJ, Nitz DA (2004) Improvements in the signal-to-noise ratio of motor cortex cells distinguish early versus late phases of motor skill learning. *J. Neurosci.* 24:5560-5569

Kawano F, Nomura T, Takeno Y, Nakano N, Ishihara A, Ohira Y (2002) Role of gravitational loading in the development of rat soleus muscle fibers. *J. Gravit. Physiol.* 9:P149-150

Kawano F, Takeno Y, Nakai N, Higo Y, Terada M, Ohira T, Nonaka I, Ohira Y (2008) Essential role of satellite cells in the growth of rat soleus muscle fibers. *Am. J. Physiol., Cell Physiol.* 295:C458-467

Keir PJ, Rempel DM (2005) Pathomechanics of peripheral nerve loading. Evidence in carpal tunnel syndrome. *J. Hand Ther.* 18:259-269

Kelly S, Dunham JP, Donaldson LF (2007) Sensory nerves have altered function contralateral to a monoarthritis and may contribute to the symmetrical spread of inflammation. *Eur. J. Neurosci.* 26:935-942

Kleim JA, Barbay S, Nudo RJ (1998) Functional reorganization of the rat motor cortex following motor skill learning. *J. Neurophysiol.* 80:3321-3325

Kleim JA, Barbay S, Cooper NR, Hogg TM, Reidel CN, Remple MS, Nudo RJ (2002) Motor learning-dependent synaptogenesis is localized to functionally reorganized motor cortex. *Neurobiol. Learn Mem.* 77:63-77

Kleim JA, Hogg TM, VandenBerg PM, Cooper NR, Bruneau R, Remple M (2004) Cortical synaptogenesis and motor map reorganization occur during late, but not early, phase of motor skill learning. *J. Neurosci.* 24:628-633

Kourtidou-Papadeli C, Kyparos A, Albani M, Frossinis A, Papadelis CL, Bamidis P, Vivas A, Guiba-Tziampiri O (2004) Electrophysiological, histochemical, and hormonal adaptation of rat muscle after prolonged hindlimb suspension. *Acta Astronaut.* 54:737-747

Kuiper JI, van Dieën JH, Everts V, Verbeek JHAM, Frings-Dresen MHW (2004) Associations between serum markers of collagen metabolism and spinal shrinkage. *Clin. Biomech.* (Bristol, Avon) 19:209-212

Lance JW, McLeod JG (1981) A physiological approach to clinical neurology. Butterworths, London.

Land PW, de Blas AL, Reddy N (1995) Immunocytochemical localization of GABAA receptors in rat somatosensory cortex and effects of tactile deprivation. *Somatosens Mot. Res.* 12:127-141

Langlet C, Canu MH, Falempin M (1999a) Short-term reorganization of the rat somatosensory cortex following hypodynamia-hypokinesia. *Neurosci. Lett.* 266:145-148

Langlet C, Canu MH, Picquet F, Falempin M (1999b) Short-term plasticity in primary somatosensory cortex of the rat after hindlimb suspension. *J. Gravit. Physiol.* 6:P59-60

Larsson B, Björk J, Elert J, Gerdle B (2000) Mechanical performance and electromyography during repeated maximal isokinetic shoulder forward flexions in female cleaners with and without myalgia of the trapezius muscle and in healthy controls. *Eur. J. Appl. Physiol.* 83:257-267

Latremoliere A, Woolf CJ (2009) Central sensitization: a generator of pain hypersensitivity by central neural plasticity. *J. Pain* 10:895-926

Leterme D, Falempin M (1998) EMG activity of three rat hindlimb muscles during microgravity and hypergravity phase of parabolic flight. *Aviat Space Environ. Med.* 69:1065-1070

Lieber RL (1986) Skeletal muscle adaptability. I: Review of basic properties. *Dev. Med.. Child Neurol.* 28:390-397

Liepert J, Gorsler A, van Eimeren T, Münchau A, Weiller C (2003) Motor excitability in a patient with a somatosensory cortex lesion. *Clin. Neurophysiol.* 114:1003-1008

Lindboe CF, Platou CS (1982) Disuse atrophy of human skeletal muscle. An enzyme histochemical study. *Acta Neuropathol.* 56:241-244

Liptak GS, Accardo PJ (2004) Health and social outcomes of children with cerebral palsy. *J. Pediatrics* 145:S36–S41

Ljung BO, Lieber RL, Fridén J (1999) Wrist extensor muscle pathology in lateral epicondylitis. *J. Hand Surg. Br.* 24:177-183

Luime JJ, Kuiper JI, Koes BW, Verhaar JAN, Miedema HS, Burdorf A (2004) Work-related risk factors for the incidence and recurrence of shoulder and neck complaints among nursing-home and elderly-care workers. *Scand J. Work Environ. Health* 30:279-286

Lundy DW, Ganey TM, Ogden JA, Guidera KJ (1998) Pathologic morphology of the dislocated proximal femur in children with cerebral palsy. J. *Pediatr. Orthop.* 18:528-534

Marbini A, Ferrari A, Cioni G, Bellanova MF, Fusco C, Gemignani F (2002) Immunohistochemical study of muscle biopsy in children with cerebral palsy. *Brain Dev.* 24:63-66

Marcuzzo S, Dutra MF, Stigger F, do Nascimento PS, Ilha J, Kalil-Gaspar PI, Achaval M (2008) Beneficial effects of treadmill training in a cerebral palsy-like rodent model: walking pattern and soleus quantitative histology. *Brain Res.* 1222:129-140

Marcuzzo S, Dutra MF, Stigger F, do Nascimento PS, Ilha J, Kalil-Gaspar PI, Achaval M (2010) Different effects of anoxia and hind-limb immobilization on sensorimotor development and cell numbers in the somatosensory cortex in rats. *Brain Dev.* 32:323-331

Martin JH, Friel KM, Salimi I, Chakrabarty S (2007) Activity- and use-dependent plasticity of the developing corticospinal system. *Neurosci. Biobehav. Rev.* 31:1125-1135

Martinez M, Delcour M, Russier M, Zennou-Azogui Y, Xerri C, Coq JO, Brezun JM (2010) Differential tactile and motor recovery and cortical map alteration after C4-C5 spinal hemisection. *Exp. Neurol.* 221:186-197

McCarson KE (1999) Central and peripheral expression of neurokinin-1 and neurokinin-3 receptor and substance P-encoding messenger RNAs: peripheral regulation during formalin-induced inflammation and lack of neurokinin receptor expression in primary afferent sensory neurons. *Neuroscience* 93:361-370

McKenzie AL, Nagarajan SS, Roberts TPL, Merzenich MM, Byl NN (2003) Somatosensory representation of the digits and clinical performance in patients with focal hand dystonia. *Am. J. Phys. Med. Rehabil.* 82:737-749

Milligan ED, Twining C, Chacur M, Biedenkapp J, O'Connor K, Poole S, Tracey K, Martin D, Maier SF, Watkins LR (2003) Spinal glia and proinflammatory cytokines mediate mirror-image neuropathic pain in rats. *J. Neurosci.* 23:1026-1040

Moalem G, Tracey DJ (2006) Immune and inflammatory mechanisms in neuropathic pain. *Brain Res. Rev.* 51:240-264

Moffitt JA, Grippo AJ, Beltz TG, Johnson AK (2008) Hindlimb unloading elicits anhedonia and sympathovagal imbalance. *J. Appl. Physiol.* 105:1049-1059

Moucha R, Kilgard MP (2006) Cortical plasticity and rehabilitation. *Prog. Brain Res.* 157:111-122

Narici MV, de Boer MD (2010) Disuse of the musculo-skeletal system in space and on earth. *Eur. J. Appl. Physiol., July 9*

Ohira Y, Yoshinaga T, Nomura T, Kawano F, Ishihara A, Nonaka I, Roy RR, Edgerton VR (2002a) Gravitational unloading effects on muscle fiber size, phenotype and myonuclear number. *Adv. Space Res.* 30:777-781

Ohira Y, Kawano F, Ishihara A (2002b) Role of afferent input in muscle atrophy. *Biol. Sci. Space* 16:147-148

Ohtori S, Takahashi K, Moriya H, Myers RR (2004) TNF-alpha and TNF-alpha receptor type 1 upregulation in glia and neurons after peripheral nerve injury: studies in murine DRG and spinal cord. *Spine* 29:1082-1088

Pakula AT, Van Naarden Braun K, Yeargin-Allsopp M (2009) Cerebral palsy: classification and epidemiology. Phys Med Rehabil *Clin. N Am.* 20:425-452

Pan Z, Yang J, Guo C, Shi D, Shen D, Zheng Q, Chen R, Xu Y, Xi Y, Wang J (2008) Effects of hindlimb unloading on ex vivo growth and osteogenic/adipogenic potentials of bone marrow-derived mesenchymal stem cells in rats. *Stem Cells Dev.* 17:795-804

Perry SM, McIlhenny SE, Hoffman MC, Soslowsky LJ (2005) Inflammatory and angiogenic mRNA levels are altered in a supraspinatus tendon overuse animal model. *J. Shoulder Elbow Surg.* 14:79S-83S

Pitcher GM, Henry JL (2004) Nociceptive response to innocuous mechanical stimulation is mediated via myelinated afferents and NK-1 receptor activation in a rat model of neuropathic pain. *Exp. Neurol.* 186:173-197

Plautz EJ, Milliken GW, Nudo RJ (2000) Effects of repetitive motor training on movement representations in adult squirrel monkeys: role of use versus learning. *Neurobiol. Learn Mem.* 74:27-55

Prechtl HF (1997) State of the art of a new functional assessment of the young nervous system. An early predictor of cerebral palsy. *Early Hum. Dev.* 50:1-11

Raineteau O, Schwab ME (2001) Plasticity of motor systems after incomplete spinal cord injury. *Nat. Rev. Neurosci* 2:263-273

Rani S, Barbe MF, Barr AE, Litivn J (2010) Role of TNF alpha and PLF in bone remodeling in a rat model of repetitive reaching and grasping. *J. Cell. Physiol.* 225:152-167

Rani S, Barbe MF, Barr AE, Litvin J (2009a) Periostin-like-factor and Periostin in an animal model of work-related musculoskeletal disorder. *Bone* 44:502-512

Rani S, Barbe MF, Barr AE, Litvin J (2009b) Induction of periostin-like factor and periostin in forearm muscle, tendon, and nerve in an animal model of work-related musculoskeletal disorder. *J. Histochem. Cytochem.* 57:1061-1073

Reed JL, Pouget P, Qi H, Zhou Z, Bernard MR, Burish MJ, Haitas J, Bonds AB, Kaas JH (2008) Widespread spatial integration in primary somatosensory cortex. *Proc. Natl. Acad. Sci. U.S.A* 105:10233-10237

Rempel D, Dahlin L, Lundborg G (1999) Pathophysiology of nerve compression syndromes: response of peripheral nerves to loading. *J. Bone Joint Surg. Am.* 81:1600-1610

Rempel DM, Diao E (2004) Entrapment neuropathies: pathophysiology and pathogenesis. *J. Electromyogr. Kinesiol.* 14:71-75

Remple MS, Bruneau RM, VandenBerg PM, Goertzen C, Kleim JA (2001) Sensitivity of cortical movement representations to motor experience: evidence that skill learning but not strength training induces cortical reorganization. *Behav. Brain Res.* 123:133-141

Rioult-Pedotti MS, Friedman D, Donoghue JP (2000) Learning-induced LTP in neocortex. *Science* 290:533-536

Romanini L, Villani C, Meloni C, Calvisi V (1989) Histological and morphological aspects of muscle in infantile cerebral palsy. *Ital. J. Orthop. Traumatol.* 15:87-93

Rose J, Haskell WL, Gamble JG, Hamilton RL, Brown DA, Rinsky L (1994) Muscle pathology and clinical measures of disability in children with cerebral palsy. *J. Orthop. Res.* 12:758-768

Rosenbaum P, Paneth N, Leviton A, Goldstein M, Bax M, Damiano D, Dan B, Jacobsson B (2007) A report: the definition and classification of cerebral palsy April 2006. *Dev. Med. Child Neurol. Suppl.* 109:8-14

Rothman SM, Kreider RA, Winkelstein BA (2005) Spinal neuropeptide responses in persistent and transient pain following cervical nerve root injury. *Spine* 30:2491-2496

Sanes JN, Donoghue JP (2000) Plasticity and primary motor cortex. *Annu. Rev. Neurosci.* 23:393-415

Schäfers M, Sorkin L (2008) Effect of cytokines on neuronal excitability. *Neurosci. Lett.* 437:188-193

Schäfers M, Sorkin LS, Sommer C (2003a) Intramuscular injection of tumor necrosis factor-alpha induces muscle hyperalgesia in rats. *Pain* 104:579-588

Schäfers M, Svensson CI, Sommer C, Sorkin LS (2003b) Tumor necrosis factor-alpha induces mechanical allodynia after spinal nerve ligation by activation of p38 MAPK in primary sensory neurons. *J. Neurosci.* 23:2517-2521

Schaible H, Ebersberger A, Von Banchet GS (2002) Mechanisms of pain in arthritis. *Ann. N. Y. Acad. Sci* 966:343-354

Schieber MH (2002) Training and synchrony in the motor system. *J. Neurosci.* 22:5277-5281

Schuenke MD, Reed DW, Kraemer WJ, Staron RS, Volek JS, Hymer WC, Gordon S, Perry Koziris L (2009) Effects of 14 days of microgravity on fast hindlimb and diaphragm muscles of the rat. *Eur. J. Appl. Physiol* 106:885-892

Shenkman BS, Nemirovskaya TL, Belozerova IN, Mazin MG, Matveeva OA (2002) Mitochondrial adaptations in skeletal muscle cells in mammals exposed to gravitational unloading. *J. Gravit. Physiol.* 9:P159-162

Shimano MM, Volpon JB (2009) Biomechanics and structural adaptations of the rat femur after hindlimb suspension and treadmill running. *Braz. J. Med. Biol. Res.* 42:330-338

Shubayev VI, Myers RR (2002) Anterograde TNF alpha transport from rat dorsal root ganglion to spinal cord and injured sciatic nerve. *Neurosci. Lett.* 320:99-101

Silverstein B, Welp E, Nelson N, Kalat J (1998) Claims incidence of work-related disorders of the upper extremities: Washington state, 1987 through 1995. *Am. J. Public Health* 88:1827-1833

Silverstein BA, Fine LJ, Armstrong TJ (1986) Hand wrist cumulative trauma disorders in industry. *Br. J. Ind. Med.* 43:779-784

Sommerich CM, Lavender SA, Buford JA, J Banks J, Korkmaz SV, Pease WS (2007) Towards development of a nonhuman primate model of carpal tunnel syndrome: performance of a voluntary, repetitive pinching task induces median mononeuropathy in Macaca fascicularis. *J. Orthop. Res.* 25:713-724

Sorkin LS, Yaksh TL (2009) Behavioral models of pain states evoked by physical injury to the peripheral nerve. *Neurotherapeutics* 6:609-619

Stein T, Schluter M, Galante A, Soteropoulos P, Tolias P, Grindeland R, Moran M, Wang T, Polansky M, Wade C (2002) Energy metabolism pathways in rat muscle under conditions of simulated microgravity. *J. Nutr. Biochem.* 13:471

Stevens L, Mounier Y, Holy X, Falempin M (1990) Contractile properties of rat soleus muscle after 15 days of hindlimb suspension. *J. Appl. Physiol* 68:334-340

Stevens L, Bastide B, Bozzo C, Mounier Y (2004) Hybrid fibres under slow-to-fast transformations: expression is of myosin heavy and light chains in rat soleus muscle. *Pflugers Arch.* 448:507-514

Stevenson EJ, Giresi PG, Koncarevic A, Kandarian SC (2003) Global analysis of gene expression patterns during disuse atrophy in rat skeletal muscle. J. Physiol. (Lond.) 551:33-48

Strata F, Coq JO, Byl N, Merzenich MM (2004) Effects of sensorimotor restriction and anoxia on gait and motor cortex organization: implications for a rodent model of cerebral palsy. *Neuroscience* 129:141-156

Sweitzer SM, Schubert P, DeLeo JA (2001) Propentofylline, a glial modulating agent, exhibits antiallodynic properties in a rat model of neuropathic pain. J. *Pharmacol. Exp. Ther* 297:1210-1217

Szabo SJ, Savoie FH, Field LD, Ramsey JR, Hosemann CD (2006) Tendinosis of the extensor carpi radialis brevis: an evaluation of three methods of operative treatment. *J. Shoulder Elbow Surg.* 15:721-727

Talmadge RJ, Roy RR, Bodine-Fowler SC, Pierotti DJ, Edgerton VR (1995) Adaptations in myosin heavy chain profile in chronically unloaded muscles. *Basic Appl. Myol* 5:117-137

Teskey GC, Monfils MH, Flynn C, Young NA, van Rooyen F, Henry LC, Ozen LJ, Henderson AK, Reid AY, Brown AR (2008) Motor maps, seizures, and behaviour. *Can. J. Exp. Psychol.* 62:132-139

Topp KS, Byl NN (1999) Movement dysfunction following repetitive hand opening and closing: anatomical analysis in Owl monkeys. *Mov. Disord.* 14:295-306

Treffort N, Dubreucq G, Canu MH, Guérardel Y, Falempin M, Picquet F (2006) Variations in amino acid neurotransmitters in the rat ventral spinal cord after hindlimb unloading. *Neurosci. Lett.* 403:147-150

Treffort N, Picquet F, Petit J, Falempin M (2005) The structure and response properties of Golgi tendon organs in control and hypodynamia-hypokinesia rats. *Exp. Neurol.*195:313-321

Vannucci RC, Connor JR, Mauger DT, Palmer C, Smith MB, Towfighi J, Vannucci SJ (1999) Rat model of perinatal hypoxic-ischemic brain damage. *J. Neurosci. Res.* 55:158-163

Vannucci RC, Vannucci SJ (2005) Perinatal Hypoxic-Ischemic Brain Damage: *Evolution of an Animal Model. Dev. Neurosci.* 27:81-86

Vermaelen M, Marini J, Chopard A, Benyamin Y, Mercier J, Astier C (2005) Ubiquitin targeting of rat muscle proteins during short periods of unloading. *Acta Physiol. Scand.* 185:33-40

Viikari-Juntura E, Silverstein B (1999) Role of physical load factors in carpal tunnel syndrome. *Scand. J. Work Environ. Health* 25:163-185

Viikari-Juntura ER (1997) The scientific basis for making guidelines and standards to prevent work-related musculoskeletal disorders. *Ergonomics* 40:1097-1117

Wallin J, Schött E (2002) Substance P release in the spinal dorsal horn following peripheral nerve injury. *Neuropeptides* 36:252-256

Walton K (1998) Postnatal development under conditions of simulated weightlessness and space flight. *Brain Res. Rev.* 28:25-34

Walton KD, Harding S, Anschel D, Harris YT, Llinás R (2005) The effects of microgravity on the development of surface righting in rats. *J. Physiol.* (Lond.) 565:593-608

Wang X, Merzenich MM, Sameshima K, Jenkins WM (1995) Remodelling of hand representation in adult cortex determined by timing of tactile stimulation. *Nature* 378:71-75

Wang XD, Kawano F, Matsuoka Y, Fukunaga K, Terada M, Sudoh M, Ishihara A, Ohira Y (2006) Mechanical load-dependent regulation of satellite cell and fiber size in rat soleus muscle. *Am. J. Physiol., Cell Physiol.* 290:C981-989

Warren R, Tremblay N, Dykes RW (1989) Quantitative study of glutamic acid decarboxylase-immunoreactive neurons and cytochrome oxidase activity in normal and partially deafferented rat hindlimb somatosensory cortex. *J. Comp. Neurol.* 288:583-592

Westerga J, Gramsbergen A (1993) The effect of early movement restriction: an EMG study in the rat. *Behav. Brain Res.* 59:205-209

Whishaw IQ, Pellis SM, Gorny BP (1992) Skilled reaching in rats and humans: evidence for parallel development or homology. *Behav. Brain Res.* 47:59-70

Willems MET, Miller GR, Stauber FD, Stauber WT (2010) Effects of repeated lengthening contractions on skeletal muscle adaptations in female rats. *J. Physiol. Sci.* 60:143-150

Wingert JR, Burton H, Sinclair RJ, Brunstrom JE, Damiano DL (2008) Tactile sensory abilities in cerebral palsy: deficits in roughness and object discrimination. *Dev. Med. Child Neurol.* 50:832-838

Wingert JR, Burton H, Sinclair RJ, Brunstrom JE, Damiano DL (2009) Joint-position sense and kinesthesia in cerebral palsy. *Arch, Phys, Med, Rehabil,* 90:447-453

Wingert JR, Sinclair RJ, Dixit S, Damiano DL, Burton H (2010) Somatosensory-evoked cortical activity in spastic diplegic cerebral palsy. *Hum. Brain Mapp.* 31:1772-1785

Winkelstein BA, Rutkowski MD, Weinstein JN, DeLeo JA (2001) Quantification of neural tissue injury in a rat radiculopathy model: comparison of local deformation, behavioral outcomes, and spinal cytokine mRNA for two surgeons. *J. Neurosci. Methods* 111:49-57

Wittenberg GF (2010) Experience, cortical remapping, and recovery in brain disease. *Neurobiol. Dis* 37:252-258

Woolf CJ, Salter MW (2000) Neuronal plasticity: increasing the gain in pain. *Science* 288:1765-1769

Xerri C, Bourgeon S, Coq J (2005) Perceptual context-dependent remodeling of the forepaw map in the SI cortex of rats trained on tactile discrimination. *Behav. Brain Res* 162:207-221

Yu ZB, Gao F, Feng HZ, Jin J (2007) Differential regulation of myofilament protein isoforms underlying the contractility changes in skeletal muscle unloading. *Am. J. Physiol., Cell Physiol* 292:C1192-1203

In: Movement Disorders: Causes, Diagnoses and Treatments
Editor: Barbara J. Larsen
ISBN 978-1-61209-200-3

Chapter III

Restless Legs Syndrome and Periodic Limb Movements of Sleep

Levent Ediz
Department of Physical Medicine Rehabilitation and Rheumatology.
Yuzuncu Yil University Medical Faculty,
65200 Van, Turkey

Abstract

Restless legs syndrome (RLS) is a common, chronic, sensorimotor, hyperkinetic movement disorder, which is characterized by significant uncomfortable creeping, crawling or cramping sensations at rest and irresistable urge to move for alleviating the symptoms focused primarily on the lower extremities and sometimes also other parts of the body. RLS symptoms may occur intermittently or daily. Symptoms begin or are exacerbated in the evening or at night and also interfere with sleep and may result in reduced sleep efficiency and even serious insomnia. PLMS are brief jerks (repetitive stereotypic movements), a flexion at the ankle, knee, and hip with an extension of the toes during sleep lasting between 0.5 to 5.0 seconds, typically occur at 20- to 40-second intervals. PLMS affect one or both legs and rarely involve the arms. PLMS usually occur during non-REM sleep and may be associated with awakening. In addition, PLMS that reduce sleep quality are common with a prevelance of 80% during sleep in patients with RLS. RLS affects about 3% to 12% of the general population, and is more common in females with a female-to-male ratio of 2:1. Although RLS could be seen from 2 to >80 years of age, the mean age at the diagnosis time is 35–40 years. RLS can be primary (idiopathic) or secondary (sporadic or symptomatic) as a result of iron deficiency (with or without anemia), chronic renal and hepatic failure, pregnancy, rheumatic diseases (especially rheumatoid arthritis and fibromyalgia), neuropathies and radiculopathies, neurodegenerative diseases such as Parkinson's disease and drugs such as antihistamines, dopamine antagonists, mirtazapine, tricyclic antidepressants, serotonergic reuptake inhibitors. Idiopathic RLS is suggested to be a complex polygenic disorder with possible genetic heterogeneity because of variations in penetrance and anticipation. Genomewide linkage analysis studies showed at least 3 major susceptibility loci on chromosomes 12q13-23, 14q13-21 and 9p24-22 regions in large families. Genes and loci associated with RLS on 2q, 20p and 16p have also been identified. While the pathophysiology of RLS and PLMS has not yet been fully understood, dopamine dysfunction locally within the central nervous system appears to have a central role in the pathophysiology of both conditions. Moderate aerobic exercise, hot baths, massage, and stretching are nonpharmacologic treatment options with some benefit. Carbidopa/levodopa, dopamine agonists particularly ropinirole and pramipexole, opioids, benzodiazepines, antiepileptic drugs (carbamazepine, gabapentine, pregabaline) and iron supplements are recommended with nonpharmacologic treatment options as primary treatments.

Introduction

Restless Legs Syndrome (RLS), also known as Ekbom's syndrome, is a common hyperkinetic sensory-motor movement disorder that is characterized by an irresistable urge to move the lower limbs that is usually accompanied or caused by peculiar/unpleasant sensations deep in the lower limbs (rarely also in the upper limbs) [1,2]. These sensations (paraesthesias) appear or are worsened during periods of rest or inactivity, particularly in the evening and at night, and are typically, partially or totally relieved by movement [3]. RLS symptoms may occur intermittently or daily. Intolerable RLS symptoms also interfere with sleep and may result in reduced sleep efficiency and even serious insomnia [4].

The syndrome was probably first described in 1672 by British anatomist and physician Thomas Willis who suggested treating it with opioids [5,6]. But nearly three centuries passed before RLS was more completely described and characterized by the Swiss neurologist Karl-Axel Ekbom in 1945 [7,8]. Then, half a century later, with the recent increased recognition and understanding of RLS, the International RLS Study Group (IRLSSG) published diagnostic criteria [9] that has been revised and expanded at an IRLSSG/National Institutes of Health consensus conference in 2002 [10,11] (Table 1).

Epidemiology

RLS appears to be a common disorder. The estimated prevalence of RLS in the general population is reported about 3–12% in western societes with one third affected to a moderate or severe degree [12-19]. Of 16,202 people surveyed, perhaps the largest to date, 7% screened positively for RLS in the United States and 5 European countries [20]. A study of 1803 adults in rural Kentucky found an age-adjusted RLS prevalence of 10% [21]. In another study including a random population of more than 10000 French adults, the prevalence of RLS was estimated to be 8.5%, with a higher prevalence observed in females (10.8%) than in males (5.8%) [22]. No difference in RLS prevalence was found between black and white individuals [23]. The prevalence of RLS is markedly lower in some Asian populations than western countries, ranging from 0.1% to 4.6% [24,25]. Although RLS could be seen from 2 to >80 years of age, it is generally a disorder of middle to old age. The prevalence increases with age. Therefore, 19% of the population older than 80 years was affected in a study [14]. In the same study, the mean age at onset was 27 years. But at least 30% of the RLS sufferers experience their first complaints before the age of 20 years [25,26]. Symptoms get worse with time, so that the patients seek treatment in middle ages. Remission is rare, observed in about

15% of RLS sufferers [27]. Sex difference in RLS has been somewhat controversial. Although there are inconsistent results in the literature, studies suggest RLS is more common in women. Usually a higher prevalence was found in women than in men in the previous studies [12,14-17,28-31]. However, no sex difference was found in some studies [24,32,33]. And the prevalence was higher in males in a Japanese study [34]. RLS also could be seen in children and adolescents [35-38]. Consensus criteria for the diagnosis of pediatric RLS were also published in 2003 [10,35] (Table 2).

Table 1. Diagnostic criteria for RLS [10]

Essential diagnostic criteria; All of the following four criteria are necessary for a diagnosis Irresistable urge to move the legs, usually associated with, or induced by, uncomfortable and unpleasant sensations in the lower limbs. Irresistable urge to move or unpleasant sensations (symptom complex) begin or worsen during periods of rest or inactivity (when sitting or lying down). 3. Symptom complex is partially or totally relieved by movement, for instance when walking or stretching, at least as long as the activity continues. 4. Symptom complex is worse during the evening or night than during the day or only occurs in the evening or at night. Supportive clinical criteria of RLS *Family history; *Response to dopaminergic therapy; *Periodic limb movements at rest or during sleep; Associated features *Natural clinical course of the disorder; Clinical course is variable but typically chronic and often progressive *Normal neurologic and physical exam findings in idiopathic/familial forms *Sleep disturbance; Sleep disorders are common in patients with severe restless legs syndrome

A large, population-based study, involving over 10,000 families has recently reported 1.9% and 2% prevalence of definite RLS in children (8–11 year olds) and adolescents (12–17 year olds), respectively [39]. About 2 to 4 in 60 to 100 adults have RLS symptoms adequately severe to be worthy of treatment. Of those, only one fourth have been diagnosed, and maybe fewer treated [40].

Clinical Signs and Symptoms

The clinical course of RLS varies substantially, but it is usually regarded as a chronic disease with a successive increase of symptoms [2]. Patients with RLS who seek medical aid usually describe both the urge to move and unpleasant, creeping or crawling sensations, calling them simply uncomfortable and deep within the lower limbs rather than on the surface. These intolerable sensations usually are felt in the muscles or bones.

Table 2. Diagnostic Criteria for RLS in Children and Adolescents (2003 NIH Workshop) [10,37]

Criteria for definite RLS in children (2 to 12 years old) Child meets all of the following four adult essential criteria: 1. An urge to move the lower limbs, usually associated with, or induced by, uncomfortableand unpleasant sensations in the lower limbs (symptoms). 2. Symptoms begin or worsen when sitting or lying down 3. Symptoms are partially or completely relieved by movement 4. Symptoms are worse in the evening or at night than during the day or occur only in the evening or at night AND Children use their own words to describe lower limb discomfort. For instance: tingle, hurt, bugs, tickle, spiders, want to run, ants, a lot of energy in his/her legs, static etc. OR Following 2 or 3 of the supporting features are met: _ Inappropriate sleep disturbance for age _ Definite RLS history of biological parent or sibling. _ The child has a sleep examination reporting a periodic limb movement index >5 per hour of sleep. Exceeding 5/h is an acceptable alternative ending index. Diagnosis of definite RLS in adolescents (13 -18 years old) All of the 4 essential adult RLS criteria are met. For all: the symptoms are not better explained by mental disorder, medical or neurologic disorder, another current sleep disorder, medication use, or substance use disorder.

They might be unilateral but are generally bilateral and symmetrical. The discomfort is often difficult to describe. Common descriptive terms used for RLS sensations by the patients are crawling, ants crawling, creeping, pulling, itching, drawing, stretching, jittery, burning, pain, true pain, worms moving, electric current, tearing, the gotta moves, fidgets, grabbing sensation, heebie jeebies, crazy legs, throbbing, tight feeling or itching bones [41].

RLS symptoms may occur intermittently or daily [1,42]. The unpleasant sensations are experienced only during periods of inactivity (when the extremities are at rest for any length of time, e.g., while sitting down or lying down, getting into bed in the late evening, train and car journeys, flights, meetings, social dinners or at the cinema) and typically alleviated totally or partially by moving the legs [2,43]. RLS sufferers experience an almost irresistible urge to move the lower extremities and they usually walk around in order to get relief [42,44]. Symptoms begin or are exacerbated in the evening or at night and also interfere with sleep and may result in reduced sleep efficiency and even serious insomnia [45]. The fourth prime cause of insomnia is RLS [2,42,45]. Loss of sleep is a serious problem both to RLS sufferers and their spouses [46].

These uncomfortable sensations of RLS are most commonly experienced between the knees and ankles, but may also be localised in the thighs, and sometimes in the feet. Despite the name of restless legs syndrome, the upper limbs may also be involved, but symptoms are usually more severe in the legs. The trunk involvement is very rare [42].

Periodic limb movements of sleep (PLMS) which reduce sleep quality and may cause multiple nocturnal arousals are common with a prevelance of 80-85% during sleep in patients with RLS [2]. The incidence of the combined syndrome of RLS and PLMS increases with age especially in adulthood and late life. There are also individuals with PLMS who do not complain of RLS. PLMS usually do not cause complaint in most cases and are observed incidentally in sleep laboratories during sleep studies [2,11,47].

RLS and PLMS are beleived 2 clinical manifestations of the same central nervous system dysfunction. PLMS are brief involuntary, rhythmic muscular jerks in the legs (repetitive stereotypic movements), a flexion at the ankle, knee, and hip with an extension of the toes and this initial jerk followed by a tonic spasm during sleep. Such events last between 0.5 to 5.0 seconds, typically occur at 20- to 40-seconds intervals for minutes or hours. PLMS affect one or both legs and rarely involve the arms. PLMS usually occur during non-REM sleep and may be associated with awakening. The severity of PLMS may be occational mild or severe occurring every night. Sometimes, the whole lower extremity or both lower extremities flex [11,48] (Table 3).

Apart from RLS which is a clinical diagnosis, the diagnosis of PLMS requires polysomnography [11,47-49]. Although polysomnography is not essential in patients with RLS, it provides information on sleep disturbances, as well as documents PLMS by tibialis anterior muscle electromyography (movements lasting between 0.5 to 5 seconds occur at 20- to 40-seconds intervals; a sequence of 4 movements between 4 to 90 seconds apart are necessary to diagnose PLMS [2,48,49]. PLMS also can be seen in a variety of sleep disturbances and in healthy individuals without sleep complaints. Nocturnal blood pressure has been reported to increase in association with PLMS [50].

In most cases, RLS sufferers are unaware of their own PLMS which disturb sleep. Periodic limb movement disorder (PLMD) is diagnosed when there are (1) PLMS documented by polysomnography, (2) PLMS exceeding norms for age, (3) clinical sleep disturbance, and (4) the absence of another primary sleep disorder or reason for the PLMS (including RLS) [11,47,51].

Patients with RLS may also complain of fatigue, diminished concentration, and psychomotor agitation. These symptoms may be directly due to the sleep disorder, or secondary depression [10,28]. A great deal of studies reported also significantly higher rates of depression symptoms in patients with RLS than in healthy controls [52]. Just before falling asleep, some patients with RLS may also have propriospinal myoclonus (PSM) which is a motor phenomenon observed in RLS different from PLMS during sleep. PSM could be defined as axial jerks involving muscles innervated by different segments of the spinal cord [53].

Etiology and Pathophysiology

RLS can occur either as a primary (idiopathic) disease or as a secondary (symptomatic) condition. Many causes have been suggested in the etiology of primary RLS. But it still remains unknown [54]. The most common hypothesis in the pathophysiology of both idiopathic RLS and PLMS is abnormal dopaminergic system function in the nigro-striatal areas of the brain [55,56]. Decreased dopamine D2 receptor binding has been shown in the striatum of patients with RLS by advanced brain imaging [56]. Cervenka et al. has demonstrated hypoactive dopaminergic neurotransmission in both striatal and extrastriatal brain regions in patients with RLS [57].

Table 3. Basic properties of periodic movements of sleep

1. The prevelence of PLMS increases with age. The prevelance is 30% in individuals over 50 years old, while %5 in persons 30 to 50 years old; and it is infrequent in those under 30 years old.
2. Indivudials with PLMS are usually asymptomatic or unaware of their own PLMS and also PLMS may wake his/her sleeping partner or sometimes the patient himself/herself.
3. Brief (0.5- to 5-seconds) jerks of one or both lower extremities in every 20 to 40 seconds, consisting of, basically, dorsiflexion of the big toe and foot. (a flexion at the ankle, knee, and hip with an extension of the toes.).
4. This initial jerk followed by a sustained tonic spasm.
5. Brief jerks may occur in an awake or drowsy person.
6. Brief jerks usually occur during arousal (stage I and II sleep-Non-REM sleep).
7. Brief jerks decrease during sleep in stages III and IV and unusual during REM sleep.

The low brain iron is a well recognized pathology of RLS. Iron is a necessary cofactor in the dopamine-producing cells for the synthesis of dopamine. The regulation of dopamine receptors in the brain is also iron-dependent [1]. Low iron and ferritin levels have been found in the cerebrospinal fluid of RLS patients [58,59]. Increased severity of RLS symtoms have also been found at serum ferritin levels below 50 ng/mL [60,61]. Brain iron deficiency particularly affects the dopamine-producing cells in the substantia nigra and their terminal regions in the striatum resulting in dopaminergic system dysfunction. Since iron is a co-factor for tyrosine hydroxilase, decreased brain iron would be an expected result in decreased tyrosine hydroxilase, contrary to this assumption, iron deficiency in the brain interestingly increases tyrosine hydroxilase activity in the substantia nigra which then increases extracellular dopamine [62-64]. Iron deficiency also decreases dopamine D1 and D2 receptors [65]. A recent autopsy study of RLS patients by Connor et al. showed increased tyrosine hydroxylase in the substantia nigra and decreased D2 receptors in the putamen [63]. Iron insufficiency in the brain produces a dopaminergic abnormality characterized as an overly activated dopaminergic system as part of the RLS pathology. Iron decrease in the brain also increases extracellular striatal dopamine levels approximately 4 times in the day compared with the levels at night [66]. This effect of the brain iron deficiency may explain the phasic motor symptoms observed in RLS. Earley and colleagues have found low cerebrospinal ferritin levels and high transferrin levels in the idiopathic form of the disorder [58]. Brain iron deficiency may also lead decreased dopamine transporter (DAT) functioning on the cell surface [67].

Cerebrospinal ferritin levels in patients with RLS have been found lower at night than during the day. Only the early onset RLS patients have had low cerebrospinal ferritin levels. No difference has been found in serum ferritin and transferrin levels of these patients [68].

Autopsy, initial cerebral spinal fluid (CSF) and brain imaging studies clearly showed also the relationship between brain iron deficiency and dopaminergic pathology in RLS [69,70]. Both abnormally increased CSF 3-Omethyldopa and abnormally increased CSF homovanillic acid indicating increased dopamine production in patients with RLS is proportional to the severity of the disorder [62].

SPECT and PET studies showed decreased iodobenzamide and decreased raclopide binding to D2 receptors in the striatum and in the putamen, and decreased DOPA binding to the striatum in patients with RLS [46,71]. Brain iron deficiency may also increase acute and chronic pain responses by increasing sensitivity to C-fiber-mediated chronic pain in patients with RLS [72]. In conclusion, the iron deficiency in the brain causes dopaminergic dysfunction by increasing tyrosine hydroxylase which subsequently increases extracellular dopamine levels, resulting in a decrease in DAT functioning on the cell surface and also causes a decrease in D2 receptors [1].

In addition to the dopaminergic dysfunction trials in RLS pathogenesis, genetic aspects of RLS and PLMS have been investigated [73]. The RLS literature has reported 40% to 92% of early-onset (individuals with symptoms first experiencing before 35 to 40 years of age) cases having family history, with much lower rates in patients with late-onset and secondary RLS [74,75].

RLS is 3–5 times more common amongst first degree relatives of individuals with RLS than in individuals without RLS suggesting an autosomal-dominant transmission with high penetrance. However, idiopathic RLS is suggested a complex polygenic disorder with possible genetic heterogeneity because of variations in penetrance and anticipation [10,76-78] (10,76,77,78). A study of 12 monozygotic twins in which at least 1 member in ten out of 12 monozygotic (MZ) twin pairs expressed RLS indicates the importance of genetic influence and also suggests high concordance and penetrance [79]. Genomewide linkage analysis studies showed at least 3 major susceptibility loci on chromosomes 12q13-23, 14q13-21 and 9p24-22 regions in large families [80-87]. Genes and loci associated with RLS on 2q33, 20p13 and 16p12 have also been identified [73,88-92]. A variant on chromosome 6p21has also been identified in patients with RLS and this variant is also a possible genetic determinant of PLMS [73,93].

Adenosine and dopaminergic systems regulate cortical sensorimotor responses. The disruptions in the adenosine and dopaminergic systems have been reported for brain iron deficiency. Cortical function studies via movement-related beta and mu rhythm reactivity showed that the symptoms of RLS are also associated with cortical sensorimotor dysfunction [94].

Secondary RLS

RLS may also occur or exacerbate in association with several medical conditions or taking of substances (such as caffeine, alcohol, or nicotine) or drugs. Secondary RLS is still an underrecognized and underdiagnosed disorder.

Causes of Secondary RLS

1. Iron deficiency and Iron deficiency anaemia; Nordlander is the first who reported on RLS and iron deficiency anaemia association. He also found that the RLS symtoms ceased with IV iron therapy in patients with iron deficiency anaemia and RLS [95]. Some studies have found up to 25% of iron deficiency among patients with RLS [40]. In another study 24.7% of the female blood donors and 14.7% of the male blood donors were affected by RLS [96]. RLS were present in 34.37% of patients with iron deficiency patients in India [97].
2. Pregnancy; During pregnancy, up to 26% of women can be affected by RLS, especially during the last trimester [98,99]. Deficiency of iron and vitamins during pregnancy is suggested to be a major cause. Leg restlessness disappears in most pregnant women soon after childbirth.
3. Renal Failure; The prevalence of RLS symptoms appears to be greater than in the general population with a wide variation ranging from 6.6% to 83% in patients with end stage renal disease (ESRD) and uraemia [100]. RLS symptoms may be experienced both before and after dialysis treatment. RLS symptoms can be improved after renal transplantation [101].
4. Rheumatic diseases; The prevelance of RLS symptoms may increase amongst those who suffer from rheumatic diseases such as rheumatoid arthritis, fibromyalgia syndrome and Sjögren's syndrome. The reduced iron status in these patients may be related to the RLS symtoms [102-104].
5. Drugs; Some drugs have the ability to provoke or exacerbate RLS. Examples of these drugs are tricyclic antidepressants, serotonergic reuptake inhibitors, mirtazapine, antihistamines and dopamine antagonists (including some antineusea medications) [105,106].
6. Neurologic conditions; Decresaed iron stores in the substantia nigra have been reported in patients with migraine [107]. RLS is five times more common in migraine patients who have dopaminergic premonitory symptoms (such as nausea, somnolence) [108]. Multiple sclerosis and Parkinson's disease could be associated with an increased risk of RLS [109,110]. The prevalence of RLS is also higher among patients with hereditary neuropathy, but not in those with acquired peripheral neuropathies [111].

Diagnosis

RLS remains a clinical diagnosis. Diagnosis of RLS is based upon a careful clinical history and a detailed physical and neurological examination. Diagnostic criteria have been established by the international RLS study group (IRLSSG) [9]. Then it has been revised and expanded at an IRLSSG/National Institutes of Health consensus conference in 2002 [10].

For definite diagnosis, 4 essential criteria for RLS are all required, 3 additional features are defined that may support but are not essential for the diagnosis and also associated features of RLS are defined [10]. As mentioned above the diagnosis of RLS is based on the following 4 essential criteria from a careful clinical history of the patient and a detailed physical and neurological examination (Table 1). (1) Irresistable urge to move the lower extremities, usually accompanied by uncomfortable/unpleasant sensations deep in the legs, (2) symptom complex are worse during periods of rest or inactivity, (3) symptom complex are totally or partially relieved by movement, and (4) symptom complex are worse in the evening or at night. Other supporting and associated features commonly found in individuals with RLS include a positive family history of RLS, sleep disturbance, decreased quality-of-life ratings, daytime fatigue, and attention deficits. Supporting criteria and associated features are also definitely helpful in the differential diagnosis.

The physical examination is generally normal in individuals with RLS except for those having a secondary form of RLS or a comorbid disorder. A neurologic examination with emphasis on peripheral nerve function, central nervous system and spinal cord are performed to rule out hereditary neuropathies and other neurologic causes of secondary RLS. A vascular examination of lower extremities is also performed to rule out vascular disorders especially superficial venous insufficiency (SVI). Polysomnography study is not routinely indicated.

Although there is currently no specific laboratory test to confirm the diagnosis of RLS, patients with RLS can be evaluated by some laboratory tests that can identify possible secondary causes of RLS include anaemia, iron deficiency (serum ferritin level of less than 50 μg per litre), blood biochemistry tests to rule out uremia and diabetes, low vitamin B12 and folate levels.

Differential Diagnosis

There are a few conditions may be confused with RLS. Potential mimics of RLS should be considered during examination [112] (Table 4). Akathisia which is a common side effect of neuroleptic medications describes the sense of motor restlessness of general body and need to move. In contrast with RLS, akathisia does not vary with rest or time of day [112].

Nocturnal leg cramps are painful involuntary muscular contractions that occur suddenly. They are usually unilateral and involve a specific muscle. Unlike RLS, nocturnal leg cramps require stretching of the affected muscle more than moving of the extremity to alleviate symptoms. Furthermore, residual pain or sensitivity after the nocturnal leg cramp helps to differentiate it from RLS [113]. Painful legs and moving toes syndrome is characterized by repetitive movements of the toes, burning sensation and moderate or severe pain in one or both feet. In contrast with RLS, pain is not necessarily alleviated by movement or increased at night [112].

Vascular intermittent claudication is one of the causes of leg discomfort and pain, but, unlike RLS, vascular intermittent claudication worsens during walking and is alleviated by rest. Peripheral neuropathies may also be misdiagnosed as RLS. However, symptoms are generally present throughout the day and not completely releived by movement [112].

Hypnic jerks (or sleep starts) are short, massive body movements during the sleep-wake transition; But unlike PLMS which is seen in RLS, the movements may involve both extremities without periodicity. The conditions that should be considered in the differential diagnosis of RLS are listed in Table 4.

Table 4. Differential diagnosis of RLS

Conditions may be confused with RLS
-Positional discomfort due to transient nerve compression -Hypnic jerks -Myopathy -Myelopathy -Nocturnal leg cramps -Painful legs and moving toes syndrome -Sore muscles -Neuroleptic-induced akathisia -Vascular intermittent claudication -Radiculopathy -Peripheral neuropathy

Treatment

Treatment of Primary RLS

Patients with mild symptoms may benefit from nonpharmacological treatment approaches such as establishing good sleep habits, exercises during daytime. Hot baths, massage of extremities, and stretching may also improve symptoms [114-117]. However, pharmacological treatment is needed in most patients with moderate or severe RLS symptoms. The dopaminergic agents, anticonvulsants, benzodiazepines and opioids are the major pharmacological classes that currently used to treat RLS.

Dopaminergic agents: Dopaminergic drugs have been used successfully for management of RLS. Various studies have showed that levodopa combined with a dopa decarboxylase inhibitor in a dosage of 50–250 mg once a day before the sleep time is effective to treat RLS and PLMS [118]. But, a major limitation of dopaminergic agent therapy is rebound and augmentation of symptoms. Augmentation refers to worsening of RLS symptoms in late afternoon or in early evening before the evening levodopa dose, requiring additional levodopa dosing. Rebound is the return of RLS symptoms especially in the morning after a dose of dopaminergic agent and appears to be directly related to the half-life of the drug [119,120]. As mentioned above, unfortunately the effect of regular levodopa last only 4 h, because of short half-life of the drug, and 25–50% of patients experience rebound symptoms during the night or in the morning [121]. Especially at a dosage exceeding 200 mg levodopa per night, augmentation was observed in over 80% of RLS patients [122,123]. Augmentation symptoms is more severe in low serum ferritin levels [124]. The pathomechanism of augmentation is suggested to be D1 receptor overstimulation while comperatively D2 and D3 receptors understimulation [125]. Combining sustained-release levodopa with regular levodopa before sleep time improves these limitations. Becauese the plasma peak occurs too late, sustained-release levodopa should not be used alone. Other previously unaffected parts of the body such as arms and trunk may progressively be involved during the treatment with levodopa [123].

These side effects of dopaminergic agents in RLS limit long-term usefulness of levodopa therapy.

Dopamine agonists: Dopamine receptor agonists have largely substituted dopaminergic agents for the first-line treatment of RLS. Augmentation is less observed with dopamine agonists than levodopa [126]. Double-blind placebo controlled clinical trials showed that nonergoline dopamine agonists pramipexole (0.125-0.75 mg range) and ropinirole (1-2 mg range) are both effective to treat symptoms of RLS and to suppress PLMS [127-133]. They are also efficacious and well tolerated in long-term treatment of RLS [134,135]. Rotigotine, another nonergot dopamine receptor agonist, formulated as a silicone-based transdermal patch (1–3 mg/24 h), has recently shown to improve both night-time and daytime symptoms in adults with idiopathic, moderate to severe RLS. Interestingly, no signs of augmentation was observed with 24 h transdermal low dose rotigotine treatment [136,137].

Ergoline derived dopamine agonists pergolide and cabergoline are both effective in RLS treatment in doses of 0.4–0.55 mg and 0.5–3 mg, respectively [138]. However, ergot dopamine agonists are no longer in first-line treatment options given the risks of cardiac valvulopathy [139]. There is also insufficient evidence and data to make treatment recommendations about other ergot dopamine agonists bromocriptine, dihydroergocriptine, and lisuride [140,141].

Opioid:; Opioids are used with increasing frequency in RLS treatment. In severe cases, especially in patients with significant daily symptoms and refractory RLS, opioids may be considered as a second-choice treatment after dopamine agonists. Opioids may also be considered a therapy choice for patients presenting with neuropathy or painful dysthesias [141-143]. Oxycodone (mean dose 15.9 mg), methadone (15.5 ± 7.7 mg/day), and tramadol (50–150 mg/day) have shown to be efficacious to treat RLS symptoms [144-146]. Augmentation has also been found with long-term tramadol treatment [147].

Short-acting opiates such as codein, oxycodone and hydrocodone may be considered for intermittent symptoms or symptoms occurring only at night [1]. Long-acting agents such as methadone, oxycodone, or the fentanyl patch may be used for more severe disease [1]. A recent meta-analysis has also focused on placebo effect of opioids in RLS and has found a large placebo effect for primary outcome measures [148]. Adverse effects such as development or exacerbation of sleep apnea, sedation, fatigue, constipation, Q-T interval prolongation and addiction issues may limit the role and use of opioids in the treatment of RLS [54].

Sedative-hypnotics (benzodiazepines)**:** The benzodiazepines, (especially clonazepam which is the best studied benzodiazepine in RLS), work mostly in improving sleep quality and have no effect on other symptoms of RLS. Therefore, they are no longer usually recommended in the treatment of RLS [54,149,150]. Adverse effects of clonazepam include addiction, tolerance, confusion and drowsiness particularly in older patients [54].

Anticonvulsants: Antiepileptics may improve RLS symptoms via augmenting gamma-aminobutyric acid (GABA) expression. Gabapentin, carbamazepine, pregabaline and valproic acid have been reported to be efficacious in treating RLS in placebo-controlled trials

Gabapentin (mean dosage ranging 800-1800 mg) has been shown to be efficacious in improving RLS-related sensorimotor symptoms and alleviating PLMS [151,152]. Augmentation has not been observed in gabapentine treated RLS sufferers [151].

Pregabalin, also a modulator of the alpha-2 delta receptor, is a promising agent in the treatment of RLS. In the recent studies, a majority of the patients with RLS achieved symptom remission with this agent (flexible dose 150-600 mg range) [153,154]. Gabapentin enacarbil (XP13512/GSK1838262), a gabapentin prodrug, 1.200 mg taken once daily, has also been recently found to alleviate RLS symptoms [155,156]. Carbamazepine (200–300 mg) improves nocturnal sensory disturbances and also decreases the number of RLS episodes reported by the patients [157,158]. In another study, valproic acid (600 mg) has also improved intensity and duration of RLS symptoms [159].

Iron supplementation: Oral iron given over a 12 week period in idiopathic RLS sufferers with low/normal ferritin values, may improve RLS symptoms [160]. However, iron therapy is only effective if patient have an iron storage deficiency. Intravenous iron sucrose has also been found effective on symptoms in patients with idiopathic RLS [161].

Treatment of Secondary RLS

Secondary RLS treatment includes both nonpharmacologic and pharmacologic approaches as mentioned above for primary RLS treatment. As well as secondary RLS symptoms may improve by treatment of the primary condition.

Iron deficiency is a common cause of secondary RLS. RLS may be seen in 30% to 35% of patients with conditions associated with iron deficiency, including anemia, renal failure and pregnancy [162]. The cause of iron deficiency should be investigated because serious diseases such as cancer (especially gastrointestinal tract) may first manifest itself as iron deficiency. Iron supplementation should be sustained until serum levels of ferritin are above 50 lg/L [162,163]. RLS symptoms may be seen in association with vitamin B12 and folic acid deficiency. RLS is common during pregnancy, and will likely resolve with delivery. Vitamin B12 or folic acid supplementations are necessary in these patients [164,165]. There is usually no improvement of RLS symptoms in patients with chronic renal failure. They generally need pharmacological treatment (with dopamine receptor agonists etc). Kidney transplantation may improve RLS symptoms [2].

Alternative Treatments

Although there is insufficient evidence in the literature to determine whether acupuncture and transcutaneous electrical nerve stimulation (TENS) are efficacious treatment options for RLS, patients may seek treatment with acupuncture and TENS [166,167]. Electromagnetic therapy and repetitive transcranial magnetic stimulation may offer some therapeutic perspectives for RLS treatment [168,169]. A herbal prescription which contains several herbals (Atractylodis Lanceae rhizoma, Hoelen, Cnidii rhizoma, Angelicae radix, Bupleuri radix, Glycyrrhizae radix and Uncariae ramulus et uncus) appears to be useful in RLS treatment [170]. Endovenous laser ablation (ELA) may alleviate RLS symptoms in patients with concurrent RLS and duplex-proven superficial venous insufficiency (SVI) [171].

Conclusion

RLS is still an underrecognized and underdiagnosed hyperkinetic movement disorder. The most common hypothesis in the pathophysiology of both idiopathic RLS and PLMS is abnormal dopaminergic system function in the nigro-striatal areas of the brain. Few guidelines have been proposed for RLS treatment [172]. The European Federation of Neurological Societies (EFNS) has developed a guideline for RLS management [41,54,173]. In this guideline, levodopa, transdermal delivery rotigotine, ropinirole and gabapentin were recommended. Of note, the most recent trials of pregabaline, gabapentin enacarbil, pramipexole and so on had not been published at the time of this guideline. However, management of RLS should be individualized with considerations for frequency of symptoms, history of augmentation and/or rebound, age, comorbid disease states and concomitant medications [41,54]. A comprehensive assessment of the multiple symptom domains associated with RLS and the impact of RLS on multidimensional aspects of function should form a routine part of the care of RLS patients. There are currently no generally accepted objective clinical findings, radiographic abnormalities or laboratory tests to assess the presence of RLS and to measure RLS severity. Therefore, the validated IRLSSG questionnaire measuring a patient's subjective responses has continued to be important in evaluation of RLS severity so far [174].

References

[1] Salas, RE; Gamaldo, CE; Allen, RP. Update in restless legs *Curr. Opin. Neurol.* 2010;23:401-406.

[2] Ekbom, K; Ulfberg, J. Restless legs *J Intern Med.* 2009;266:419-431.

[3] Ondo, WG. Restless legs *Neurol Clin.* 2009;27:779-799.

[4] Avidan, AY. Parasomnias and movement disorders *Semin Neurol.* 2009;29:372-392.

[5] Willis, T. *De anima brutorum.* London: Wells and Scot;1672.

[6] Critchley, M. The pre-dormitum. *Rev. Neurol.* 1955;93:101–106.

[7] Ekbom, KA. Restless legs: a clinical study. *Acta Med Scand.* 1945;58:1-123.

[8] Ekbom, KA. Restless legs syndrome. *Neurology.* 1960;10:868–873.

[9] The International Restless Legs Syndrome Study Group. Walters , AS. Toward a better definition of the restless legs syndrome. *Mov. Disord.* 1995;10:634–642.

[10] Allen, RP; Picchietti, D; Hening, WA; Trenkwalder, C; Walters, AS; Montplaisi, J. Restless legs syndrome: diagnostic criteria, special considerations, and epidemiology. A report from the restless legs syndrome diagnosis and epidemiology workshop at the National Institutes of Health. *Sleep Med.* 2003;4:101-119.

[11] Hening, W. The clinical neurophysiology of restless legs syndrome and periodic limb movements/ Part I: diagnosis, assessment, and characterization. *Clin. Neurophysiol.* 2004;115:1965–1974.

[12] Ghorayeb, I; Tison, F. Restless legs. *Presse Med.* 2010;39:564-570.

[13] Allen, RP; Walters, AS; Montplaisir, J; Hening, W; Myers, A; Bell, TJ; Ferini-Strambi, L. Restless legs syndrome prevalence and impact: REST general population study. *Med.* 2005;165:1286-1292.

[14] Berger, K; Luedemann, J; Trenkwalder, C; John, U; Kessler, C. Sex and the risk of restless legs syndrome in the general population. *Arch. Intern. Med.* 2004;164:196-202.

[15] Bjorvatn, B; Leissner, L; Ulfberg, J; Gyring, J; Karlsborg, M; Regeur, L; Skeidsvoll, H; Nordhus, IH; Pallesen, S. Prevalence, severity and risk factors of restless legs syndrome in the general adult population in two Scandinavian countries. *Sleep Med.* 2005;6:307-312.

[16] Lavigne, GJ; Montplaisir, JY. Restless legs syndrome and sleep bruxism: prevalence and association among Canadians. *Sleep.* 1994;17:739–743.

[17] Hogl, B; Kiechl, S; Willeit, J; Saletu, M; Frauscher, B; Seppi, K; Müller, J; Rungger, G; Gasperi, A; Wenning, G; Poewe, W. Restless legs syndrome: A community based study of prevalence, severity, and risk factors. *Neurology.* 2005;64:1920-1924.

[18] Ulfberg, J; Nystrom, B; Carter, N; Edling, C. Prevalence of restless legs syndrome among men aged 18 to 64 years: An association with somatic disease and neuropsychiatric symptoms. *Mov. Disord.* 2001;16:1159-1163.

[19] Ulfberg, J;Nystrom, B; Carter, N; Edling, C. Restless Legs Syndrome among working-aged women. *Eur. Neurol.* 2001;46:17-19.

[20] McCrink, L; Allen, RP; Wolowacz, S; Sherrill, B; Connolly, M; Kirsch, J. Predictors of health-related quality of life in sufferers with restless legs syndrome: a multi-national study. *Sleep Med.* 2007;8:73-83.

[21] Phillips, B; Young, T; Finn, L; Asher, K; Hening, WA; Purvis, C. Epidemiology of restless legs symptoms in adults. *Arch. Int. Med.* 2000;160:2137-2141.

[22] Tison, F; Crochard, A; Leger, D; Bouee, S; Lainey, E; El Hasnaoui, A. Epidemiology of restless legs syndrome in French adults: a nationwide survey. The INSTANT study. *Neurology* 2005;65:239–46.

[23] Lee, HB; Hening, WB; Allen, RP; Earley, CJ; Eaton, WW; Lyketsos, CG. Race and restless legs syndrome symptoms in an adult community sample in east Baltimore. *Sleep Med.* 2006;7:642-645.

[24] Tan, EK; Seah, A; See, SJ; Lim, E; Wong, MC; Koh, KK. Restless legs syndrome in an Asian population: A study in Singapore. *Mov. Disord.* 2001;16:577–579.

[25] Mizuno, S; Miyaoka, T; Inagaki, T; Horiguchi, J. Prevalence of restless legs syndrome in non-institutionalized Japanese elderly. Psychiatry Clin Neurosci. 2005;59:461–465.

[26] Kotagal, S; Silber, MH. Childhood-onset restless legs syndrome. *Ann. Neurol.* 2004;56:803–807.

[27] Walters, AS; Hickey, K; Maltzman , J; Verrico, T; Joseph, D; Hening, W; Wilson, V; Chokroverty, S. A questionnaire study of 138 patients with restless legs syndrome: The "Night-Walkers" survey. *Neurology.* 1996;46:92–95.

[28] Earley, CJ. Clinical practice. Restless legs syndrome. *N. Engl. J. Med.* 2003;348:2103-2109.

[29] Conti, CF; deOliveira, MM; Andriolo, RB; Saconato, H; Atallah, AN; Valbuza, JS; Coin de Carvalho, LB; do Prado, GF. Levodopa for idiopathic restless legs syndrome: Evidence-based review. *Movement Disorders.* 2007;22:1943-1951.

[30] Zucconi, M; Ferini-Strambi, L. Epidemiology and clinical findings of restless legs syndrome. *Sleep Medicine.* 2004;5:293-299.

[31] Rothdach, AJ; Trenkwalder, C; Haberstock, J; Keil, U; Berger, K. Prevalence and risk factors of RLS in an elderly population. *Neurology.* 2000;54:1064-1068.

[32] Winkelman, JW; Finn, L; Young, T. Prevalence and correlates of restless legs syndrome symptoms in the Wisconsin Sleep Cohort. *Sleep Med.* 2006;7:545-552.

[33] Phillips, B; Young, T; Finn, L; Asher, K; Hening, WA; Purvis, C. Epidemiology of restless legs symptoms in adults. *Arch. Int. Med.* 2000;160:2137-2141.

[34] Kageyama, T; Kabuto, M; Nitta, H; Kurokawa, Y; Taira, K; Suzuki, S; Takemoto, T. Prevalences of periodic limb movement-like and restless legs-like symptoms among Japanese adults. *Psychiatry Clin. Neurosci.* 2000;54:296-298.

[35] Picchietti, MA; Picchietti, DL. Restless Legs Syndrome and Periodic Limb Movement Disorder in Children and Adolescents. *Seminars in Pediatric Neurology.* 2008;15:91-99.

[36] Picchietti, MA; Picchietti, DL. Advances in pediatric restless legs *Sleep Med.* 2010 ;11:643-651.

[37] Picchietti, DL; Rajendran, RR; Wilson, MP; Picchietti, MA. Pediatric restless legs *Sleep Med.* 2009;10:925-931.

[38] Picchietti, DL; Stevens, HE. Early manifestations of restless legs *Sleep Med.* 2008;9:770-781.

[39] Picchietti, D; Allen, RP; Walters, AS; Davidson, JE; Myers, A; Ferini-Strambi, L. Restless legs syndrome: prevalence and impact in children and adolescents—The Peds REST study. *Pediatrics.* 2007;120:253-266.

[40] Hening, W; Walters, A; Allen, R; Montplaisir, J; Myers, A; Ferini-Strambi, L. Impact, diagnosis and treatment of restless legs syndrome (RLS) in a primary care population: The REST (RLS epidemiology, symptoms, and treatment) primary care study. *Sleep Medicine.* 2004;5:237-246.

[41] Ryan, M; Slevin, JT. Restless legs *Am. J. Health Syst. Pharm.* 2006:63:1599-1612.

[42] Vecchierini, MF, Léger, D. Restless legs. *Presse Med.* 2010;39:556-563.

[43] Moyer, DE; Zayas-Bazan, J; Reese, G. Restless legs syndrome: diagnostic time-savers, Tx tips. *J. Fam. Pract.* 2009;58:415-423.

[44] Truter, I. Restless Legs Syndrome. *SA Pharmaceutical Journal.* 2008;75:12-20.

[45] Wellbery, CE. Getting the facts on restless legs. *American Family Physician.* 2000;62: 51.

[46] Vergne-Salle, P; Coyral, D; Dufauret, K; Bonnet, C; Bertin, P; Trèves, R. Is restless legs *Joint Bone Spine.* 2006;73:369-373.

[47] Trenkwalder, C; Walters, AS; Hening, W. Periodic limb movements and restless legs syndrome. *Neurol. Clin.* 1996;14:629–650.

[48] Pollmacher, T; Schulz, H. Periodic leg movements (PLM): Their relationship to sleep stages. *Sleep.* 1993;16:572–577.

[49] Bae, CJ; Lee, JK; Foldvary-Schaefer, N. The use of sleep studies in neurologic practice. *Semin Neurol.* 2009;29:305-319.

[50] Pennestri, MH; Montplaisir, J; Colombo, R; Lavigne, G; Lanfranchi, PA. Nocturnal blood pressure changes in patients with restless legs syndrome. *Neurology.* 2007;68:1213-1218.

[51] American Academy of Sleep Medicine. *International Classification of Sleep Disorders,* Second Edition: Diagnostic and Coding Manual. Westchester, IL, American Academy of Sleep Medicine, 2005.

[52] Picchietti, D; Winkelman, JW. Restless legs *Sleep.* 2005;28:891-898.

[53] Vetrugno, R; Provini, F; Plazzi, G; Cortelli, P; Montagna, P. Propriospinal myoclonus: A motor phenomenon found in restless legs syndrome different from periodic limb movements during sleep. *Mov. Disord.* 2005;20:1323–1329.

[54] Ryan, M; Slevin, JT. Restless Legs Syndrome. *Journal of Pharmacy Practice.* 2007;20: 430-448.

[55] Montplaisir, J; Lorrain, D; Godbout, R. Restless legs syndrome and periodic leg movements in sleep: the primary role of dopaminergic mechanism. *Eur Neurol.* 1991;31:41–43.

[56] Trenkwalder, C; Paulus, W; Walters, AS. The restless legs syndrome. *Lancet Neurol.* 2005;4:465–475.

[57] Cervenka, S; Palhagen, SE; Comley, RA; Panagiotidis, G; Cselenyi, Z; Matthews , JC; Lai, RY; Halldin, C; Farde, L. Support for dopaminergic hypoactivity in restless legs syndrome: a PET study on D2-receptor binding. *Brain.* 2006;129:2017–2028.

[58] Earley, CJ; Connor, JR; Beard, JL; Malechi, EA; Epstein, DK; Allen, RP. Abnormalities in CSF concentrations of ferritin and transferin in restless legs syndrome. *Neurology.* 2000;54:1698–1700.

[59] Mizuno, S; Mihara, T; Miyaoka, T; Inagahi, T; Horiguchi, J. CSF iron, ferritin and transferrin levels in restless legs syndrome. *J. Sleep Res.* 2005;14:43–47.

[60] O'Keeffe, ST; Gavin, K; Lavan, JN. Iron status and restless legs syndrome in the elderly. *Age Ageing.* 1994;23:200-203.

[61] Sun, ER; Chen, CA; Ho, G; Earley, CJ; Allen, RP. Iron and the restless legs syndrome. *Sleep.* 1998;21:371-377.

[62] Allen, RP; Connor, JR; Hyland, K; Earley, CJ. Abnormally increased CSF 3-Ortho-methyldopa (3-OMD) in untreated restless legs syndrome (RLS) patients indicates more severe disease and possibly abnormally increased dopamine synthesis. *Sleep Med.* 2009;10:123-128.

[63] Connor, JR; Wang, XS; Allen, RP; Beard, JL; Wiesinger, JA; Felt, BT; Earley, JC. Altered dopaminergic profile in the putamen and substantia nigra in restless leg syndrome. *Brain.* 2009;132:2403–2412.

[64] Winkelman, JW. Considering the causes of RLS. *Eur. J. Neurol.* 2006;13:8-14.

[65] Erikson, KM; Jones, BC; Hess, EJ; Zhang, Q; Beard, JL. Iron deficiency decreases dopamine D1 and D2 receptors in rat brain. *Pharmacol. Biochem .Behav.* 2001;69:409–418.

[66] Bianco, LE; Unger, EL; Earley, CJ; Beard, JL. Iron deficiency alters the day night variation in monoamine levels in mice. *Chronobiol. Int.* 2009; 26:447– 463.

[67] Erikson, KM; Jones, BC; Beard, JL. Iron deficiency alters dopamine transporter functioning in rat striatum. *J. Nutr.* 2000;130:2831–2837.

[68] Earley, CJ; Connor, JR; Beard, JL; Clardy, SL; Allen, RP. Ferritin levels in the cerebrospinal fluid and restless legs syndrome: Effects of different clinical phenotypes. *Sleep.* 2005;28:1069–1075.

[69] Earley, CJ; Barker, PB; Horska, A; Allen, RP. MRI-determined regional brain iron concentrations in early- and late-onset restless legs syndrome. *Sleep Med.* 2006;7:458-461.

[70] Connor, JR; Boyer, PJ; Menzies, SL; Dellinger, B; Allen, RP; Ondo, WG; Earley, CJ. Neuropathological examination suggests impaired brain iron acquisition in restless legs syndrome. *Neurology.* 2003;61:304-309.

[71] Trenkwalder, C; Walters, AS; Hening, WA; Chokroverty, S; Antonini, A; Dhawan, V. Positron emission tomographic studies in the restless legs syndrome. *Mov. Disord.* 1999;1:141–145.

[72] Dowling, P; Klinker, F; Amaya, F; Paulus, W; Liebetanz, D. Iron-deficiency sensitizes mice to acute pain stimuli and formalin-induced nociception. *J. Nutr.* 2009;139:2087-2092.

[73] Winkelmann, J; Polo, O; Provini, F; Nevsimalova, S; Kemlink, D; Sonka, K. Genetics of restless legs syndrome (RLS): State-of-the-art and future directions. *Mov. Disord.* 2007;22:449-458.

[74] Winkelmann, J; Wetter, TC; Collado-Seidel, V; Gasser, T; Dichgans, M; Yassouridis, A. Clinical characteristics and frequency of the hereditary restless legs syndrome in a population of 300 patients. *Sleep.* 2000;23:597-602.

[75] Bassetti, Cl; Mauerhofer, D; Gugger, M; Mathis, J; Hess, CW. Restless legs syndrome: a clinical study of 55 patients. *Eur Neurol.* 2001;45:67-74.

[76] Winkelmann, J; Muller-Myhsok, B; Wittchen, HU; Hock, ***B;*** Prager, M; Pfister, H. Complex segregation analysis of restless legs syndrome provides evidence for an autosomal dominant mode of inheritance in early age at onset families. *Ann Neurol.* 2002;52:297-302.

[77] Trenkwalder, C; Seidel, VC; Gasser, T; Oertel, WH. Clinical symptoms and possible anticipation in a large kindred of familial restless legs syndrome. *Mov. Disord.* 1996;11: 389–394.

[78] Lazzarini, A; Walters, AS; Hickey, K; Coccagna, G; Lugaresi, E; Ehrenberg, BL; Picchietti, DL; Brin, MF; Stenroos, ES; Verrico, T; Johnson, WG. Studies of penetrance and anticipation in five autosomal-dominant restless legs syndrome pedigrees. *Mov. Disord.* 1999;14:111–116.

[79] Ondo, WG; Dat Vuong, K; Wang, Q. Restless legs syndrome in monozygotic twins: clinical correlates. *Neurology.* 2000;55:1404-1406.

[80] Winkelmann , J; Schormair, B; Lichtner, P; Ripke, S; Xiong, L; Jalilzadeh, S; Fulda, S; Pütz, B. Genome-wide association study of restless legs syndrome identifies common variants in three genomic regions. *Nat Genet.* 2007;39:1000–1006.

[81] Desautels, A; Turecki, G; Montplaisir, J; Sequeira, A; Verner, A; Rouleau, GA. Identification of a major susceptibility locus for restless legs syndrome on chromosome 12q. *Am. J. Hum. Genet.* 2001;69:1266-1270.

[82] Desautels, A; Turecki, G; Montplaisir, J; Xiong, L; Walters, AS; Ehrenberg, BL; Brisebois, K. Restless legs syndrome: confirmation of linkage to chromosome 12q, genetic heterogeneity, and evidence of complexity. *Arch. Neurol.* 2005;62:591-596.

[83] Kock, N; Culjkovic, B; Maniak, S; Schilling, K; Müller, B; Zühlke, C; Ozelius, L; Klein, C; Pramstaller, PP; Kramer, PL. Mode of inheritance and susceptibility locus for restless legs syndrome, on chromosome 12q. *Am. J. Hum. Genet.* 2002;71:205-208.

[84] Bonati, MT; Ferini-Strambi, L; Aridon, P; Oldani, A; Zucconi, M; Casari, G. Autosomal dominant restless legs syndrome maps on chromosome 14q. *Brain.* 2003;126:1485-1492.

[85] Winkelmann, J; Ferini-Strambi, L. Genetics of restless legs syndrome. *Sleep Med. Rev.* 2006;10:179-183.

[86] Chen, S; Ondo, WG; Rao, S; Li, L; Chen, Q; Wang, Q. Genomewide linkage scan identifies a novel susceptibility locus for restless legs syndrome on chromosome 9p. *Am. J. Hum. Genet.* 2004;74:876-885.

[87] Levchenko, A; Montplaisir, J; Dubé MP; Riviere, JB; St-Onge, J; Turecki, G; Xiong, L; Thibodeau, P; Desautels, A; Verlaan, DJ; Rouleau, GA. The 14q restless legs syndrome locus in the French Canadian population. *Ann. Neurol.* 2004;55:887-891.

[88] Levchenko, A; Montplaisir, JY; Asselin,G; Provost, S; Girard, SL; Xiong, L; Lemyre, E; St-Onge, J. Autosomal dominant locus for restless legs syndrome in French-Canadians on chromosome 16p12.1. *Mov. Disord.* 2009;24:40–50.

[89] Pichler, I; Hicks, AA; Pramstaller, PP. Restless legs syndrome: an update on genetics and future perspectives. *Clin. Genet.* 2008;73:297–305.

[90] Winkelmann, J; Lichtner, P; Schormair, B; Uhr, M; Hauk, S; Stiasny-Kolster, K; Trenkwalder, C; Paulus, W. Variants in the neuronal nitric oxide synthase (nNOS, NOS1) gene are associated with restless legs syndrome. *Mov. Disord.* 2008;23:350–358.

[91] Lohmann-Hedrich, K; Neumann, A; Kleensang, A; Lohnau, T; Muhle, H; Djarmati, A; König, IR; Pramstaller, PP; Schwinger, E. Evidence for linkage of restless legs syndrome to chromosome 9p: are there two distinct loci? *Neurology.* 2008;70:686–694.

[92] Young, JE; Vilarino-Guell, C; Lin, S-C; Wszolek, ZK; Farrer, M. Clinical and genetic description of a family with a high prevalence of autosomal dominant restless legs syndrome. *Mayo Clin. Proc.* 2009;84: 134–138.

[93] Stefansson, H; Rye, DB; Hicks, A; Petursson, H; Ingason, A; Thorgeirsson, TE; Palsson, S, Sigmundsson, T, Sigurdsson, AP. A genetic risk factor for periodic limb movements in sleep. *N. Engl. J. Med.* 2007;357:639-647.

[94] Tyvaert, L; Houdayer, E; Devanne, H; Bourriez, JL; Derambure, P; Monaca, C. Cortical involvement in the sensory and motor symptoms of primary restless legs syndrome. *Sleep Med.* 2009;10:1090–1096.

[95] Nordlander, NB. Therapy in restless legs. Acta Med Scand. 1953;145:453–457.

[96] Ulfberg, J; Nystrom, B. Restless legs syndrome in blood donors. *Sleep Med.* 2004;5:115–118.

[97] Rangarajan, S; D'Souza, GA. Restless legs syndrome in Indian patients having iron deficiency anemia in a tertiary care hospital. *Sleep Med.* 2007;8:247-251.

[98] Manconi, M; Govoni, V; De Vito, A; Economou, NT; Cesnik, E; Casetta, I; Mollica, G; Ferini-Strambi, L; Granieri, E. Restless legs syndrome and pregnancy. *Neurology* 2004; 63:1065–9.

[99] Hensley, JG. Leg cramps and restless legs syndrome during pregnancy. *J. Midwifery Womens Health.* 2009;54:211-218.

[100] Cavallini, L; Impedovo, A; Abaterusso, C; Loschiavo, C; Lupo, A. *G. Ital. Nefrol.* 2010;27:37-46.

[101] Winkelmann, J; Stautner, A; Samtleben, W; Trenkwalder, C. Long-term course of restless legs syndrome in dialysis patients after kidney transplantation. *Mov. Disord.* 2002; 17:1072–1076.

[102] Hening, WA; Caivano, CK. Restless legs syndrome: a common disorder in patients with rheumatologic conditions. *Semin. Arthritis Rheum.* 2008;38:55–62.

[103] Taylor-Gjevre, RM; Gjevre, JA; Skomro, R; Nair, B. Restless legs syndrome in a rheumatoid arthritis patient cohort. *J. Clin. Rheumatol.* 2009;15:12–15.

[104] Stehlik, R; Arvidsson, L; Ulfberg, J. Restless legs syndrome is common among female patients with fibromyalgia. *Eur. Neurol.* 2009;61:107–111.

[105] Trenkwalder, C; Paulus, W. Restless legs syndrome: pathophysiology, clinical presentation and management. *Nat. Rev. Neurol.* 2010;6:337-346.

[106] Ondo, WG. Restless legs syndrome. Curr Neurol Neurosci Rep. 2005;5:266–274.

[107] Welch, KM; Nagesh, V; Aurora, SK; Gelman, N. Periaqueductal gray matter dysfunction in migraine: cause or the burden of illness? *Headache* 2001; 41:629–637.

[108] Cologno, D; Cicarelli, G; Petretta, V; d'Onofrio, F; Bussone, G. High prevalence of dopaminergic premonitory symptoms in migraine patients with restless legs syndrome: a pathogenetic link? *Neurol. Sci.* 2008;29:166–168.

[109] Manconi, M; Rocca, MA; Ferini-Strambi, L; Tortorella, P; Agosta, F; Comi, G; Filippi, M. Restless legs syndrome is a common finding in multiple sclerosis and correlates with cervical cord damage. *Mult. Scler.* 2008;14:86–93.

[110] Ondo, WG; Vuong, KD; Jankovic, J. Exploring the relationship between Parkinson disease and restless legs syndrome. *Arch. Neurol.* 2002;59:421–424.

[111] Hattan, E; Chalk, C; Postuma, RB. Is there a higher risk of restless legs syndrome in peripheral neuropathy? *Neurology.* 2009;72:955–960.

[112] Ferini-Strambi, L. RLS-like symptoms: differential diagnosis by history and clinical assessment. *Sleep Med.* 2007;8:3-6.

[113] Riley, JD; Antony, SJ. Leg cramps: differential diagnosis and management. *Am. Fam. Physician.* 1995;52:1794-1798.

[114] Lakasing, E. Exercise beneficial for restless legs *Practitioner.* 2008;252:43-45.

[115] McManama Aukerman, M; Aukerman, D. Exercise and restless legs syndrome: a randomized controlled trial. *J. Am. Board Fam. Med.* 2006;19:487-493.

[116] Parker, KP; Rye, DB. Restless legs syndrome and periodic limb movement disorder. *Nurs Clin. N. Am.* 2002;37:655-673.

[117] Hening, W; Allen, R; Earley, C; Kushida, C; Picchietti, D; Silber, M. The treatment of restless legs syndrome and periodic limb movement disorder. *Sleep.* 1999;22:970-999.

[118] Conti, CF; de Oliviera, MM; Andriolo, RB; Saconato, H; Atallah, AN; Valbuza, JS; Coin de Carvalho, LB; do Prado, GF. Levodopa for idiopathic restless legs syndrome: evidence-based review. *Mov Disord.* 2007;22:1943–1951.

[119] Schapira, AH. Restless legs syndrome: an update on treatment options. *Drugs.* 2004;64:149-158.

[120] Paulus, W; Trenkwalder, C. Less is more: pathophysiology of dopaminergic-therapy-related augmentation in restless legs syndrome. *Lancet Neurol.* 2006;5:878-886.

[121] Comella, CL. Restless legs syndrome. Treatment with dopaminergic agents. *Neurology.* 2002;58:S87–92.

[122] Allen, RP; Earley, CJ. Augmentation of the restless legs syndrome with carbidopa / levodopa. *Sleep.* 1996;19: 205–213.

[123] Garcia-Borreguero, D. Augmentation: understanding a key feature of RLS. *Sleep Med.* 2004;5:5–6.

[124] Trenkwalder, C; Hogl, B; Benes, H; Kuhnen, R. Augmentation in restless legs syndrome is associated with low ferritin. *Sleep Med.* 2008;9:572–574.

[125] Paulus, W; Trenkwalder, C. Less is more: pathophysiology of dopaminergic-therapy-related augmentation in restless legs syndrome. *Lancet Neurol.* 2006;5:878-886.

[126] Happe, S; Trenkwalder, C. Role of dopamine receptor agonists in the treatment of restless legs syndrome. *CNS Drugs*. 2004;18:27–36.

[127] Oertel, WH; Stiasny-Kolster, K; Bergtholdt, B. Pramipexole RLS Study Group. Efficacy of pramipexole in restless legs syndrome: a six week, multicenter, randomized, double-blind study (effect-RLS study). *Mov Disord*. 2007;22:213–219.

[128] Winkelman, JW; Sethi, KD; Kushida, CA; Becker, PM; Koester, J; Cappola, JJ; Reess, J. Efficacy and safety of pramipexole in restless legs syndrome. *Neurology*. 2006;67:1034–1039.

[129] Partinen, M; Hirvonen, K; Jama, L; Alakuijala, A; Hublin, C; Tamminen, I; Koester, J; Reess, J. Efficacy and safety of pramipexole in idiopathic restless legs syndrome: a polysomnographic dose-finding study – the PRELUDE study. *Sleep Med.* 2006;7: 407–417.

[130] Brindani, F; Vitetta, F; Gemignani, F. Restless legs syndrome: differential diagnosis and management with pramipexole. *Clinical Interventions in Aging*. 2009:4;305–313.

[131] Trenkwalder C, Garcia-Borreguero D, Montagna P et al. Ropinirole in the treatment of restless legs syndrome: results from the TREAT RLS 1 study, a 12 week, randomised, placebo controlled study in 10 European countries. *J. Neurol. Neurosurg Psychiatry*. 2004; 75: 92–97.

[132] Allen, R; Becker, PM; Bogan, R; Schmidt, M; Kushida, CA; Fry, JM; Poceta, JS; Winslow, D. Ropinirole decreases periodic leg movements and improves sleep parameters in patients with restless legs syndrome. *Sleep*. 2004;27:839-841.

[133] Bogan, RK; Fry, JM; Schmidt, MH; Carson, SW; Ritchie, SY; for the TREAT RLS US Study Group. Ropinirole in the treatment of patients with restless legs syndrome: a US-based randomized, double-blind, placebo-controlled clinical trial. *Mayo Clin. Proc.* 2006;81:17–27.

[134] Garcia-Borreguero, D; Grunstein, R; Sridhar, G; Dreykluft, T; Montagna, P; Dom, R; Lainey, E; Moorat, A; Roberts, J. A 52-week open-label study of the long-term safety of ropinirole in patients with restless legs syndrome. *Sleep Med*. 2007;8:742–752.

[135] Montplaisir, J; Fantini, ML; Desautels, A; Michaud, M; Petit, D; Filipini, D. Long-term treatment with pramipexole in restless legs syndrome. *Eur. J. Neurol.* 2006;13:1306–1311.

[136] Trenkwalder, C; Benes, H; Poewe, W; Oertel, WH; Garcia-Borreguero, D; de Weerd, AW; and SP790 Study Group. Efficacy of rotigotine for treatment of moderate-to-severe restless legs syndrome: a randomised, double-blind, placebo-controlled trial. *Lancet Neurol*. 2008;7:595–604.

[137] Hening, WA; Allen, RP; Ondo, WG; Walters, AS; Winkelman, JW; Becker, P; Bogan, R; Fry, JM; Kudrow, DB; Lesh, KW; Fichtner, A; Schollmayer, E; on behalf of the SP792 Study Group. Rotigotine improves restless legs *Mov. Disord.* 2010. DOI: 10.1002/mds.23157.

[138] Allen, RP; Earley, CJ. Restless legs syndrome: a review of clinical and pathophysiologic features. *J. Clin. Neurophysiol.* 2001;18:128–147.

[139] Worthington, A; Thomas, L.Valvular heart disease *Eur. J. Echocardiogr.* 2008;9:828-830.

[140] Comella, CL. Restless legs syndrome. Treatment with dopaminergic agents. *Neurology*. 2002;58:87–92.

[141] Trenkwalder, C; Hening, WA; Montagna, P; Oertel, WH; Allen, RP; Walters, AS; Costa, J. Treatment of restless legs syndrome: an evidence-based review and implications for clinical practice. *Mov. Disord.* 2008;23:2267–2302.

[142] Gamaldo, CE; Earley, CJ. Restless legs syndrome: a clinical update. *Chest.* 2006; 130:1596–1604.

[143] Walters, AS; Winkelmann, J; Trenkwalder, C; Fry, JM; Kataria, V; Wagner, M; Sharma, R; Hening, W; Li, L. Long-term follow-up on restless legs syndrome patients treated with opioids. *Mov. Disord* 2001; 16: 1105–1109.

[144] Lauerma, H; Markkula, J. Treatment of restless legs syndrome with tramadol: an open study. *J. Clin. Psychiatry.* 1999;60:241–244.

[145] Walters, AS; Wagner, ML; Hening, WA; Grasing, K; Mills, R; Chokroverty, S; Kavey, N. Successful treatment of the idiopathic restless legs syndrome in a randomized double-blind trial of oxycodone versus placebo. *Sleep.* 1993;16:327–332.

[146] Ondo, WG. Methadone for refractory restless legs syndrome. *Mov. Disord.* 2005;20:345–348.

[147] Vetrugno, R; La Morgia, C; D'Angelo, R; Loi, D; Provini, F; Plazzi, G; Montagna, P. Augmentation of restless legs syndrome with long-term tramadol treatment. *Mov. Disord.* 2007;22:424–427.

[148] Fulda, S; Wetter, T. Where dopamine meets opioids: a metaanalysis of the placebo effect in restless legs syndrome. *Brain.* 2008;131:902–917.

[149] Saletu, M; Anderer, P; Saletu-Zyhlarz, G; Prause, W; Semler, B; Zoghlami, A. Restless legs syndrome (RLS) and periodic limb movements disorder (PLMD): acute placebo-controlled sleep laboratory studies with clonazepam. *Eur. Neuropsychopharmacol.* 2001;11:153–161.

[150] Mitler, MM; Browman, CP; Menn, SJ; Gujavarty, K; Timms, RM. Nocturnal myoclonus: treatment efficacy of clonazepam and temazepam. Sleep. 1986;9:385-392.

[151] Happe, S; Sauter, C; Klösch, G; Saletu, B; Zeitlhofer, J. Gabapentin versus ropinirole in the treatment of idiopathic restless legs syndrome. *Neuropsychobiology.* 2003;48:82–86.

[152] Garcia-Borreguero, D; Larrosa, O; de la Llave, Y; Verger, K; Masramon, X; Hernandez, G. Treatment of restless legs syndrome with gabapentin. *Neurology.* 2002; 59:1573–1579.

[153] Goodman, A. Pregabalin reported to improve restless legs symptoms and sleep. *Neurol. Today.* 2009;9:25–27.

[154] Garcia-Borreguero, D; Larrosa, O; Williams, AM; Albares, J; Pascual, M; Palacios, JC; Fernandez, C.Treatment of restless legs *Neurology.* 2010;74:1897-1904.

[155] Imamura, S; Kushida, C. Gabapentin enacarbil (XP13512/GSK1838262) as an alternative treatment to dopaminergic agents for restless legs syndrome. *Expert Opin. Pharmacother.* 2010;11:1925-1932.

[156] Kushida, CA; Becker, PM; Ellenbogen, AL; Canafax, DM; Barrett, R; for the XP052 Study Group. Randomized, double blind, placebo-controlled study of XP13512/ GSK1838262 in patients with RLS. *Neurology.* 2009;72:439–446.

[157] Telstad, W; Sorensen, O; Larsen, S; Lillevold, PE; Stensrud, P; Nyberg-Hansen, R. Treatment of the restless legs syndrome with carbamazepine: a double blind study. *BMJ.*1984;288:444–446.

[158] Lundvall, O; Abom, PE; Holm, R. Carbamazepine in restless legs: a controlled pilot study. *Eur. J. Clin. Pharmacol.* 1983;25:323–324.

[159] Eisensehr, I; Ehrenberg, BL; Solti, SR; Noachtar, S. Treatment of idiopathic restless legs syndrome (RLS) with slow-release valproic acid compared with slow-release levodopa/benserazid: a randomized, placebo-controlled, double-blind, cross-over study. *J .Neurol.* 2004;251:579-583.

[160] Wang, J; O'Reilly, B; Venkataraman, R; Mysliwiec, V; Mysliwiec, A. Efficacy of oral iron in patients with restless legs syndrome and a low-normal ferritin: a randomized, double-blind, placebo-controlled study. *Sleep Med.* 2009;doi:10.1016/j. *sleep.* 2008.11.003.

[161] Grote, L; Leissner, L; Hedner, J; Ulfberg, J. A randomized, double-blind, placebo controlled, multi-center study of intravenous iron sucrose and placebo in the treatment of restless legs syndrome. *Mov .Disord.* 2009;24:1445-1452.

[162] Sun, ER; Chen, CA; Ho, G; Earley, CJ; Allen, RP. Iron and the restless legs syndrome. *Sleep.* 1998;21:371-377.

[163] Krieger, J; Schroeder, C. Iron, brain and restless legs syndrome. *Sleep Med. Rev.* 2001; 5:277–286.

[164] Patrick, LR. Restless legs syndrome: pathophysiology and the role of iron and folate. *Altern. Med Rev.* 2007;12:101–12.

[165] Tunc, T; Karadaq, YS; Dogulu, F; Inan, LE. Predisposing factors of restless legs syndrome in pregnancy. *Mov. Disord.* 2007;22:627–631.

[166] Cui, Y; Wang, Y; Liu, Z. Acupuncture for restless legs syndrome. *Cochrane Database Syst. Rev.* 2008 Oct 8;(4):CD006457.

[167] Waldinger, MD; de Lint, GJ; Venema, PL; van Gils, AP; Schweitzer, DH. Successful transcutaneous electrical nerve stimulation in two women with restless genital syndrome: the role of adelta- and C-nerve fibers. *J. Sex Med.* 2010;7:1190-1199.

[168] Civardi, C; Collini, A; Monaco, F; Cantello, R. Applications of transcranial magnetic stimulation in sleep medicine. *Sleep Med. Rev.* 2009;13:35-46.

[169] Nilsson, SE. Electromagnetic therapy in restless legs syndrome and nocturnal leg muscle cramps. Same effect of pulsating electromagnetic fields and placebo. *Lakartidningen.* 2008;105:2167-2170.

[170] Shinno, H; Yamanaka, M; Ishikawa, I; Danjo, S; Nakamura, Y; Inami, Y; Horiguchi, J. Successful treatment of restless legs syndrome with the herbal prescription Yokukansan. *Prog. Neuropsychopharmacol Biol. Psychiatry.* 2010;34:252-253.

[171] Hayes, CA; Kingsley, JR; Hamby, KR; Carlow, J. The effect of endovenous laser ablation on restless legs syndrome. *Phlebology.* 2008;23:112-117.

[172] Hening, WA.Current guidelines *Am. J. Med.* 2007;120:22-27.

[173] Vignatelli, L; Billiard, M; Clarenbach, P; Garcia-Borreguero, D; Kaynak, D; Liesiene, V; Trenkwalder, C. EFNS guidelines on management of restless legs syndrome and periodic limb movement disorder in sleep. *Eur. J. Neurol.* 2006;13:1049-1065.

[174] Walters, AS; and the International Restless Legs Syndrome Study Group. Validation of the International Restless Legs Syndrome Study Group rating scale for restless legs syndrome. *Sleep Med.* 2003;4:121–132.

Reviewed by Ibrahim Tekeoglu, Professor Doctor, MD, Yuzuncu Yil University, Department of Physical Medicine and Rehabilitation and Rheumatology.

In: Movement Disorders: Causes, Diagnoses and Treatments
Editor: Barbara J. Larsen
ISBN 978-1-61209-200-3

Chapter IV

Psychiatric Comorbidities in Parkinson's Disease

***Ingrid de Chazeron**, *I. Chéreau-Boudet*† *and P. M. Llorca*‡**
Univ Clermont 1, UFR Medecine, EA3845, Clermont-Ferrand, F-63001 France, CHU Clermont-Ferrand, Psychiatry B, Clermont-Ferrand, F-63003, France

Abstract

Besides the classical motor symptoms, Parkinson's disease (PD) also leads to cognitive, behavioral and mood symptoms. Among them, impulsiveness disorders or addictive behaviors such as addiction to antiparkinsonian medications, compulsive behaviors, pathological gambling, hypersexuality and compulsive shopping have been reported. Hypersexuality in PD was first described in 1983 [1] and Molina et al. reported in 2000 [2] pathological gambling (PG). The same year, Giovannoni et al. [3] described Hedonistic Homeostatic Dysregulation (HHD), the original term for Dopamine Dysregulation Syndrome (DDS). Many recent studies have reported this syndrome suggesting that it could be more frequent than assumed [3-6] Recently in the field of impulsive disorders spectrum, binge-eating has also been described. Some patients may even develop addiction problems or behavioral symptoms in association with DDS and this co-occurrence has been already demonstrated by Laurence et al. in 2003 [5]. Depression, anxiety, apathy, anhedonia, mania/hypomania and hallucinations are among psychiatric disorders that also constitute the dark side of PD. Specific scales in each domain can be helpful in detecting not only severe but early cases.

Concerning the risk factors for addiction, several studies have now demonstrated an association with antiparkinsonian medications and behavioral disorders such as HS, PG and DDS. L-dopa in monotherapy and more specifically in higher doses can induce or worsen these disorders [7]. Dopamine agonists were also associated with DDS (4), PG and HS [8, 9]. The predominant role of dopamine agonists has been emphasized by Mamkinian et al (10). Recent studies [11, 12] show that dopamine agonists increase the

* Corresponding address: Rue Montalembert, 63000 Clermont-Ferrand, France, Phone +33 4 73 75 45 80, Fax +33 4 73 75 21 29, Email: idechazeron@chu-clermontferrand.fr.
† ichereau@chu-clermontferrand.fr
‡ pmllorca@chu-clermontferrand.fr

sensation of a "better than expected" outcome and impair the negative reinforcing effect of losing. However, controversy exists over the role and importance of L-dopa in relation to addiction/repetitive behaviors/impulse control disorders. Risk factors for depression, anxiety, apathy, anhedonia, mania/hypomania and hallucinations have been much debate and only recently considered to be a whole part of the disease. Global approach of psychiatric comorbidities in PD can be a good strategy for good management of this disease resulting in an improvement in the quality of life and suitable conditions for treatment by neurosurgery when indicated.

Introduction

Although the classical illustration of Parkinson's disease (PD) is tremor and motor symptoms, PD also leads to cognitive, behavioral and mood symptoms. Among them, some have defined addictive behaviors, characterized by impaired control over drug use/behavior, preoccupation with addictive behaviors, displaying addictive behavior despite adverse consequences, and having distortions in thinking [13]. This definition has psychological characteristics because the individual has an obsessive preoccupation with the substance/behavior which leads to another classification, frequently used by others: impulsive disorders. The incidence of addictive is estimated in PD between 10-15% [14, 15].

Depression, anxiety, apathy, anhedonia, mania/hypomania and hallucinations are among these disorders that constitute the dark side of PD. These non-motor aspects of PD like many other degenerative brain diseases [16] are not psychological reactions to the experience of having a devastating neurological disease. Psychiatric disorders are a complete part of the disease.

Addictions/ Impulse Disorders

These include pathological gambling, hypersexuality, compulsive shopping and addiction to antiparkinsonian medications. Recently, binge eating disorders have been also described [15].

Pathological Gambling

A number of studies have already associated pathological gambling with PD, suggesting that it is a frequent impulse control disorder characterized by excessive gambling [7]. Molina et al. [2] first reported pathological gambling (PG) in 2000. Pathological gamblers tend to report experience with many types of gambling (for example, casinos, lotteries ...), as well as losses that can range from several hundred to many thousands of dollars. Gambling persists despite pleas from others, as do the decimation of bank accounts and the destruction of careers and families. Sleeplessness, irritability and tension are often only relieved by gambling. For pathological gamblers in general, there is a high risk of suicide [17], but it is not known whether this association is true for people with PD.

The prevalence of pathological gambling in Parkinson's disease range from 2.2% [18] to 10% in patients taking dopamine agonists [15, 19-26]. By contrast, the lifetime prevalence of pathological gambling in the general population in Europe is around 1% to 2% [27, 28].

The identification of pathological gamblers was generally undertaken by the same screening tool (South Oaks Gambling Screen (SOGS)) [29]. The SOGS has been demonstrated to provide a reliable tool for identifying people who are currently problem gamblers [29]. The SOGS is scored by calculating the number of items endorsed out of 20 (20 items) but different cut-off point referencing could be taken [29, 30]. Caution must be taken concerning the time explored (lifetime or past-30-day) when using this tool. Massachusetts Gambling Screen [31] can also be used to identify problem or pathological gambling (pathological gambling, 5 criteria endorsed; problem gambling, 3-4 criteria endorsed).

Researchers are reporting a number of factors that appear to be associated with an increased risk of developing pathological gambling in response to treatment with dopamine agonists among Parkinson's disease (PD) patients. Their findings suggest that PD patients who have a younger age at PD onset, higher novelty-seeking traits, or a personal or family history of alcohol abuse have a greater risk of developing this sometimes-devastating response to therapy [14, 15]. A review in Movement Disorders in 2007 [32] found that pathological gambling behavior was diagnosed two to eight times more frequently among Parkinson's patients taking these agonists than among the general population. The predominant role of dopamine agonists has been emphasized by many authors [9, 10, 27] due to the reversibility of PG after stopping taking a dopamine agonist and adjusting the L-dopa daily dose. Other studies [8, 11, 12, 24, 25] show that dopamine agonists increase the sensation of a "better than expected" outcome and impair the negative reinforcing effect of losing. In the study of Giladi et al. 2007 [33], the longer duration of dopamine agonists treatment seems to influence the outcome.

Hypersexuality

Hypersexuality in PD was first described in 1983 [1]. It involves recurrent and excessive time consumed by sexual fantasies and urges, and by planning for and engaging in sexual behavior, and sexual behavior in association with repetitive but unsuccessful efforts to control or significantly reduce these sexual fantasies, urges, and behavior. Hypersexual behaviors range from intrusive sexual thoughts, urges or remarks, to overt, inappropriate and often offensive sexual behaviors [34]. There may be increased demands for sexual activity in an established context or attempts at indiscriminate sexual activity in random contexts. Some patients continually make inappropriate remarks in public while others - in a departure from previous behaviors - may begin to use pornography, patronize prostitutes, engage in internet-based sexual activity or develop paraphilias (intense, sexually arousing fantasies, urges or behaviors such as exhibitionism, cross-dressing or sado-masochism). There is clinically significant personal distress or impairment in social, occupational or other important areas of functioning associated with the frequency and intensity of these sexual fantasies, urges, and behaviors. These forms of hypersexuality may be accompanied by such disruptive experiences as irritability, anger, mood instability and disturbed sleep. Hypersexual behavior typically entails an increase in premorbid sexual activities as well as an increase in the variety of sexual behaviors [35].

Voon et al. study 2006 [7] suggest a current prevalence at 2.0%, lifetime prevalence at 2.4%; 2.6% to 3.5% for Weintraub et al. [15, 18]; 4.3% for Cooper et al. [36] and around 10% for Singh et al. [21, 26].

Even if, at first sight, pathological hypersexuality appears to be difficult to estimate because people may be embarrassed by its possible impact to social disability, self-assessment seems to be a good method to diagnose hypersexuality. Patients could be asked directly if they have participated in hypersexual behavior in a questionnaire. The Sexual Addiction Screening Test (SAST) [37] has been designed and validated to discriminate between addictive and non-addictive behavior. It is an early assessment tool for clinicians although it can be improved.

Several risk factors appear to be associated with an increased risk of developing hypersexuality in patients with PD [36, 38]: male gender, younger age at PD onset, current major depression and novelty-seeking behaviors. Pontone and colleagues [39] found an association with depressed mood, disinhibition, irritability, and appetite disturbance. Hypersexuality has been associated with dopaminergic drug therapy [7, 15, 35]. The role of dopamine agonists has been emphasized by Mamkinian et al [10] due to the reversibility of HS after stopping dopamine agonists and adjustment of the L-dopa daily dose. DA treatment was implicated in the emergence of the sexual behavior for Klos et al. 2005 [40]; rather than its longer duration for Giladi et al 2007 [33].

Compulsive Shopping

Although compulsive shopping/buying disorders (CBD) is not specifically described in DSM-IV, diagnostic criteria have been proposed. These include being frequently preoccupied with buying or subject to irresistible, intrusive, and/or senseless impulses to buy [41]; frequently buying unneeded items or more than can be afforded; shopping for periods longer than intended; and experiencing adverse consequences, such as marked distress, impaired social or occupational functioning, and/or financial problems [42)]which can even lead to suicide attempts [42-44] Four distinct phases of CBD have been identified [45]: 1) anticipation; 2) preparation; 3) shopping; and 4) spending.

Compulsive shopping prevalence in PD has been previously estimated between 0.4% - 2% [7, 18, 24, 43, 46-48] but it rises to more than 7% in other works: 10% of a sample of 50 consecutively evaluated PD patients who met criteria for compulsive buying in Isaias et al. study (26) and 7.2% in the recent Weintraub et al. study [15].

The diagnostic criteria for CBD proposed by McElroy et al. (42) has received widespread acceptance among researchers and has been used in several studies as a threshold for the disorder. The core elements of the criteria include: [1] Frequent preoccupation with shopping or intrusive, irresistible, 'senseless' buying impulses; (2) clearly buying more than is needed or can be afforded; [3] distress related to buying behavior; and [4] significant interference with work or social functioning. Compulsive Buying Scale can also been used [49]. The seven scale items reflect a need to spend money (items 1 and 6), awareness that spending behavior is aberrant (item 2), loss of control (items 3 and 4), buying things to improve mood (item 5), and probable financial problems (item 7). Some limitations in this screening tool are false positive and false negative rates. However, because CBD currently lacks definitive criteria, tools to identify it must be adapted to this evolution.

No specific factors have been associated with a higher risk for CBD because it is often contained within the wide spectrum of impulse control disorders. However, the longer duration of DA treatment [33] was suggested.

Addiction to Antiparkinsonian Medications

Abuse of anti-parkinsonian medications is another impulse-control disorder that can occur in people with PD. It consists of a pattern of inappropriate and excessive use of anti-parkinsonian medications (e.g., escalating daily dosages) along with drug-seeking behavior, tolerance and psychological dependence. The core features of DDS hoards in association with disabling mood and behavioral changes. Even early on in the course of their Parkinson's disease, affected patients will insist upon increases in dopaminergic medications to treat "unbearable" motor symptoms as well as psychological feelings. Increasingly, patients have a distorted view of "on-off" motor and mental states - that is, they describe an intense "high" and increased energy or well-being in the "on" state and irritability, anxiety, or even despair or suicidality in the "off" state. In 2000, Giovannoni et al. [3] described Hedonistic Homeostatic Dysregulation (HHD), the original term for Dopamine Dysregulation Syndrome (DDS).

Many recent studies have reported this syndrome suggesting that it could be more frequent than supposed [3-6]. One previous report [6] found DDS prevalence at 3-4%.

DDS can be investigated with the short screening questionnaire designed by Pezzella et al. [50]. It is based on the diagnostic criteria for DDS published originally in Givonnani study [3]. The questionnaire is directed at both patients and their caregivers and comprises the overuse of dopaminergic treatment and mood or behavioral changes.

The risk of developing DDS in PD patients with a history of affective disorder seems to be major. So, anxiety is a risk factor generally admitted and comprised in diagnostic criteria proposed for DDS syndrome by Pezzella et al. 2005 [6]. Anxiety could be a causal factor in the decision to use antiparkinsonian drugs in order to ameliorate symptoms and relive experiences bestowed by its beneficial motor effect. Other known risk factors have been described: young age at PD onset, male gender, heavy alcohol consumption, and illegal/experimental drug use [4-6, 51]. A recent study suggests that people in creative or artistic professions may be at additional risk of developing DDS [52].

Binge Eating Disorders

Binge-eating disorder (BED) is a syndrome that resembles bulimia nervosa and is characterized by episodes of uncontrolled eating, eating more rapidly than normal, eating alone, feeling disgusted, depressed or guilty after over-eating and eating large amounts of food when not feeling physically hungry. BED differs from bulimia nervosa in that sufferers do not engage in purging activities, like vomiting or laxative abuse. Eating disorders can be expressed by an increased appetite for noticeably sweet food (e.g., chocolate, cake, ice cream…). There was no organization in acute episodes of rapid ingestion but patients reported continuous and uncontrollable nibbling occurring randomly between meals, during the day, and sometimes at night when combined with insomnia. The amount and the ingredients of the regular meals were not altered. They used strategies to continue inappropriate eating behavior.

Compulsive or binge eating has been reported in PD, but its prevalence until recently was not known [3, 53]. Recent reports [15, 54] found compulsive eating in around 4.3% to 6% of Parkinson's disease patients

Diagnostic and Statistical Manual of Mental Disorders research criteria for binge-eating disorder [15] the Diagnostic and Statistical Manual of Mental Disorders (Fourth Edition, Text Revision) [13] proposed research criteria for binge-eating disorder (positive response to both gateway questions and 3 secondary questions). A self- questionnaire: Questionnaire on Eating and Weight Patterns-Revised (QEWP-R) [55] assesses a range of features associating the presence or absence of binge episodes and features related to BED. Another part of this questionnaire deals with obesity and eating disorders, such as dieting and weight history. The QEWP-R performed satisfactorily as initial screens for the diagnosis of BED [56, 57].

A longer duration of DA treatment [33] was associated with the new-onset heightened interest in or motivation for eating. Nirenberg and Waters [53] described the case of 7 PD patients who presented eating compulsions and concurrent weight gain as a result of being on Pramipexole medication. Four of these patients concomitantly exhibited other compulsive behaviors. Khan and Rana [58] confirm this by a case description of a patient who developed a compulsive eating disorder when treated with a dopamine agonist, pramipexole.

Punding

Punding is characterized by typical behaviors including an intense fascination with repetitive manipulations of technical equipment, the continual examining, handling; sorting of common objects, hoarding (e.g., collecting, arranging, or taking apart objects), excessive grooming and walkabout, defined as excessive, aimless wandering [3, 59-62]. Originally described by Rylander in 1972 [63] in amphetamine and cocaine addicts, the first description of punding in an L-dopa treated patient was in 1994 [61].

Regarding punding, in one series examining PD patients on higher L-dopa equivalent daily dosages (LEDDs), 14% met criteria for punding (59), but another, wider study of unselected PD patients reported a prevalence rate of 1.4% (64). This prevalence in more recent studies was intermediate in the range of those described previously:

8.2% in the Nguyen's cohort [65] and 4.2% in Lee et al. study [66].

Punding behaviors can be assessed by a self-reporting questionnaire: the Punding Scale that has been recently developed by Lawrence [67] in relation with Evans criteria for punding [59]. This questionnaire was scored separately for each activity giving a value between 0 and 42, with higher scores indicative of punding. The punding can be also evaluated using the Ardouin Scale [68]. This is a new scale based on the concept of hypo- and hyperdopaminergic mood and behavior is in validation. It is a semi-structured interview and one part addresses hyperdopaminergic behaviors including one item on punding. Open-ended questions introduce each item, allowing patients to express themselves as freely as possible. Close-ended questions permit the rating of severity and intensity.

Factors associated with punding include younger disease onset, impulsivity, and higher dopamine agonist dose [59, 64, 67] or higher LEDDs (59) or L-dopa [69].

Other Addictions?

In general population, alcohol, cigarettes and marijuana appear to remain the first three abuse/dependence substances. However, these substances have been investigated in risk factors for Parkinson disease but poorly during the disease.

If tobacco smokers have a well-documented lowered incidence of PD compared to general population, tobacco dependency in PD patients is consequently not studied. A lower prevalence of smokers in PD compared to general population has been previously observed in other studies [70, 71]. The range of smokers in PD patients is from 5.2% to 34.0% [70-72].

Both alcohol misuse and dependence may in general be less common in PD than in general population [72, 73]. Significantly fewer PD patients drink alcohol compared to control population; around 30% are fully abstinent [73].

For these two substances, more than the prevalence, the dependence profile for PD patients has not been studied.

Little is known on prevalence of marijuana consumption in PD. Only the study of Venderová et al. [74] evaluates this possible experience. Cannabis use was reported by 25% of PD patients, most of them using approximately half a teaspoon of fresh or dried leaves orally. None of the patients had any experience with recreational use of cannabis before taking it to alleviate PD symptoms. Patients mostly decide to take cannabis based on information presented in the media. So, recently, among cannabis compounds, cannabidiol (CBD) has been presented to be a very promising agent in neuroprotective actions and with the highest prospect for therapeutic use [75].

Concerning available tools for assessing tobacco dependency, the Fagerström Test for Nicotine Dependence (FTND) [76] is a screening tool for physical nicotine dependence and is used extensively in various countries. It consists of six items and is easily understood and rapidly applied. The scores obtained enable classification of nicotine dependence into five levels: none (0-2 points); low (3-4 points); medium (5-6 points); high (7-8 points); and very high (9-10 points).

The Alcohol Use Disorders Identification Test (AUDIT) consists of 10 items. Each question is scored from 0 to 4. It was originally designed for use in primary health care settings to detect early hazardous or harmful drinking [77]. Participants diagnosed as "alcohol dependent" have an AUDIT cut-off point of 11 and 8 for "harmful users".

An initial validation of the Cannabis Use Problems Identification Test (CUPIT), a brief self-reporting screen developed to expedite detection of currently and potentially problematic cannabis use has been described [78]. The 16 CUPIT items measure the DSM/ICD three-dimensional concept of risky use, dependence/using behavior, health and social problems, requiring a reading level of approximately 7/8 years' schooling and about 5 minutes administration time. Scores can range from 0 (no use at all) to 82 (daily/more than daily use, severely problematic). Rapidly scored and interpreted, self- or other-administered, the CUPIT can be use as a population screener.

Co-Addictions

Co-addictions have been little explored in Parkinson's disease even if there is a growing recognition that synergistically chronic dependence on multiple physiologically addictive substances and/or behaviors may occur. All classes of addiction could share a possible common physiopathology. Consistent with a possible dissociation between natural reward and drugs of abuse, the study of Lardeux et al. 2008 [79] has recently shown that sub-populations of subthalamic nucleus neurons exhibit specific responses to either cocaine or sucrose rewards, suggesting that reward-dependent microcircuits may also exist within the subthalamic nucleus.

In the large study of over 3000 PD patients [15], current cigarette smoking has been found as additional variables independently associated with compulsive behaviors. Frequently, more than one impulse-control disorder is present for 4 percent of patients, sometimes accompanied by psychotic symptoms (that is, hallucinations or delusions) or a mood disorder (depression or anxiety) [15]. Evans et al. [59] conclude that punding and DDS often co-occur. Pathological gambling can be associated with the presence of other compulsive disorders such as the compulsive use of dopaminergic drugs [3], compulsive shopping, and hypersexuality [23].

Hallucinations

The latter definition distinguishes hallucinations from the related phenomena of dreaming, which does not involve wakefulness; illusion, which involves distorted or misinterpreted real perception; imagery, which does not mimic real perception and is under voluntary control. Hallucinations can occur in any sensory modality (visual, auditory, olfactory, gustatory, tactile, proprioceptive…). Studies on psychosis have mostly focused on visual hallucinations, the most common type of psychotic symptom in PD. Commonly reported experiences are visions of animals, persons, and other figures going about normal and appropriate activities. These hallucinations tend to present in a repetitive and stereotyped fashion and frequently become familiar to the patient. Simpler hallucinations may be flashes of light, swirling shapes, or a transient, vague image in the peripheral field (passage hallucination) [80]. Mixed hallucinations combining different modalities may also occur [81]. Some PD patients report a frequent sensation of an unidentified presence, often called a "guardian angel" [82]. Psychotic symptoms (hallucinations) may be mild or severe, occur together or single. Patient can be able to appreciate its false nature (good insight) but some patients may try to interact with its (loss of insight). Hallucinations are more common in the evening and at night, usually favored by dim light, low competing sensory stimulation, or reduced vigilance [82, 83].

In a recent meta-analysis [84] of prospective studies, visual hallucinations were reported in 16–37% of patients and auditory in less than 2–22%. Therefore, the total lifetime prevalence of hallucinations of all types was around 46% [82].

There are several rating scales in use, although no generally accepted ones. Item 2 of the Unified Parkinson's Disease Rating Scale (UPDRS) (85) subscale 1 can be used, and also the neuropsychiatric inventory (NPI) [86]. Recent reviews [87, 88] have compared the different scales, listed their strengths and weaknesses and provided some guidelines regarding recommendations.

Dementia has been the single most commonly identified risk factor for psychotic symptoms [82, 84, 89-91]. Day time somnolence, but not severe sleep disorders, was an independent predictive factor for visual hallucinations [82]. Older age, and disease duration are associated with hallucinations [82, 84]. Sufferers of coexisting depression has been suggested to be at risk of developing hallucinations [82, 83]. Drug treated patients are at much higher risk than non-treated patients even if the exact role of the medications in causing psychotic symptoms is unclear [92]. Other studies concluded that there are no effects of chronic drug dosage or drug class (L-dopa or agonists) that impact on the risk of developing visual hallucinations [82, 83, 93].

Depression / Anxiety

Anxiety and depression frequently occur and often coexist in patients with Parkinson disease. The most common anxiety disorders in PD are panic attacks (often during off-periods), generalized anxiety disorder (GAD), simple and social phobias [87]. Distinctive features of depression in PD include elevated levels of dysphoria, irritability, relative absence of guilt or feelings of failure and a low suicide rate despite a high frequency of suicidal ideation [94]. The key characteristics of depression are low mood and lack of interest or pleasure (anhedonia), one of which is required for a diagnosis of depression in most classifications. Other features of depression may be present in varying combinations but many of these, such as altered appetite or sleep, weight change, loss of libido, psychomotor retardation, reduced memory, and loss of energy may overlap with the symptoms of PD, making diagnosis of depression in PD difficult [87]. Whereas major depression, defined by DSM-IV [13], is uncommon and accounts for 10% of these cases, the remaining have less severe symptoms, but experience feelings of sadness with loss of energy and reduced vitality (95). These symptoms are not usually chronic, but occur at two temporal points in PD, early in the disease near the time of diagnosis and late in the disease as disability and impairment increase [96, 97].

Anxiety and depression are both common in people with PD and there is a wide range in results for their prevalence in PD patients: 5.3% - 40% for anxiety disorders [87, 98] and 2.7% - 90% for depression [87, 94, 99-101]. This large variation is probably due to the variability of scale used and the severity of depressive/anxiety symptoms. More probably, anxiety affects around one third percent to 40% of PD patients [102-108] and approximately 40%-45% of PD patients had mild to moderate depressive symptoms (97, 101, 109, 110). Current depressive illness is significantly more prevalent in PD sufferers (11.3%) compared with age and sex matched non-sufferers (3.5%), in agreement with other works [94]. In studies using structured interviews and standardized diagnostic criteria, the prevalence of major depressive disorder in patients with PD ranges from 2.3% to 55.6% [101].

Concerning scales, Beck Anxiety Inventory, the BAI, is a self report questionnaire that consists of 21 items meant to measure the severity of somatic, affective, and cognitive symptoms associated with panic attacks and generalized anxiety in a psychiatric population [111]. A higher score indicates more severe anxiety symptoms. In the recent publication comparing properties of anxiety rating scales in PD, the BAI is probably a good scale to study the epidemiology and markers of anxiety symptoms, and for monitoring changes in symptom severity as a result of treatment [105]. A problem still remain, as in many anxiety scale, it has symptoms that overlap with somatic and cognitive symptoms of PD as well. It is the same for depression scales. As differentiation of overlapping symptoms of depression and PD remains difficult, clinical rating scales should be used only with adjustment for severity and change in PD symptoms using appropriate scales [112]. For screening purposes, the Hamilton Depression Rating Scale (HAM-D) [113] and the Montgomery-Åsberg Depression Rating Scale (MADRS) [114] have better psychometric properties. However interviewers must have clinical psychiatric training in the specification of symptoms [97].

The 17-item version of the HAM-D, interviewer-administered, is more commonly used, nine of the items are scored on a five-point scale, ranging from zero to four and eight items are scored on a three-point scale, from zero to two. The total score can range from 0 to 54. One formulation suggests that scores between 7 and 17 indicate mild depression, between 18 and 24 indicate moderate depression, and scores over 24 indicate severe depression.

The MADRS is a ten-item diagnostic questionnaire. It has a fixed scaling of seven points (from 0 through 6). A MADRS cut-off score of 6 is frequently used to detect the presence of depression in PD [115, 116] but some define a cut-off score of 10 [117].

Experience of dyskinesias or on/off fluctuations showed positive associations with anxiety, while L-dopa dosage had no effect [103, 118]. Other "subtypes" of PD have been previously shown to be associated with anxiety as gait dysfunction and freezing [103, 119-121]. Anxiety disorders and depressive disorders may share familial susceptibility factors (genetic or non-genetic) with PD [122].

Concerning depression disorders risk factor, there is no linear correlation with duration or severity of PD (94) even if there's a higher risk of depression in patients with younger age at onset of PD [123]. Previous studies have reported that cognitive impairment and apathy are significantly associated with depression [124, 125].

Apathy

"Parkinson's apathy" includes difficulty initiating projects, inability to follow complex instructions, short-term memory loss, and difficulty in switching gears midstream. The symptoms of apathy are closely related to anhedonia and depression, and are sometimes difficult to recognize. Apathy may occur as part of another disorder (notably depression and dementia) or as an isolated syndrome. For example it can exist in the absence of depression [126]. The distinction to separate depression from apathy is that the key characteristic of depression is sadness and is perceived by the patient as negative, whereas apathy is affectively neutral to the patient [109]. Apathy has been associated with more severe cognitive dysfunction and a decrease in performing activities of daily living (ADL) [127-130].

Apathy is reported in 17% to 70% of all PD patients [126-132] influenced by the extent of cognitive impairment and depressive symptoms in the sample, the assessment tools used, and the person undertaking the rating (i.e., a clinician, family member, or patient) [87].

Apathy symptoms in the absence of depression occur in 4%–30% (14% average prevalence) and reported prevalence for the combination of apathy and depression is 12%–47% [126-129, 131, 133].

The lack of generally accepted diagnostic criteria for apathy as a syndrome means that there is no gold standard to assess such psychometric properties in the sensitivity and specificity of scales [105]. The Lille Apathy Rating Scale Assessment [134] was especially designed for patients with PD and validated in a group of PD patients with and without dementia. The LARS is a recently developed scale that consists of 33 items divided into nine domains. It is undertaken as a structured interview with the patient. The LARS has been validated against a clinical judgment of apathy; it showed good sensitivity and specificity of apathy in non-demented patients.

Because apathy is often associated with cognitive decline, the assessment of apathy in demented patients may prove especially problematic. It is for this reason that the Dementia Apathy Interview and Rating scale (DAIR) seems to be a good tool [135]. DAIR is a 16-item structured interview with the primary caregiver designed to assess illness-related changes in motivation, emotional responsiveness, and engagement. The apathy score is a sum of all items reflecting change, divided by the number of items completed, with higher scores representing greater average apathy. Apathy scores can range from 0 (patient shows apathetic behavior almost never or less than once a week) to 3 (patient shows apathetic behavior almost always or almost every day).

Dementia at baseline and a more rapid decline in speech and axial impairment during follow-up were independent risk factors for incident apathy [132]. Previous studies have shown that dopaminergic treatment may decrease apathy in patients with PD without dementia and major depression [136] and a recent study [132] suggests that dopaminergic dysfunction does not play a major role in the pathophysiology of apathy in more advanced PD with comorbid depression and dementia.

Anhedonia

In psychology and psychiatry, anhedonia is an inability to experience pleasurable emotions from normally pleasurable life events such as eating, exercise or social interaction. Anhedonia is generally seen as a symptom and not a syndrome. Anhedonia is often seen as a core symptom of major depressive disorder. Its broad definition does not deal with the full symptom picture [137]. Treadway and Zald [138] evoked and the clinician may adopt specific terms like "motivational anhedonia" ("anticipatory" pleasure) and "consumer anhedonia" (emotion or pleasure "in-the-moment"). The adoption of specific terms like "motivational" and "consumer" are recommended as a means of refining the description of anhedonic symptoms. This has already begun to occur in the schizophrenia literature [137, 139] and should be extended to other disorders that feature alterations in reward processing. Thus, this distinction between different forms of anhedonia could have a strong heuristic value in PD patients [140].

Lemke et al. [141] found that 45.7% of all patients, in agreement with the prior study of Isella [142]. Lemke et al. [141] also observed that 79.7% of depressed Parkinson's disease patients suffered from anhedonia.

The self-rating Snaith-Hamilton Pleasure Scale (SHAPS) [141, 143, 144] is a practical, reliable instrument to assess anhedonia in patients with Parkinson's disease. Although only the transcultural validity of the SHAPS has been validated in PD patients [141, 145], it is the most frequently used scale to assess anhedonia in this population and has clinically proven its usefulness [105]. The SHAPS range scores from 0 to 14, higher values representing more severe anhedonia; cut-off score for anhedonia is ≥ 3).

Independent of the clear and established importance of anhedonia in depression, its clinical characteristics (disease duration, disease severity, motor disability) appear not to affect anhedonia in patients with Parkinsonism [142, 145]. Neuropsychological and quantitative neuroradiological features also do not show any significant correlation with physical anhedonia [142].

Mania /Hypomania

Impulsive behaviors in people with Parkinson's can also be a feature of hypomanic or manic disturbances, which are typically characterized by persistently elevated, expansive, grandiose or irritable mood states. Hypomanic episodes differ from manic ones by the absence of psychotic symptoms and in that they do not cause significant distress or impair one's work, family, or social life in an obvious way.

Theses behaviors tend to be associated in time in PD with motor fluctuations manifested by "on" and "off" phases. For example, patients experience elevated mood (euphoria and hypomania) during the "on" phase [146]. However, mood fluctuations may also occur without evident motor fluctuations in some patients [147]. Hypomania can be seen in patients with DDS [3].

The prevalence of mania and hypomania in PD is not known. It is probably due to the difficulty of diagnosing them in PD because of the overlap of symptoms between PD and hypomania. These complex problems require detailed assessment and diagnosis by specialist PD services, with input from psychiatrists and/or clinical psychologists. Mood fluctuations (profound mood changes from depression to hypomania that can occur several times a day) have been estimated to occur in 7%–21% of patients with Parkinson's disease [147].

For mania, the most frequently used scale is the Young Mania Rating Scale (YMRS) [148]. This scale is used however to assess illness severity in patients already diagnosed with mania. The Altman Mania Rating Scale (ASRM) [149] may be a good tool in the diagnosis of manic symptoms and for assessing both the presence and the severity of the symptoms. It is a professional scale used that consists of five items. It may be used as a screening tool to detect manic symptoms for clinical or research purposes. It correlates with the (YMRS) [148] and it is compatible with the DSM-IV criteria [13].

The Hypomania/Mania Symptom Checklist (HCL-32) [150] is a self-screening tool to diagnose people with bipolar disorder. It comprises a checklist of possible symptoms of hypomania that are rated yes (present or typical of me) or no (not present or not typical) by the subject. Although the HCL-32 is a sensitive instrument for hypomanic symptoms, it does not distinguish between bipolar disorders (from axis I or II) [150].

Previous reports associate mania with excess dopaminergic stimulation or hyperkinetic movement disorders [151, 152]. Moreover, since depression and mania are the opposite poles of a continuum of mood changes, some case-reports describe development of a manic episode following treatment of depression in PD [153, 154]..

Conclusion

Addictions and other psychiatric complications are frequent and must not be underestimated. Clinical assessment using specific questions or scales can be useful for their management and should be done as soon as possible. If treatment-related risk factors including the use of L-dopa or agonist therapy have been evoked in many cases, multifactor etiology remains a matter of debate.

Psychiatric comorbidities in Parkinson's disease are important factors that can impair quality of life, affect disease prognosis, and even impede treatment by over-consuming treatment or compromising medication adherence.

References

[1] Vogel HP, Schiffter R. Hypersexuality--a complication of dopaminergic therapy in Parkinson's disease. *Pharmacopsychiatria* 1983;16(4):107-10.

[2] Molina JA, Sainz-Artiga MJ, Fraile A, Jimenez-Jimenez FJ, Villanueva C, Orti-Pareja M, et al. Pathologic gambling in Parkinson's disease: a behavioral manifestation of pharmacologic treatment? *Mov. Disord.* 2000;15(5):869-72.

[3] Giovannoni G, O'Sullivan JD, Turner K, Manson AJ, Lees AJ. Hedonistic homeostatic dysregulation in patients with Parkinson's disease on dopamine replacement therapies. *J. Neurol. Neurosurg. Psychiatry* 2000;68(4):423-8.

[4] Evans AH, Lawrence AD, Potts J, Appel S, Lees AJ. Factors influencing susceptibility to compulsive dopaminergic drug use in Parkinson disease. *Neurology* 2005; 65(10):1570-4.

[5] Lawrence AD, Evans AH, Lees AJ. Compulsive use of dopamine replacement therapy in Parkinson's disease: reward systems gone awry? Lancet Neurol 2003;2(10):595-604.

[6] Pezzella FR, Colosimo C, Vanacore N, Di Rezze S, Chianese M, Fabbrini G, et al. Prevalence and clinical features of hedonistic homeostatic dysregulation in Parkinson's disease. *Mov. Disord.* 2005;20(1):77-81.

[7] Voon V, Hassan K, Zurowski M, de Souza M, Thomsen T, Fox S, et al. Prevalence of repetitive and reward-seeking behaviors in Parkinson disease. *Neurology* 2006;67(7):1254-7.

[8] Dodd ML, Klos KJ, Bower JH, Geda YE, Josephs KA, Ahlskog JE. Pathological gambling caused by drugs used to treat Parkinson disease. *Arch. Neurol.* 2005; 62(9):1377-81.

[9] Driver-Dunckley E, Samanta J, Stacy M. Pathological gambling associated with dopamine agonist therapy in Parkinson's disease. *Neurology* 2003;61(3):422-3.

[10] Mamikonyan E, Siderowf AD, Duda JE, Potenza MN, Horn S, Stern MB, et al. Long-term follow-up of impulse control disorders in Parkinson's disease. *Mov. Disord.* 2008; 23(1):75-80.

[11] van Eimeren T, Ballanger B, Pellecchia G, Miyasaki JM, Lang AE, Strafella AP. Dopamine agonists diminish value sensitivity of the orbitofrontal cortex: a trigger for pathological gambling in Parkinson's disease? *Neuropsychopharmacology* 2009; 34(13):2758-66.

[12] Voon V, Pessiglione M, Brezing C, Gallea C, Fernandez HH, Dolan RJ, et al. Mechanisms underlying dopamine-mediated reward bias in compulsive behaviors. *Neuron* 2010;65(1):135-42.

[13] Association AP. Diagnostic and statistical manual of mental disorders. Fourth Edition ed. Washington: APA; 1994.

[14] Voon V, Thomsen T, Miyasaki JM, de Souza M, Shafro A, Fox SH, et al. Factors associated with dopaminergic drug-related pathological gambling in Parkinson disease. *Arch. Neurol.* 2007;64(2):212-6.

[15] Weintraub D, Koester J, Potenza MN, Siderowf AD, Stacy M, Voon V, et al. Impulse control disorders in Parkinson disease: a cross-sectional study of 3090 patients. *Arch. Neurol.* 2010;67(5):589-95.

[16] Liszewski CM, O'Hearn E, Leroi I, Gourley L, Ross CA, Margolis RL. Cognitive impairment and psychiatric symptoms in 133 patients with diseases associated with cerebellar degeneration. *J. Neuropsychiatry Clin. Neurosci.* 2004;16(1):109-12.

[17] Hodgins DC, Mansley C, Thygesen K. Risk factors for suicide ideation and attempts among pathological gamblers. *Am. J. Addict.* 2006;15(4):303-10.

[18] Weintraub D. Impulse control disorders in Parkinson's disease: prevalence and possible risk factors. *Parkinsonism Relat Disord.* 2009;15 Suppl 3:S110-3.

[19] Avanzi M, Baratti M, Cabrini S, Uber E, Brighetti G, Bonfa F. Prevalence of pathological gambling in patients with Parkinson's disease. *Mov. Disord.* 2006; 21(12):2068-2072.

[20] Crockford D, Quickfall J, Currie S, Furtado S, Suchowersky O, El-Guebaly N. Prevalence of problem and pathological gambling in Parkinson's disease. *J. Gambl. Stud* .2008; 24(4):411-422.

[21] Singh A, Kandimala G, Dewey RB, Jr., O'Suilleabhain P. Risk factors for pathologic gambling and other compulsions among Parkinson's disease patients taking dopamine agonists. *J. Clin. Neurosci* .2007;14(12):1178-81.

[22] Volberg RA, Banks SM. A review of two measures of pathological gambling in the United States. *J. Gambl. Stud.* 1990;6:153-63.

[23] Voon V, Hassan K, Zurowski M, Duff-Canning S, de Souza M, Fox S, et al. Prospective prevalence of pathologic gambling and medication association in Parkinson disease. *Neurology* 2006;66(11):1750-2.

[24] Lu C, Bharmal A, Suchowersky O. Gambling and Parkinson disease. *Arch. Neurol.* 2006;63(2):298.

[25] Grosset KA, Macphee G, Pal G, Stewart D, Watt A, Davie J, et al. Problematic gambling on dopamine agonists: Not such a rarity. *Mov. Disord* .2006;21(12):2206-8.

[26] Isaias IU, Siri C, Cilia R, De Gaspari D, Pezzoli G, Antonini A. The relationship between impulsivity and impulse control disorders in Parkinson's disease. *Mov. Disord.* 2008;23(3):411-5.

[27] Tyne HL, Medley G, Ghadiali E, Steiger MJ. Gambling in Parkinson's disease. *Mov. Dis.* 2004;19((suppl 9)).

[28] Biganzoli A, Capelli M, Capitanucci D, Smaniotto R, Alippi M. [An investigation into pathological gambling. Epidemiological study of gambling attitudes and prevalence of pathological gambling in the Pavia province (Italy)]. 2004.

[29] Lesieur HR, Blume SB. The South Oaks Gambling Screen (SOGS): a new instrument for the identification of pathological gamblers. *Am. J. Psychiatry* 1987;144(9):1184-8.

[30] Shaffer HJ, Hall MN. Estimating prevalence of adolescent gambling disorders: A quantitative synthesis and guide toward standard gambling nomenclature. *J. Gambling Stud.* 1996;12:193-214.

[31] Shaffer HJ, LaBrie R, Scanlan KM, Cummings TN. Pathological gambling among adolescents: Massachusetts gambling screen (MAGS*). J. Gambl. Stud* 1994.

[32] Gallagher DA, O'Sullivan SS, Evans AH, Lees AJ, Schrag A. Pathological gambling in Parkinson's disease: risk factors and differences from dopamine dysregulation. An analysis of published case series. *Mov. Disord.* 2007;22(12):1757-63.

[33] Giladi N, Weitzman N, Schreiber S, Shabtai H, Peretz C. New onset heightened interest or drive for gambling, shopping, eating or sexual activity in patients with Parkinson's disease: the role of dopamine agonist treatment and age at motor symptoms onset. *J. Psychopharmacol.* 2007;21(5):501-6.

[34] Kafka MP. Hypersexual disorder: a proposed diagnosis for DSM-V. *Arch. Sex Behav.* 2010;39(2):377-400.

[35] Shaw P, Blockley A, Clough C, Chaudhuri R, Weeks R, David AS. Hypersexuality and Parkinson's disease. *J. Neurol. Neurosurg. Psychiatry* 2003;74(6):834.

[36] Cooper CA, Mikos AE, Wood MF, Kirsch-Darrow L, Jacobson CE, Okun MS, et al. Does laterality of motor impairment tell us something about cognition in Parkinson disease? Parkinsonism Relat Disord 2009;15(4):315-7.

[37] Carnes PJ. Out of the Shadows.Understanding sexual addiction. 3rd Revised edition ed. Center City; 2001.

[38] Jeffrey S. Factors Associated with Hypersexuality in PD Patients. In. International Congrcss of Parkinson's Disease and Movement Disorders (Poster presentation); 2007.

[39] Pontone G, Williams JR, Bassett SS, Marsh L. Clinical features associated with impulse control disorders in Parkinson disease. *Neurology* 2006;67(7):1258-61.

[40] Klos KJ, Bower JH, Josephs KA, Matsumoto JY, Ahlskog JE. Pathological hypersexuality predominantly linked to adjuvant dopamine agonist therapy in Parkinson's disease and multiple system atrophy. *Parkinsonism Relat. Disord.* 2005;11(6):381-6.

[41] Black DW. Compulsive buying disorder: definition, assessment, epidemiology and clinical management. *CNS Drugs* 2001;15(1):17-27.

[42] McElroy SL, Keck PE, Jr., Pope HG, Jr., Smith JM, Strakowski SM. Compulsive buying: a report of 20 cases. *J. Clin. Psychiatry* 1994;55(6):242-8.

[43] Koran LM, Faber RJ, Aboujaoude E, Large MD, Serpe RT. Estimated prevalence of compulsive buying behavior in the United States. *Am. J. Psychiatry* 2006; 163(10):1806-12.

[44] O'Guinn TC, Faber RJ. Compulsive buying: a phenomenological exploration. *J. Consum. Res.* 1989;16:147-57.

[45] Black DW. A review of compulsive buying disorder. *World Psychiatry* 2007;6(1):14-8.

[46] Ceravolo R, Frosini D, Rossi C, Bonuccelli U. Impulse control disorders in Parkinson's disease: definition, epidemiology, risk factors, neurobiology and management. *Parkinsonism Relat Disord.* 2009;15 Suppl 4:S111-5.

[47] Christenson GA, Faber RJ, de Zwaan M, Raymond NC, Specker SM, Ekern MD, et al. Compulsive buying: descriptive characteristics and psychiatric comorbidity. *J. Clin. Psychiatry* 1994;55(1):5-11.

[48] Kenangil G, Ozekmekci S, Sohtaoglu M, Erginoz E. Compulsive behaviors in patients with Parkinson's disease. *Neurologist* 2010;16(3):192-5.

[49] Faber RJ, O'Guinn TC. A clinical screener for compulsive buying. *J. Consumer Res.* 1992;19:459-69.

[50] Pezzella FR, Di Rezze S, Chianese M, Fabbrini G, Vanacore N, Colosimo C, et al. Hedonistic homeostatic dysregulation in Parkinson's disease: a short screening questionnaire. *Neurol .Sci* .2003;24(3):205-6.

[51] Voon V. Repetition, repetition, and repetition: compulsive and punding behaviors in Parkinson's disease. *Mov. Disord.* 2004;19(4):367-70.

[52] Schwingenschuh P, Katschnig P, Saurugg R, Ott E, Bhatia KP. Artistic profession: a potential risk factor for dopamine dysregulation syndrome in Parkinson's disease? *Mov. Disord* .2010;15(25(4)):493-6.

[53] Nirenberg MJ, Waters C. Compulsive eating and weight gain related to dopamine agonist use. *Mov. Disord.* 2006;21(4):524-9.

[54] Weintraub D. Dopamine and impulse control disorders in Parkinson's disease. Ann Neurol 2008;64 Suppl 2:S93-100.

[55] Spitzer RL, Yanovski SZ, Marcus MD. The Questionnaire on Eating and Weight Patterns-Revised (QEWP-R). 1993.

[56] Celio AA, Wilfley DE, Crow SJ, Mitchell J, Walsh BT. A comparison of the binge eating scale, questionnaire for eating and weight patterns-revised, and eating disorder examination questionnaire with instructions with the eating disorder examination in the assessment of binge eating disorder and its symptoms. *Int. J. Eat Disord.* 2004;36(4):434-44.

[57] Elder KA, Grilo CM, Masheb RM, Rothschild BS, Burke-Martindale CH, Brody ML. Comparison of two self-report instruments for assessing binge eating in bariatric surgery candidates. *Behav. Res. Ther.* 2006;44(4):545-60.

[58] Khan W, Rana AQ. Dopamine agonist induced compulsive eating behaviour in a Parkinson's disease patient. *Pharm. World Sci.* 2010;32(2):114-6.

[59] Evans AH, Lees AJ. Dopamine dysregulation syndrome in Parkinson's disease. *Curr. Opin. Neurol.* 2004;17(4):393-8.

[60] Fernandez HH, Friedman JH. Punding on L-dopa. Mov Disord 1999;14(5):836-8.

[61] Friedman JH. Punding on levodopa. *Biol. Psychiatry* 1994;36(5):350-1.

[62] Miwa H, Morita S, Nakanishi I, Kondo T. Stereotyped behaviors or punding after quetiapine administration in Parkinson's disease. Parkinsonism *Relat. Disord.* 2004;10(3):177-80.

[63] Rylander G. Psychoses and the punding and choreiform syndromes in addiction to central stimulant drugs. *Psychiatr. Neurol .Neurochir* .1972;75(3):203-12.

[64] Miyasaki JM, Al Hassan K, Lang AE, Voon V. Punding prevalence in Parkinson's disease. *Mov. Disord.* 2007;22(8):1179-81.

[65] Nguyen FN, Chang YL, Okun MS, Rodriguez RL, Shapiro MA, Jacobson CE, et al. Prevalence and characteristics of punding and repetitive behaviors among Parkinson patients in North-Central Florida. *Int. J. Geriatr. Psychiatry* 2010;25(5):540-1.

[66] Lee JY, Kim JM, Kim JW, Cho J, Lee WY, Kim HJ, et al. Association between the dose of dopaminergic medication and the behavioral disturbances in Parkinson disease. *Parkinsonism Relat Disord* .2010;16(3):202-7.

[67] Lawrence AJ, Blackwell AD, Barker RA, Spagnolo F, Clark L, Aitken MR, et al. Predictors of punding in Parkinson's disease: results from a questionnaire survey. *Mov. Disord.* 2007;22(16):2339-45.

[68] Ardouin C, Chereau I, Llorca PM, Lhommee E, Durif F, Pollak P, et al. [Assessment of hyper- and hypodopaminergic behaviors in Parkinson's disease]. *Rev. Neurol.* (Paris) 2009;165(11):845-56.

[69] Kumar S. Punding in Parkinson's disease related to high-dose levodopa therapy. *Neurol. India* 2005;53(3):362.

[70] Alves G, Kurz M, Lie SA, Larsen JP. Cigarette smoking in Parkinson's disease: influence on disease progression. *Mov. Disord.* 2004;19(9):1087-1092.

[71] Scott WK, Zhang F, Stajich JM, Scott BL, Stacy MA, Vance JM. Family-based case-control study of cigarette smoking and Parkinson disease. *Neurology* 2005;64(3):442-7.

[72] Benedetti MD, Bower JH, Maraganore DM, McDonnell SK, Peterson BJ, Ahlskog JE, et al. Smoking, alcohol, and coffee consumption preceding Parkinson's disease: a case-control study. *Neurology* 2000;55(9):1350-1358.

[73] Hernan MA, Chen H, Schwarzschild MA, Ascherio A. Alcohol consumption and the incidence of Parkinson's disease. *Ann .Neurol.* 2003;54(2):170-5.

[74] Venderova K, Ruzicka E, Vorisek V, Visnovsky P. Survey on cannabis use in Parkinson's disease: subjective improvement of motor symptoms. *Mov. Disord.* 2004;19(9):1102-6.

[75] Iuvone T, Esposito G, De Filippis D, Scuderi C, Steardo L. Cannabidiol: a promising drug for neurodegenerative disorders? *CNS Neurosci. Ther.* 2009;15(1):65-75.

[76] Fagerstrom KO, Heatherton TF, Kozlowski LT. Nicotine addiction and its assessment. *Ear Nose Throat J.* 1990;69(11):763-5.

[77] Saunders JB, Aasland OG, Babor TF, de la Fuente JR, Grant M. Development of the Alcohol Use Disorders Identification Test (AUDIT): WHO Collaborative Project on Early Detection of Persons with Harmful Alcohol Consumption--II. *Addiction* 1993;88(6):791-804.

[78] Bashford J, Flett R, Copeland J. The Cannabis Use Problems Identification Test (CUPIT): development, reliability, concurrent and predictive validity among adolesce nts and adults. *Addiction* 2010;105(4):615-25.

[79] Lardeux S, Paleressompoulle D, Pernaud R, Cador M, Baunez C. Selective encoding of natural reward versus cocaine by subthalamic nucleus neurons. *Soc. Neurosci. Abs* 2008(34):88-94.

[80] Goetz CG. Scales to evaluate psychosis in Parkinson's disease. Parkinsonism Relat Disord 2009;15 Suppl 3:S38-41.

[81] Goetz CG, Wuu J, Curgian L, Leurgans S. Age-related influences on the clinical characteristics of new-onset hallucinations in Parkinson's disease patients. *Mov. Disord.* 2006;21(2):267-70.

[82] Fenelon G, Mahieux F, Huon R, Ziegler M. Hallucinations in Parkinson's disease: prevalence, phenomenology and risk factors. *Brain* 2000;123 (Pt 4):733-45.

[83] Sanchez-Ramos JR, Ortoll R, Paulson GW. Visual hallucinations associated with Parkinson disease. *Arch. Neurol.* 1996;53(12):1265-8.

[84] Fenelon G, Alves G. Epidemiology of psychosis in Parkinson's disease. *J. Neurol. Sci.* 2010;289(1-2):12-7.

[85] Fahn S, Elton RL, Committee UD. The Unified Parkinson's Disease Rating Scale. In: Recent developments in Parkinson's disease. Florham Park ed. New Jersey; 1987. p. 153-63.

[86] Cummings JL, Mega M, Gray K, Rosenberg-Thompson S, Carusi DA, Gornbein J. The Neuropsychiatric Inventory: comprehensive assessment of psychopathology in dementia. *Neurology* 1994;44(12):2308-14.

[87] Aarsland D, Marsh L, Schrag A. Neuropsychiatric symptoms in Parkinson's disease. *Mov. Disord.* 2009;24(15):2175-86.

[88] Fernandez HH, Aarsland D, Fenelon G, Friedman JH, Marsh L, Troster AI, et al. Scales to assess psychosis in Parkinson's disease: Critique and recommendations. *Mov. Disord.* 2008;23(4):484-500.

[89] Aarsland D, Ballard C, Larsen JP, McKeith I. A comparative study of psychiatric symptoms in dementia with Lewy bodies and Parkinson's disease with and without dementia. *Int. J. Geriatr. Psychiatry* 2001;16(5):528-36.

[90] Kitayama M, Wada-Isoe K, Nakaso K, Irizawa Y, Nakashima K. Clinical evaluation of Parkinson's disease dementia: association with aging and visual hallucination. *Acta Neurol. Scand.* 2007;116(3):190-5.

[91] Papapetropoulos S, Mash DC. Psychotic symptoms in Parkinson's disease. From description to etiology. *J. Neurol.* 2005;252(7):753-64.

[92] Diederich NJ, Fenelon G, Stebbins G, Goetz CG. Hallucinations in Parkinson disease. *Nat .Rev. Neurol.* 2009;5(6):331-42.

[93] Biglan KM, Holloway RG, Jr., McDermott MP, Richard IH. Risk factors for somnolence, edema, and hallucinations in early Parkinson disease. *Neurology* 2007;69(2):187-95.

[94] Cummings JL. Depression and Parkinson's disease: a review. *Am. J. Psychiatry* 1992;149(4):443-454.

[95] Marsh L, McDonald WM, Cummings J, Ravina B. Provisional diagnostic criteria for depression in Parkinson's disease: report of an NINDS/NIMH Work Group. *Mov. Disord* .2006;21(2):148-58.

[96] Ravina B, Camicioli R, Como PG, Marsh L, Jankovic J, Weintraub D, et al. The impact of depressive symptoms in early Parkinson disease. *Neurology* 2007;69(4):342-7.

[97] Inoue T, Kitagawa M, Tanaka T, Nakagawa S, Koyama T. Depression and major depressive disorder in patients with Parkinson's disease. Mov Disord 2010;25(1):44-9.

[98] Ehrt U, Aarsland D. Psychiatric aspects of Parkinson's disease. *Curr. Opin. Psychiatry* 2005;18(3):335-41.

[99] Schrag A. Quality of life and depression in Parkinson's disease. *J. Neurol. Sci.* 2006;248(1-2):151-7.

[100] Weintraub D, Moberg PJ, Duda JE, Katz IR, Stern MB. Effect of psychiatric and other nonmotor symptoms on disability in Parkinson's disease. *J. Am. Geriatr. Soc.* 2004;52(5):784-8.

[101] Reijnders JS, Ehrt U, Weber WE, Aarsland D, Leentjens AF. A systematic review of prevalence studies of depression in Parkinson's disease. *Mov. Disord.* 2008;23(2):183-9; quiz 313.

[102] Rodriguez-Blazquez C, Frades-Payo B, Forjaz MJ, de Pedro-Cuesta J, Martinez-Martin P. Psychometric attributes of the Hospital Anxiety and Depression Scale in Parkinson's disease. *Mov. Disord.* 2009.

[103] Dissanayaka NN, Sellbach A, Matheson S, O'Sullivan JD, Silburn PA, Byrne GJ, et al. Anxiety disorders in Parkinson's disease: prevalence and risk factors. *Mov. Disord.* 2010;25(7):838-45.

[104] Richard IH. Anxiety disorders in Parkinson's disease. Adv Neurol 2005;96:42-55.

[105] Leentjens AF, Dujardin K, Marsh L, Martinez-Martin P, Richard IH, Starkstein SE, et al. Apathy and anhedonia rating scales in Parkinson's disease: critique and recommendations. *Mov. Disord.* 2008;23(14):2004-14.

[106] Stein MB, Heuser IJ, Juncos JL, Uhde TW. Anxiety disorders in patients with Parkinson's disease. *Am. J.Psychiatry* 1990;147(2):217-20.

[107] Nuti A, Ceravolo R, Piccinni A, Dell'Agnello G, Bellini G, Gambaccini G, et al. Psychiatric comorbidity in a population of Parkinson's disease patients. *Eur. J. Neurol.* 2004;11(5):315-20.

[108] Lauterbach EC, Freeman A, Vogel RL. Differential DSM-III psychiatric disorder prevalence profiles in dystonia and Parkinson's disease. *J. Neuropsychiatry Clin. Neurosci.* 2004;16(1):29-36.

[109] Goetz CG. New developments in depression, anxiety, compulsiveness, and hallucinations in Parkinson's disease. *Mov. Disord.* 2010;25 Suppl 1:S104-9.

[110] Starkstein SE, Leentjens AF. The nosological position of apathy in clinical practice. *J. Neurol. Neurosurg. Psychiatry* 2008;79(10):1088-92.

[111] Beck AT, Epstein N, Brown G, Steer RA. An inventory for measuring clinical anxiety: psychometric properties. *J. Consult. Clin. Psychol.* 1988;56(6):893-7.

[112] Schrag A, Barone P, Brown RG, Leentjens AF, McDonald WM, Starkstein S, et al. Depression rating scales in Parkinson's disease: critique and recommendations. *Mov. Disord.* 2007;22(8):1077-92.

[113] Williams JB. A structured interview guide for the Hamilton Depression Rating Scale. *Arch. Gen. Psychiatry* 1988;45(8):742-7.

[114] Montgomery SA, Asberg M. A new depression scale designed to be sensitive to change. *Br .J. Psychiatry* 1979;134:382-9.

[115] Snaith RP, Harrop FM, Newby DA, Teale C. Grade scores of the Montgomery-Asberg Depression and the Clinical Anxiety Scales. *Br. J. Psychiatry* 1986;148:599-601.

[116] Hughes TA, Ross HF, Musa S, Bhattacherjee S, Nathan RN, Mindham RH, et al. A 10-year study of the incidence of and factors predicting dementia in Parkinson's disease. *Neurology* 2000;54(8):1596-602.

[117] Silberman CD, Laks J, Capitao CF, Rodrigues CS, Moreira I, Engelhardt E. Recognizing depression in patients with Parkinson's disease: accuracy and specificity of two depression rating scale. *Arq .Neuropsiquiatr.* 2006;64(2B):407-11.

[118] Walsh K, Bennett G. Parkinson's disease and anxiety. *Postgrad Med. J.* 2001; 77(904):89-93.

[119] Giladi N, Hausdorff JM. The role of mental function in the pathogenesis of freezing of gait in Parkinson's disease. *J. Neurol. Sci.* 2006;248(1-2):173-6.

[120] Lauterbach EC, Freeman A, Vogel RL. Correlates of generalized anxiety and panic attacks in dystonia and Parkinson disease. *Cogn. Behav. Neurol.* 2003;16(4):225-33.
[121] Vazquez A, Jimenez-Jimenez FJ, Garcia-Ruiz P, Garcia-Urra D. "Panic attacks" in Parkinson's disease. A long-term complication of levodopa therapy. *Acta Neurol.* Scand. 1993;87(1):14-8.
[122] Arabia G, Grossardt BR, Geda YE, Carlin JM, Bower JH, Ahlskog JE, et al. Increased risk of depressive and anxiety disorders in relatives of patients with Parkinson disease. *Arch. Gen. Psychiatry* 2007;64(12):1385-92.
[123] Kostic VS, Filipovic SR, Lecic D, Momcilovic D, Sokic D, Sternic N. Effect of age at onset on frequency of depression in Parkinson's disease. *J. Neurol. Neurosurg. Psychiatry* 1994;57(10):1265-7.
[124] Tandberg E, Larsen JP, Aarsland D, Laake K, Cummings JL. Risk factors for depression in Parkinson disease. *Arch. Neurol* .1997;54(5):625-30.
[125] Zgaljardic DJ, Borod JC, Foldi NS, Rocco M, Mattis PJ, Gordon MF, et al. Relationship between self-reported apathy and executive dysfunction in nondemented patients with Parkinson disease. *Cogn. Behav. Neurol.* 2007;20(3):184-92.
[126] Kirsch-Darrow L, Fernandez HH, Marsiske M, Okun MS, Bowers D. Dissociating apathy and depression in Parkinson disease. *Neurology* 2006;67(1):33-8.
[127] Aarsland D, Larsen JP, Lim NG, Janvin C, Karlsen K, Tandberg E, et al. Range of neuropsychiatric disturbances in patients with Parkinson's disease. *J. Neurol .Neurosurg. Psychiatry* 1999;67(4):492-6.
[128] Isella V, Melzi P, Grimaldi M, Iurlaro S, Piolti R, Ferrarese C, et al. Clinical, neuropsychological, and morphometric correlates of apathy in Parkinson's disease. *Mov. Disord.* 2002;17(2):366-71.
[129] Levy ML, Cummings JL, Fairbanks LA, Masterman D, Miller BL, Craig AH, et al. Apathy is not depression. *J. Neuropsychiatry Clin. Neurosci.* 1998;10(3):314-9.
[130] Pluck GC, Brown RG. Apathy in Parkinson's disease. *J. Neurol. Neurosurg. Psychiatry* 2002;73(6):636-42.
[131] Starkstein SE, Mayberg HS, Preziosi TJ, Andrezejewski P, Leiguarda R, Robinson RG. Reliability, validity, and clinical correlates of apathy in Parkinson's disease. *J. Neuropsychiatry Clin. Neurosci.* 1992;4(2):134-9.
[132] Pedersen KF, Alves G, Aarsland D, Larsen JP. Occurrence and risk factors for apathy in Parkinson disease: a 4-year prospective longitudinal study. *J. Neurol. Neurosurg. Psychiatry* 2009;80(11):1279-82.
[133] Dujardin K, Sockeel P, Devos D, Delliaux M, Krystkowiak P, Destee A, et al. Characteristics of apathy in Parkinson's disease. *Mov. Disord* 2007;22(6):778-84.
[134] Sockeel P, Dujardin K, Devos D, Deneve C, Destee A, Defebvre L. The Lille apathy rating scale (LARS), a new instrument for detecting and quantifying apathy: validation in Parkinson's disease. *J. Neurol .Neurosurg. Psychiatry* 2006;77(5):579-84.
[135] Strauss ME, Sperry SD. An informant-based assessment of apathy in Alzheimer disease. *Neuropsychiatry Neuropsychol. Behav. Neurol.* 2002;15(3):176-83.
[136] Czernecki V, Pillon B, Houeto JL, Pochon JB, Levy R, Dubois B. Motivation, reward, and Parkinson's disease: influence of dopatherapy. *Neuropsychologia* 2002; 40(13):2257-67.

[137] Gard DE, Kring AM, Gard MG, Horan WP, Green MF. Anhedonia in schizophrenia: distinctions between anticipatory and consummatory pleasure. *Schizophr Res.* 2007;93(1-3):253-60.

[138] Treadway MT, Zald DH. Reconsidering anhedonia in depression: Lessons from translational neuroscience. *Neurosci .Biobehav Rev.* 2010.

[139] Gold JM, Waltz JA, Prentice KJ, Morris SE, Heerey EA. Reward processing in schizophrenia: a deficit in the representation of value. *Schizophr Bull* 2008;34(5):835-47.

[140] Loas G, Monestes JL, Yon V, Thomas P, Gard DE. Anticipatory anhedonia in schizophrenia subjects. *Encephale* 2010;36(1):85-7.

[141] Lemke MR, Brecht HM, Koester J, Kraus PH, Reichmann H. Anhedonia, depression, and motor functioning in Parkinson's disease during treatment with pramipexole. *J. Neuropsychiatry Clin. Neurosci.* 2005;17(2):214-20.

[142] Isella V, Iurlaro S, Piolti R, Ferrarese C, Frattola L, Appollonio I, et al. Physical anhedonia in Parkinson's disease. *J. Neurol. Neurosurg. Psychiatry* 2003;74(9):1308-11.

[143] Franz M, Lemke MR, Meyer T, Ulferts J, Puhl P, Snaith RP. [German version of the Snaith-Hamilton-Pleasure Scale (SHAPS-D). Anhedonia in schizophrenic and depressive patients]. *Fortschr. Neurol. Psychiatr.* 1998;66(9):407-13.

[144] Snaith RP, Hamilton M, Morley S, Humayan A, Hargreaves D, Trigwell P. A scale for the assessment of hedonic tone the Snaith-Hamilton Pleasure Scale. *Br. J. Psychiatry* 1995;167(1):99-103.

[145] Santangelo G, Morgante L, Savica R, Marconi R, Grasso L, Antonini A, et al. Anhedonia and cognitive impairment in Parkinson's disease: Italian validation of the Snaith-Hamilton Pleasure Scale and its application in the clinical routine practice during the PRIAMO study. *Parkinsonism Relat Disord.* 2009;15(8):576-81.

[146] Bayulkem K, Lopez G. Nonmotor fluctuations in Parkinson's disease: clinical spectrum and classification. *J. Neurol. Sci.* 2010;289(1-2):89-92.

[147] Richard IH, Frank S, McDermott MP, Wang H, Justus AW, Ladonna KA, et al. The ups and downs of Parkinson disease: a prospective study of mood and anxiety fluctuations. *Cogn. Behav. Neurol.* 2004;17(4):201-7.

[148] Young RC, Biggs JT, Ziegler VE, Meyer DA. A rating scale for mania: reliability, validity and sensitivity. *Br. J. Psychiatry* 1978;133:429-35.

[149] Altman EG, Hedeker D, Peterson JL, Davis JM. The Altman Self-Rating Mania Scale. *Biol. Psychiatry* 1997;42(10):948-55.

[150] Angst J, Adolfsson R, Benazzi F, Gamma A, Hantouche E, Meyer TD, et al. The HCL-32: towards a self-assessment tool for hypomanic symptoms in outpatients. *J. Affect. Disord.* 2005;88(2):217-33.

[151] Black KJ, Perlmutter JS. Septuagenarian Sydenham's with secondary hypomania. *Neuropsychiatry Neuropsychol. Behav. Neurol.* 1997;10(2):147-50.

[152] Goodwin FK. Biochemical and pharmacological studies, in Manic-Depressive Illness. In: Goodwin FK, Jamison KR, editors. New York: Oxford University Press; 1990. p. 416-502.

[153] Singh A, Althoff R, Martineau RJ, Jacobson J. Pramipexole, ropinirole, and mania in Parkinson's disease. *Am. J. Psychiatry* 2005;162(4):814-5.
[154] Verinder S, Smith A. A Case of Mania Following the Use of Pramipexole. *Am. J. Psychiatry* 2007;164:351.

In: Movement Disorders: Causes, Diagnoses and Treatments
ISBN 978-1-61209-200-3
Editor: Barbara J. Larsen

Chapter V

Parkinson Syndrome in Mitochondrial Disorders

Josef Finsterer *

Krankenanstalt Rudolfstiftung, Vienna,
Danube University Krems, Krems, Austria, Europe

Abstract

Parkinson syndrome (PS) has been repeatedly described as a clinical feature of mitochondrial disorders (MIDs). PS may be mild and only one of several other phenotypic features or PS may dominate the phenotype. PS manifestations may precede the other MID manifestations or may develop after onset of the non-PS MID manifestations. Evidence for an association between PS and MID comes also from a number of patients with PS or Parkinson disease (PD), who developed clinical or instrumental features of a MID in the absence of an immunhistochemical, biochemical or genetic defect indicative of a MID. Repeatedly, it has been also shown that some of the PD patients have an increased number of various mtDNA mutations in the nigrostriatal area. It has been also shown that mutations in genes causing hereditary PD, such as parkin, PINK1, alpha-synuclein (SCNA), leucine-rich kinase-2 (LRRK2), or DJ1, cause mitochondrial dysfunction, for which the term "mitochondrial nigropathies" has been coined. This mini-review wants to give an overview about the close relation between mitochondrial dysfunction and PS/PD at least in some of these patients.

Keywords: *mitochondrial myopathy, metabolic disease, neurodegenerative disorder, extrapyramidal disease,*

* Corresponding author: Josef Finsterer, MD, PhD, Postfach 20, 1180 Vienna, Austria, Europe, Tel. +43-1-71165-92085, Fax. +43-1-4781711, E-mail: fifigs1@yahoo.de.

Introduction

Due to the multisystem nature of most of the mitochondrial disorders (MIDs), also the CNS is frequently affected [1]. CNS manifestations of MIDs include stroke-like episodes, epilepsy, pyramidal affection, migraine, or migraine-like headache, cerebellar abnormalities, optic atrophy, cognitive impairment, dementia, psychosis, pituitary adenoma, atrophy, white matter lesions, calcifications, cysts, laminar cortical necrosis, microbleeds, paroxysmal electroencephalography (EEG) activity, aneurysms, but also Parkinson syndrome (PS) [2]. PS is due to degeneration of nigrostriatal dopaminergic neurons, which typically contain cytoplasmic aggregates termed Lewy-bodies. This review wants to give a short overview about recent advances concerning the pathogenesis, clinical and instrumental manifestations, and treatment of PS in patients with MID.

Frequency

Concerning the frequency of PS in MIDs only limited data are available. In a study of 76 MID patients 12% presented with clinical manifestations of a PS [3]. In a study of 159 Italian PD patients, none of them carried the most frequent of the MERRF mutations m.8344A>G [4].

A. Evidence for PS in MIDs

So far, a number of patients with a MID has been reported who also developed features of PS. PS in MIDs may develop before or after onset of the clinical manifestations of a MID and may be a dominant or non-dominant feature of the MID. MID with PS may be diagnosed on the immune-histochemical, biochemical, or genetic level. Further evidence for an association of PS with MID derives from the findings that some patients with PS develop clinical, histological, or biochemical features of a MID, that some PS patients carry mtDNA mutations in neurons involved in the nigro-striatal system, and that mutated genes responsible for hereditary forms of PS impair various mitochondrial functions.

1. MIDs with PS as a Non-Dominant Feature

There are several reports about MID patients who also presented with features of PS or the full-blown clinical picture and reports about PS patients in whom MID was diagnosed only after detection of PS. The first of these reports originates from Japan, in which a 55yo female with myopathy, deafness, and insulin-dependent diabetes mellitus due to the m.3243A>G mtDNA mutation additionally developed gait disturbance, slowing of movements, a masked face, a positive Meyerson's sign (inability to resist against blinking when tapped on the glabella), rigidospasticity, hypokinesia, mental impairment, vertical ophthalmoplegia, hearing loss, and limb weakness [5]. In two families with pigmentary retinopathy and levodopa-responsive tremor; rigidity, and micrographia following an autosomal dominant mode of inheritance, multiple mtDNA deletions were identified in the affected individuals [6]. Post-mortem examination showed severe neuronal loss in the substantia nigra even in a patient without Parkinsonism [6]. PS was also a feature of the phenotype in a 34yo male with bilateral subacute optic neuropathy (LHON) associated with cervical dystonia and supranuclear ophthalmoplegia who carried the 3460 mtDNA mutation [7]. In another patient, a young boy, akinetic rigid syndrome and features of MELAS syndrome were due to a 4bp deletion in the mitochondrial cytb gene [8]. PS was also a phenotypic feature in a patient with myoclonic epilepsy, ataxia and myopathy who carried the m.8344A>G mutation [9]. In a female with autosomal dominant chronic progressive external ophthalmoplegia (CPEO) due to multiple mtDNA deletions but absence of a mutation in POLG1, ANT1, or twinkle, prominent features of levodopa-responsive Parkinsonism and later levodopa-induced dyskinesias developed [10]. In a 3-generation family with autosomal dominant CPEO and Parkinsonism the heterozygous mutation n.1121G>A (R374Q) in exon 1 of the twinkle gene was detected in all family members [11]. In a large family with autosomal dominant CPEO due to multiple mtDNA deletions one additionally presented with Parkinsonism [12]. He carried the n.1532G>A mutation in exon 8 and the intronic variant c.2070 + 158G>A in cis and an additional heterozygous substitution in exon 7 in trans (1389G>T) of the POLG1 gene [12]. In a 65yo male late-onset ataxia, Parkinsonism, ophthalmoplegia, peripheral neuropathy, and sensorineural hearing loss were attributed to the W748S POLG1 mutation [13]. In a patient with autosomal recessive CPEO, followed by pseudo-orthostatic tremor, and levodopa-responsive Parkinsonism, the phenotype was attributed to two novel POLG1 mutations [14]. In a further patient with CPEO due to multiple mtDNA deletions lately evolving into severe sensory and cerebellar ataxia, peripheral neuropathy, Parkinsonism, and depression, one mutation each in the POLG1 and the ANT1 gene were detected [15]. In a patient with CPEO and Parkinsonism the disease was caused by the novel twinkle mutation R334Q [16]. In a 63yo patient with dyschromatopsia, ptosis, ophthalmoparesis, generalised weakness, hypoacusis, and cataract, due to the c.3104+3A>T OPA1 mutation in compound heterozygosity with the p.G848S mutation, levodopa-responsive PS was additionally described [17]. In a five-generation Belgien family with Leigh syndrome due to the m14487T>C mutation with heteroplasmy rates of 97-99% some of the 12 affected family members presented with progressive hypokinetic-rigid syndrome [18].

2. MIDs with PS as the Dominant Feature

The first report about PS patients carrying mtDNA mutations described three patients of whom one carried a variant at np4336 and a 5-nucleotide insertion in the 12S rRNA gene, one a variant at np3397 that converted a highly conserved methionine to a valine, and one patient a variant each at np3397 and at np3196 in a tRNA gene [19]. A few years later two patients with PS were described who both carried the m.4336A>G mutation [20]. In a study on five pairs of monocygotic twins with a long-term history of PD, two novel missense mutations, m.4925G>A in the ND2 gene and m.10192C>T in the ND3 gene, which were identical in both pairs, were detected in four of the pairs [21]. In addition, 20 known polymorphisms in genes encoding for respiratory chain complex I (RCCI) subunits or mtDNA tRNA genes were found [21]. A 40yo patient with PS additionally developed upper motor neuron signs, oculomotor dysfunction, cerebellar dysfunction, dysautonomia, hyper-CK-aemia, orthostatic hypotension, liver cirrhosis, and lactacidosis [22]. His family history was positive for liver cirrhosis, diabetes, ptosis, CPEO, lactacidosis, and hyper-CK-emia. Muscle biopsy showed 3% ragged-red-fibers and 10% COX-negative muscle fibers. Multiple mtDNA deletions were found in the skeletal muscle [22]. A 52yo patient with PS since age 38y developed multiple symmetric lipomas of the neck, shoulders and limbs, and lactacidosis 14y later. Since muscle biopsy showed ragged red fibers and COX-negative fibers, and since he carried a 5kb mtDNA deletion, a MID was diagnosed [22]. In two patients with dystonic toe curling, action tremor, masked face, bradykinesia, stooped posture, rigidity, and axonal polyneuropathy, muscle biopsy showed ragged-red and cytochrome-c-oxidase negative muscle fibers and PCR revealed multiple mtDNA deletions. Sequencing of the POLG1 gene revealed two new compound heterozygote mutations [23]. In a patient with PS and alpha-synuclein abnormalities the disorder was caused by a novel POLG1 mutation resulting in multiple mtDNA deletions [24]. Following these findings, POLG1 mutations appear to be the ones most frequently responsible for PS in MID patients. This finding is supported by a Finnish study showing that POLG1 polymorphisms were more frequent among 140 Finnish patients with PD as compared to aged- and ethnically-matched controls [25]. These results, however, could not be confirmed in a study on 641 North American Caucasian PD patients, the frequency of the non-10/11Q alleles was not significantly different from controls [26].

B. Mtdna Mutations in Neurons of the Nigro-Striatal System or Neighboring Areas

A number of PS patients has been reported, who accumulated mtDNA mutations in cerebral areas critical for PS. In a post-mortem study of three patients with PS the frequency of mtDNA substitutions was increased in the striatum [27]. In a study of 22 patients with PD, the new amino-acid exchange-causing mtDNA mutations m.3992C>T, m.4024A>G (ND1), m.11253T>C, m.12084C>T (ND4), m.13711G>A, m.13768T>C (ND5), and m.14582T>C (ND6) were found in the substantia nigra of these patients [28]. Additionally, the five known missense mutations m.3335T>C, m.3338T>C (ND1), m.5460G>A (ND2), m.10398A>G (ND3), and m.13966A>G (ND5) as well as three secondary LHON mutations (m.4216T>C, m.4917A>G, m.13708G>A) were detected [28]. In a study of 20 PD patients the homoplasmic mutations m.15950G>A in the tRNA(Thr) gene and m.15965T>C in the tRNA(Pro) gene were detected in mtDNA extracted from the substantia nigra in one patient each [29]. Additionally, 10 novel polymorphisms were detected [29]. Another autopsy study of PD patients found considerable regional heterogeneity in the heteroplasmy rates of the mtDNA mutation m.5460G>A (ND2 subunit gene) between various cerebral regions [30]. In a further study of PD patients high levels of mtDNA deletions were detected in the substantia nigra of these patients [31]. Single or multiple mtDNA deletions were also found in neurons of the substantia nigra in another cohort of PD patients but breakpoint characteristics and mechanisms leading to the formation of these deletions were not different from patients with advanced age [32].

C. Mutated Genes in Hereditary PD Impairing Mitochondrial Functions

Hereditary PD is due to mutations in five different genes, including PTEN putative kinase-1 (PINK1), parkin, DJ1, SNCA, and leucine-rich kinase-2 (LRRK2) [33]. Mutations in all these genes impair mitochondrial functions at a different level and to a variable degree [34]. The proteins involved are either mitochondrial proteins or associated with mitochondria. All of them are involved in pathways that elicit oxidative stress or ROS damage [35].

Conclusions

In patients in whom PS is associated with various other clinical presentations or in PS patients who develop multisystem disease, a MID should be suspected and an appropriate diagnostic work-up initiated. To elucidate the role of mtDNA mutations in cerebral regions critical for PD, these patients should undergo autopsy and affected and non-affected tissue should be investigated for the prevalence and distribution of these mutations. In patients in whom PD is hereditary search for mutations in the PINK1, parkin, DJ1, SNCA, or LRRK2 genes should be carried out. If such investigations are negative, linkage studies for other candidate genes should be encouraged. Therapy of PS in patients with a MID follows the guidelines for the treatment of non-mitochondrial PD. Antioxidants, lactate lowering agents, alternative energy sources, or cofactors, may be may be of additional help, although there effect in this indication is unproven. Due to the frequent multisystem nature of MIDs, the prognosis of patients with PS and MID may vary from those with PS but without an MID.

References

[1] McFarland R, Taylor RW, Turnbull DM. A neurological perspective on mitochondrial disease. *Lancet Neurol*. 2010;9:829-840.

[2] Finsterer J. Central nervous system imaging in mitochondrial disorders. *Can. J. Neurol. Sci.* 2009;36:143-53.

[3] Finsterer J. Parkinson syndrome as a manifestation of mitochondriopathy. *Acta Neurol. Scand.* 2002;105:384-9.

[4] Mancuso M, Nesti C, Petrozzi L, Orsucci D, Frosini D, Kiferle L, Bonuccelli U, Ceravolo R, Murri L, Siciliano G. The mtDNA A8344G "MERRF" mutation is not a common cause of sporadic Parkinson disease in Italian population. *Parkinsonism Relat Disord.* 2008;14:381-2.

[5] Hara K, Yamamoto M, Anegawa T, Sakuta R, Nakamura M. Mitochondrial encephalomyopathy associated with parkinsonism and a point mutation in the mitochondrial tRNA(Leu)(UUR)) gene. *Rinsho Shinkeigaku* 1994;34:361-5.

[6] Chalmers RM, Brockington M, Howard RS, Lecky BR, Morgan-Hughes JA, Harding AE. Mitochondrial encephalopathy with multiple mitochondrial DNA deletions: a report of two families and two sporadic cases with unusual clinical and neuropathological features. *J. Neurol. Sci.* 1996;143:41-5.

[7] Thobois S, Vighetto A, Grochowicki M, Godinot C, Broussolle E, Aimard G. Leber "plus" disease: optic neuropathy, parkinsonian syndrome and supranuclear ophthalmoplegia. *Rev. Neurol.* (Paris) 1997;153:595-8.

[8] De Coo IF, Renier WO, Ruitenbeek W, Ter Laak HJ, Bakker M, Schägger H, Van Oost BA, Smeets HJ. A 4-base pair deletion in the mitochondrial cytochrome b gene associated with parkinsonism/MELAS overlap syndrome. *Ann. Neurol.* 1999;45:130-3.

[9] Horvath R, Kley RA, Lochmüller H, Vorgerd M. Parkinson syndrome, neuropathy, and myopathy caused by the mutation A8344G (MERRF) in tRNALys. *Neurology* 2007;68:56-8.

[10] Wilcox RA, Churchyard A, Dahl HH, Hutchison WM, Kirby DM, Thyagarajan D. Levodopa response in Parkinsonism with multiple mitochondrial DNA deletions. *Mov. Disord.* 2007;22:1020-3.

[11] Baloh RH, Salavaggione E, Milbrandt J, Pestronk A. Familial parkinsonism and ophthalmoplegia from a mutation in the mitochondrial DNA helicase twinkle. *Arch. Neurol.* 2007;64:998-1000.

[12] Hudson G, Schaefer AM, Taylor RW, Tiangyou W, Gibson A, Venables G, Griffiths P, Burn DJ, Turnbull DM, Chinnery PF. Mutation of the linker region of the polymerase gamma-1 (POLG1) gene associated with progressive external ophthalmoplegia and Parkinsonism. *Arch. Neurol.* 2007;64:553-7.

[13] Remes AM, Hinttala R, Kärppä M, Soini H, Takalo R, Uusimaa J, Majamaa K. Parkinsonism associated with the homozygous W748S mutation in the POLG1 gene. *Parkinsonism Relat .Disord* .2008;14:652-4.

[14] Invernizzi F, Varanese S, Thomas A, Carrara F, Onofrj M, Zeviani M. Two novel POLG1 mutations in a patient with progressive external ophthalmoplegia, levodopa-responsive pseudo-orthostatic tremor and parkinsonism. *Neuromuscul. Disord.* 2008;18:460-4.

[15] Galassi G, Lamantea E, Invernizzi F, Tavani F, Pisano I, Ferrero I, Palmieri L, Zeviani M. Additive effects of POLG1 and ANT1 mutations in a complex encephalomyopathy. *Neuromuscul. Disord.* 2008;18:465-70.

[16] Vandenberghe W, Van Laere K, Debruyne F, Van Broeckhoven C, Van Goethem G. Neurodegenerative Parkinsonism and progressive external ophthalmoplegia with a Twinkle mutation. *Mov. Disord.* 2009;24:308-9.

[17] Milone M, Liewluck T, Wang J, Leavin JA, Wong L-J. A novel splice site mutation of the POLG gene in two unrelated adults with ophthalmoparesis and myopathy. *Acta Myol* .2010;29:235.

[18] Dermaut B, Seneca S, Dom L et al. Progressive myoclonic epilepsy as an adult-onset manifestation of Leigh syndrome due to m.14487T>C. *J. Neurol. Neurosurg. Psychiatry* 2010;81:90-3

[19] Shoffner JM, Brown MD, Torroni A, Lott MT, Cabell MF, Mirra SS, Beal MF, Yang CC, Gearing M, Salvo R, et al. Mitochondrial DNA variants observed in Alzheimer disease and Parkinson disease patients. *Genomics* 1993;17:171-84.

[20] Egensperger R, Kösel S, Schnopp NM, Mehraein P, Graeber MB. Association of the mitochondrial tRNA(A4336G) mutation with Alzheimer's and Parkinson's diseases. *Neuropathol Appl. Neurobiol.* 1997;23:315-21.

[21] Kösel S, Grasbon-Frodl EM, Hagenah JM, Graeber MB, Vieregge P. Parkinson disease: analysis of mitochondrial DNA in monozygotic twins. *Neurogenetics* 2000;2:227-30.

[22] Siciliano G, Mancuso M, Ceravolo R, Lombardi V, Iudice A, Bonuccelli U. Mitochondrial DNA rearrangements in young onset parkinsonism: two case reports. *J. Neurol. Neurosurg. Psychiatry* 2001;71:685-7.

[23] Davidzon G, Greene P, Mancuso M, Klos KJ, Ahlskog JE, Hirano M, DiMauro S. Early-onset familial parkinsonism due to POLG mutations. *Ann. Neurol.* 2006;59:859-62.

[24] Betts-Henderson J, Jaros E, Krishnan KJ, Perry RH, Reeve AK, Schaefer AM, Taylor RW, Turnbull DM. Alpha-synuclein pathology and Parkinsonism associated with POLG1 mutations and multiple mitochondrial DNA deletions. *Neuropathol. Appl.* Neurobiol 2009;35:120-4.

[25] Luoma PT, Eerola J, Ahola S, Hakonen AH, Hellström O, Kivistö KT, Tienari PJ, Suomalainen A. Mitochondrial DNA polymerase gamma variants in idiopathic sporadic Parkinson disease. *Neurology* 2007;69:1152-9.

[26] Eerola J, Luoma PT, Peuralinna T, Scholz S, Paisan-Ruiz C, Suomalainen A, Singleton AB, Tienari PJ. POLG1 polyglutamine tract variants associated with Parkinson's disease. *Neurosci. Lett.* 2010;477:1-5.

[27] Tanaka M, Kovalenko SA, Gong JS, Borgeld HJ, Katsumata K, Hayakawa M, Yoneda M, Ozawa T. Accumulation of deletions and point mutations in mitochondrial genome in degenerative diseases. *Ann. N Y Acad. Sci.* 1996;786:102-11.

[28] Kösel S, Grasbon-Frodl EM, Mautsch U, Egensperger R, von Eitzen U, Frishman D, Hofmann S, Gerbitz KD, Mehraein P, Graeber MB. Novel mutations of mitochondrial complex I in pathologically proven Parkinson disease. *Neurogenetics* 1998;1:197-204.

[29] Grasbon-Frodl EM, Kösel S, Sprinzl M, von Eitzen U, Mehraein P, Graeber MB. Two novel point mutations of mitochondrial tRNA genes in histologically confirmed Parkinson disease. *Neurogenetics* 1999;2:121-7.

[30] Schnopp NM, Kösel S, Egensperger R, Graeber MB. Regional heterogeneity of mtDNA heteroplasmy in parkinsonian brain. Clin Neuropathol 1996;15:348-52.

[31] Bender A, Krishnan KJ, Morris CM, Taylor GA, Reeve AK, Perry RH, Jaros E, Hersheson JS, Betts J, Klopstock T, Taylor RW, Turnbull DM. High levels of mitochondrial DNA deletions in substantia nigra neurons in aging and Parkinson disease. *Nat. Genet.* 2006;38:515-7.

[32] Reeve AK, Krishnan KJ, Elson JL, Morris CM, Bender A, Lightowlers RN, Turnbull DM. Nature of mitochondrial DNA deletions in substantia nigra neurons. *Am. J. Hum. Genet* .2008;82:228-35.

[33] Winklhofer KF, Haass C. Mitochondrial dysfunction in Parkinson's disease. *Biochim. Biophys. Acta* 2010;1802:29-44.

[34] Nuytemans K, Theuns J, Cruts M, Van Broeckhoven C. Genetic etiology of Parkinson disease associated with mutations in the SNCA, PARK2, PINK1, PARK7, and LRRK2 genes: a mutation update. *Hum. Mutat.* 2010;31:763-80.

[35] Lin TK, Liou CW, Chen SD, Chuang YC, Tiao MM, Wang PW, Chen JB, Chuang JH. Mitochondrial dysfunction and biogenesis in the pathogenesis of Parkinson's disease. Chang Gung. *Med. J.* 2009;32:589-99.

In: Movement Disorders: Causes, Diagnoses and Treatments ISBN: 978-1-61209-200-3
Editor: Barbara J. Larsen

Chapter VI

Unawareness of Movement Disorders in Parkinson's Disease

Martina Amanzio[*] and Diana M .E. Torta
University of Torino, Turin, Italy

Abstract

The concept of awareness of illness refers to the ability that people have in recognizing their disturbances. The presence of a possible unawareness of illness is well described in different clinical pathologies. The awareness of deficits may be sometimes altered in patients suffering from Parkinson's disease (PD). In order to have a greater clinical utility, theoretical models of unawareness, should allow for the possibility of integrating neurobiological and neuropsychological levels of explanation and should comprehend convergent analyses of these levels. With the aim of integrating such levels of explanations, a series of variables of interest will be considered from a convergent perspective at the neurobiological, neuropsychological and psychological-psychiatric levels.

In particular, this chapter will focus on a specific analysis of awareness of movement disorders in non-demented patients with PD and motor fluctuations. So far, only one study has analyzed differences in the awareness of deficits in PD patients by comparing the *on* and *off* states using an extensive battery of cognitive and behavioral functioning (Amanzio, Monteverdi, Giordano, Soliveri, Filippi & Geminiani; 2010). The results of this study demonstrated that PD patients have a selective reduced awareness of dyskinesias when in the *on* state, while being aware of their hypokinesias in the *off* state. Interestingly, such a reduced awareness of dyskinesia-related movement disorders was associated with executive functions in the *on* state. In contrast, no association with executive functions was found in the *off* state.

We believe that this study together with more in depth analysis of the phenomenon of unawareness of deficits may add important elements to the literature on neuropsychological impairments observed in unaware - non-demented patients with PD -

[*] Corresponding author: Department of Psychology, University of Torino, Via Verdi 10, 10123 Turin, Italy. Tel.: +39 11 6702468; E-mail: martina.amanzio@unito.it

in terms of executive dysfunctions. Besides, such elements may significantly contribute to the management of this particular class of pathology.

Our explanatory hypothesis is that the disruption of prefrontal-subcortical connections may cause impaired insight, independently of cognitive deterioration. Our model will also critically discuss the role that motivation may have in the unawareness of symptoms in the *on* medication state.

Keywords: Parkinson's disease, awareness of movement disorders, dyskinesia, hypokinesia, executive functions

1. Role and Measurement of Dyskinesias in Parkinson's Disease

The clinical diagnosis of dyskinesias and their treatment are complicated by the fact that, to date, validated diagnostic tools are scarce and poorly diffused. In the research field, dyskinesias have been quantified using a broad range of instruments: Doppler ultrasound, electromyography, dynamometer and accelerometers (Hoff, van Hilten & Roos; 1999). In the clinical practice, starting from the seventies, numerous scales have been introduced to evaluate dyskinesias in Parkinson's disease (PD) (Colosimo, Martinez-Martin, Fabbrini, Hauser, Merello, Miyasaki et al.; 2010). Among the most widely known and used scales are: the Abnormal Involuntary Movement Scale (AIMS), which evaluates the severity of dyskinesias in different body parts, such as the face, mouth, trunk and limbs (Gharabawi, Bossie, Lasser, Turkoz, Rodriguez & Chouinard; 2005). Some items of this scale address the patient's awareness of involuntary movements and the impact they have on normal daily activities (Guy; 1976); the Rush Dyskinesia Rating Scale (RDRS) created, as the more recent Parkinson's Disease Dyskinesia Scale (PDYS-26), to evaluate the impact of dyskinesias on activities of daily living (Goetz, Stebbins, Shale, Lang, Chemik, Chmura et al.; 1994); the Lang–Fahn Scale (LFS), aimed at capturing those problems that do not generally emerge during normal clinical practice and focused in particular on patients' perception of their dyskinesias (Colosimo, Martinez-Martin, Fabbrini, Hauser, Merello, Miyasaki et al.; 2010); the Clinical Dyskinesia Rating Scale (CDRS); the Unified Parkinson's Disease Rating Scale (UPDRS) Part IV which investigates the duration, intensity and level of impairment produced by dyskinesias and, lastly, the recent Unified Dyskinesia Rating Scale (UDyRS), designed to specifically assess dyskinesias in PD (Goetz, Nutt & Stebbins; 2008). This latter scale evaluates the effects of dyskinesias and dystonias separately and is made up of four parts: parts I and II are based on the patient's self-evaluation, parts III and IV are completed by an expert examiner, who rates dyskinesias objectively. Some items require the caregiver's opinion (Colosimo, Martinez-Martin, Fabbrini, Hauser, Merello, Miyasaki et al.; 2010). Among the other less-used scales are the Obeso Scale, which contains items similar to those of the RDRS, and is included in the Core Assessment Program for Intracerebral Transplantation (CAPIT) (Langston, Widner, Goetz, Brooks, Fahn & Freeman; 1992), protocol for the evaluation of parkinsonian patients to be submitted to surgical treatment (Colosimo, Martinez-Martin, Fabbrini, Hauser, Merello, Miyasaki et al.; 2010), and in its more recent version, the Core Assessment Program for Surgical Interventions in Parkinson's disease (CAPSIT) (Defer, Widner, Remy & Levivier; 1999).

All the aforementioned scales have some important limitations. First, each focuses on one or more characteristics of dyskinesias: duration, intensity, phenomenology, anatomical distribution, level of disability caused to patients and the way they are perceived (Goetz, Nutt & Stebbins; 2008). However, no one scale exhaustively captures all these issues (Goetz; 1999), perhaps also due to the fact that dyskinesias are a heterogeneous and extremely complex phenomenon (Colosimo, Martinez-Martin, Fabbrini, Hauser, Merello, Miyasaki et al.; 2010). Translation also represents a major problem: many of these scales, especially the oldest ones, have been translated into several languages, but such versions have only rarely been validated (Tonelli, Tonelli, Poiani, Vital & Andreatini; 2003; Martınez-Martın, Gil-Nagel, Gracia, Gomez, Martınez-Sarries & Bermejo; 1994). As for more recent scales (e.g. the UDyRS), the translated versions are not yet available (Colosimo, Martinez-Martin, Fabbrini, Hauser, Merello, Miyasaki et al.; 2010). Furthermore, the scales have been developed following very different strategies: some are parts of more extensive batteries for measuring the symptoms of the pathology, others have been designed specifically and exclusively to assess dyskinesias in PD, or created to evaluate dyskinesias in pathologies other than PD and only afterwards adapted to PD (Martinez-Martin & Cubo; 2007). The UPDRS is the most widely used in the current clinical practice. The UPDRS was introduced in 1987 (Fahn & Elton; 1987), and continues to be the most complete scale for evaluating parkinsonian symptomatology and rating the disease. The UPDRS is divided into four parts: the first evaluates mental activities and mood, the second the ability to carry out activities of daily living and the third investigates motor functions (Verhagen, Myre, Verwey, Hassin-Baer, Arzbaecher, Sierens, et al.; 2004). The fourth, recently revised, gathers anamnestic information relating to motor complications induced by long-term L-dopa therapy (Jankovic; 2005). Unfortunately, this scale provides little information on dyskinesias (Goetz, Stebbins, Shale, Lang, Chemik, Chmura, et al.; 1994): indeed, of its 42 items, only three are centered on the evaluation of dyskinesias. An alternative to such scales is represented by self-evaluation instruments, such as diaries, which are completed by the patients themselves by indicating the time, the therapy-dose and chronology of the appearance of involuntary movements (Hauser, Friedlander, Zesiewicz, Adler, Seeberger, & O'Brien; 2000). Self-evaluation scales have the advantage of not being limited to a specific moment. However, they may be influenced by the patient's emotional and cognitive states and thus prone to important biases (Colosimo, Martinez-Martin, Fabbrini, Hauser, Merello, Miyasaki et al.; 2010). For this reason and for the profound impact dyskinesias have on the capacity to perform daily activities, quality of life and degree of disability in parkinsonian patients, there is still the need for a unique scale to exhaustively and effectively evaluate dyskinesias.

2. Unawareness for Dyskinesias And Instruments for Neuropsychological Evaluation of the Disease

The problems associated with correct diagnostic evaluation of dyskinesias are not exclusively related to the difficulty of using adequate evaluation scales. Indeed, there is another important and interesting aspect that should be underlined: in the clinical practice it is not unusual to find patients who seem completely unaware of their dyskinesias (Vitale, Pellecchia, Grossi, Fragassi, Cuomo, Di Maio et al.; 2001; Seltzer, Vasterling, Mathias &

Brennan; 2001). Patients suffering from PD tend not to recognize these involuntary movements, especially at their onset, and usually tend not to link the phenomenon to the use of levodopa. Dyskinesias are more negatively judged by caregivers than by patients who nevertheless experience them in the first person (Marras & Lang; 2003). Indeed, patients do not complain about dyskinesias and simply tend to report a general worsening of the symptomatology. Furthermore, when L-dopa doses are suggested to reduce dyskinesias, it is not unusual to encounter resistance as patients seem to prefer the persistence of dyskinesias and a possible worsening of the parkinsonian symptomatology (Hung, Adeli, Arenovich, Fox & Lang; 2010). This resistance to a reduction in therapy is also seen in patients suffering from Hedonistic Homeostatic Dysregulation (Torta & Castelli; 2008; Pezzella, Colosimo, Vanacore, Di Rezze, Chianese, Fabbrini et al.; 2005; Pezzella, Di Rezze, Chianese, Fabbrini, Vanacore, Colosimo et al.; 2003; Giovannoni, O'Sullivan, Turner, Manson & Lees; 2000). These patients ask for ever increasing doses of treatment and only feel in the *on* state when markedly dyskinetic. However, they never report such dyskinesias as an adverse effect of their therapy. For this syndrome an impairment in reward systems has been hypothesized (Torta & Castelli; 2008).

Unawareness of disease is difficult to evaluate clinically. For this reason, as previously mentioned, caregivers often provide valuable help. In the few published works on this topic, unawareness is detected when a difference is found between the evaluation of the disease as provided by patients and by caregivers (Leritz, Loftis, Crucian, Friedman & Bowers; 2004). In this sense, it is important to consider that the possibility of the caregiver being under stress, often associated with mood changes, may constitute a relevant bias. Caregivers, especially if they look after a relative, bear an important burden which may lead them to overestimate the problems (Antoine, Antoine, Guermonprez & Frigard; 2004). An alternative approach is to create an index of lack of awareness given by the discrepancy between the score patients assign to themselves and their actual performance on a task (Antoine, Antoine, Guermonprez & Frigard; 2004). Lack of awareness of dyskinesias is an important factor to take into account as it has significant practical consequences (Seltzer, Vasterling, Mathias & Brennan; 2001). Indeed, while in some particular situations, unawareness of the disease may be an advantage for patients - for example to avoid embarrassment in social situations (Jenkinson; 2009), it has nonetheless been widely demonstrated that unawareness of an illness may seriously hamper the benefits of rehabilitative treatment and produce greater stress for caregivers (Seltzer, Vasterling, Yoder & Thompson; 1997; DeBettignies, Mahurin & Pirozzolo; 1990). Furthermore, not being aware of deficits may constitute a real danger for patients: unaware patients may undertake potentially dangerous activities or make mistakes in following therapeutic indications (Seltzer, Vasterling, Mathias & Brennan; 2001). Dyskinesias may also cause difficulties in the execution of daily living activities: not recognizing these problems also means failing in the search for alternative solutions (Jenkinson, Edelstyn, Stephens & Ellis; 2009).

3. Factors Associated with Unawareness for Dyskenisias

One interesting question, that few researchers have asked is: "Why are PD patients often unaware of their involuntary movements?" Previous research has focused on the role of the subcortical structures. Some studies have demonstrated that disturbances in the awareness of the diseases may emerge following damage to some subcortical structures of the right hemisphere, such as the thalamus, the nucleus caudatus, or the internal capsula (Hillis, Lenz, Zirth, Dougherty, Exkel & Jackson; 1998; Kumral, Kocaer, Ertubey & Kumral; 1995; Stein & Volpe; 1983). This probably occurs because the subcortical structures have numerous connections with the cortical regions, and frontal lobes. For this reason, in patients with lesions to some subcortical structures, it is reasonable to find deficits in unawareness similar to those that are found in the Alzheimer's disease (Amanzio, Torta, Sacco, Cauda, D'Agata, Duca et al.; in press; Amanzio & Torta; 2009). Subcortical lesions seem to be particularly associated with unawareness of involuntary movements (Lazzarino & Nicolai; 1991). Lack of awareness was recently observed in patients with lesions to the basal ganglia (Mikos, Springer, Nisenzon, Kellison, Fernandez, Okun et al.; 2009), such as PD patients (Albin, Young & Penney; 1989), patients suffering from Wilson's disease or Huntington's disease (HD) (Rosenblatt & Leroi; 2000). HD patients are also subject to the development of dyskinesias (Hoff, van Hilten & Roos; 1999), of which they rarely complain (Vitale, Pellecchia, Grossi, Fragassi, Cuomo, Di Maio et al.; 2001). A phenomenon similar to that in patients suffering from PD (Vitale, Pellecchia, Grossi, Fragassi, Cuomo, Di Maio et al.; 2001).

According to some authors, these difficulties may be ascribable to the numerous connections that the basal ganglia have with the frontal lobes (Seltzer, Vasterling, Mathias & Brennan; 2001). This appears to be particularly true in patients affected by HD. It is now clear that the duration and severity of illness in HD are associated with a progressive deterioration of the frontal lobe (Folstein, Folstein & Brandt; 1990). Besides cognitive impairments also seems to explain the lack of awareness of dyskinesias in patients with a long duration of illness. Indeed, in HD, the unawareness of dyskinesias seems to be directly related to the duration and severity of the illness (Vitale, Pellecchia, Grossi, Fragassi, Cuomo, Di Maio et al.; 2001). In contrast, in PD patients, lack of awareness of involuntary movements seems to be inversely correlated with the severity of the involuntary movements themselves (Vitale, Pellecchia, Grossi, Fragassi, Cuomo, Di Maio et al.; 2001). For PD patients there may thus be some alternative hypotheses to explain the phenomenon. Some authors have proposed that disturbances in awareness may be mainly correlated with neuropsychological dysfunctions in PD patients (Seltzer, Vasterling, Mathias & Brennan; 2001). Other researchers have suggested a pathophysiological hypothesis, proposing that excessive dopaminergic stimulation may, besides inducing dyskinesias, have adverse effects on awareness, by acting on the mesocorticolimbic circuit (Vitale, Pellecchia, Grossi, Fragassi, Cuomo, Di Maio et al.; 2001), which modulates various cognitive and emotional functions. In PD there is a progressive degeneration of dopaminergic, serotonergic and noradrenergic functions, with a probable overlap between these systems and the fronto-subcortical circuits that may be implicated in awareness (Seltzer, Vasterling, Mathias & Brennan; 2001). The same authors however, did not rule out a purely psychological explanation. It is a well known fact that, dyskinesias in PD are a consequence of the therapeutic dopaminergic hyperstimulation which these patients undergo to control bradykinesia. They thus fail to criticize their dyskinesias simply because they do not perceive such involuntary movements as abnormal. This hypothesis would help to explain why it is easier for these patients to report the presence of dyskinesias when they interfere with the performance of a specific motor task (Vitale, Pellecchia, Grossi, Fragassi, Cuomo, Di Maio et al.; 2001). Other authors have suggested a deficit in the capacity to distinguish between movements that are actually performed and those that were merely intended; this would lead patients to believe that they had performed the actual intended movement even if that were not the case (Jenkinson, Edelstyn, Stephens & Ellis; 2009).

A crucial point in order to fully understand the phenomenon and its clinical implications is the analysis of how affective-motivational aspects correlate with unawareness. This point, is discussed in detail in the following paragraph.

4. Emotional-Motivational Aspects of Unawareness of Dyskenisias in Parkinsons's Disease Patients

Concerning the emotional-motivational aspects of unawareness, the correlation between unawareness of illness and alterations in mood tone towards the negative pole appears intuitive. Several authors, who have studied neurodegenerative pathologies such as Alzheimer's disease, have indeed suggested that depression is more frequently present in patients with mild cognitive impairment and a good insight level (Starkstein, Sabe, Vazquez, Teson, Petracca, Chemerinski et al.; 1996; Sevush & Leve; 1993). Under this hypothesis, depression is considered as a reaction to the progression of disability which limits patients' abilities in every-day life and relationships (Wragg & Jeste; 1989; Kral; 1983). However, in PD depressive symptomatology may, in several cases, precede motor symptoms. This points to the role of neurobiological factors in the onset of emotional alterations in such pathologies. Other studies have shown a low – almost absent - correlation between good awareness of illness and depression (Antoine, Antoine, Guermonprez & Frigard; 2004; Migliorelli, Teson, Sabe, Petracca, Petracchi, Leiguarda et al.; 1995; Lopez, Becker, Somsak, Dew & DeKosky; 1994). Furthermore, if the hypothesis of depression as a psychological reaction to the discomfort produced by the illness were true, it would be reasonable to find an attenuation of the depressive symptomatology when the disease progresses. This seems not to occur. Indeed, depression is commonly found in later stages of the disease as well (Burns, Jacoby & Levy; 1990; Pearson, Teri, Reifler & Raskind; 1989). Interestingly, some authors have investigated the relationship between unawareness of illness and psychiatric and behavioral changes more in depth (Clare; 2004). Weinstein and colleagues (Weinstein, Friedland & Wagner; 1994) claim that there is a close relationship between the loss of awareness and the onset of behavioral problems. In particular, lack of awareness seems to be associated with irritability, hyperactivity, disinhibition (Seltzer, Vasterling, Mathias & Brennan; 2001; Migliorelli, Teson, Sabe, Petracca, Petracchi, Leiguarda et al.; 1995) and apathy (Derouesne, Thibault, Lagha-Petrucci, Baudouin-Madec, Ancri & Lacomblez; 1999). The relationship between unawareness of illness and apathy was already supported by previous works on AD (Ott,

Lafleche, Whellihan, Buongiorno, Albert & Fogel; 1996; Starkstein, Sabe, Vazquez, Teson, Petracca, Chemerinski et al.; 1996) and explained on the basis of a common physio-pathological hypothesis, concerning alterations of the amygdala (Derouesne, Thibault, Lagha-Petrucci, Baudouin-Madec, Ancri & Lacomblez; 1999; Braak & Braak; 1991). The correlation between unawareness and presence of hallucinations, delusions, and confabulation, does not seem to be statistically relevant (Lopez, Becker, Somsak, Dew & DeKosky; 1994). That between unawareness and cognitive impairments appears more controversial. Performance on reasoning tests (Starkstein, Sabe, Vazquez, Teson, Petracca, Chemerinski et al.; 1996; Migliorelli, Teson, Sabe, Petracca, Petracchi, Leiguarda et al.; 1995), and the ability to denominate objects also appear to be preserved in unaware patients (Sevush & Leve; 1993). Other studies have instead shown that unawareness of illness in PD patients decreases the more cognitive abilities are impaired, thus as a consequence of the cortical degeneration that appears as the disease progresses (Leritz, Loftis, Crucian, Friedman & Bowers; 2004). The hypothesis that cognitive deterioration may be a critical variable in the development of unawareness was also proposed by Seltzer and colleagues (Seltzer, Vasterling, Mathias & Brennan; 2001). Many authors have claimed that there may in particular be a correlation between lack of awareness and poor scores on tests investigating executive functions, since both depend on deficits at a cortical level. (Ott, Lafleche, Whellihan, Buongiorno, Albert & Fogel; 1996). For instance, Lopez and colleagues reported a correlation between poor awareness and low scores on the *Trial Making Test part B,* which evaluates cognitive flexibility and switching (Reitan; 1958). Similarly, correlations have been shown between poor awareness and pathological scores on the *Wisconsin Card Sorting Test,* which evaluates perseveration and categorization abilities (Nelson; 1976) and phonemic fluency tests (Michon, Deweer, Pillon, Agid & Dubois; 1994), on which frontal patients are usually impaired (Newcombe; 1969).

The relationship between unawareness of the illness and neuropsychiatric symptoms needs to be further investigated. This holds particularly true in patients suffering from PD. As suggested above, only a few studies have specifically addressed the phenomenon of unawareness of dyskinesias (Leritz, Loftis, Crucian, Friedman & Bowers; 2004) and even fewer have accurately considered the patient's psychiatric and cognitive status.

For instance, in their study investigating the lack of awareness in HD and PD patients, Vitale and colleagues (Vitale, Pellecchia, Grossi, Fragassi, Cuomo, Di Maio et al.; 2001) did not consider patients' neuropsychiatric and cognitive aspects, and thus did not exclude dementia. The same applies to the work of Seltzer and colleagues (Seltzer, Vasterling, Mathias & Brennan; 2001). Although they studied unawareness by comparing AD and PD patients (Seltzer, Vasterling, Mathias & Brennan; 2001), dementia was not an exclusion criteria and participants did not undergo a psychiatric or neuropsychological examination. Leritz and colleagues recently overcame such shortcomings (Leritz, Loftis, Crucian, Friedman & Bowers; 2004). Their study investigated unawareness in non-demented PD patients. Thorough attention was paid to the motor and psychiatric aspects of the patients included in the study. Psychiatric components were evaluated through the *Depression Inventory* (BDI, Beck, Brown, Steer, Eidelson & Riskin; 1987), *Geriatric Depression Scale* (GDS, Yesavage, Brink, Rose, Lum, Huang, Adey et al.; 1983) and *State-Trait Anxiety Inventory* (STAI, Spielbeger; 1983), however no significant results were found. In particular, they did not highlight any correlation between psychiatric symptomatology and the laterality of the disease, clinically assessed. These authors did, however, find a relationship between unawareness of motor symptoms and cognitive impairments. They claim that unawareness worsens as cognitive abilities decrease, namely in advanced stages of the disease when the deterioration involves both the subcortical and cortical structures. Their results may be explained on the basis of possible damage to the frontal lobe, as already hypothesized by other authors (Kaszniak & Zak; 1996; Schacter; 1990) or, alternatively, due to right-hemisphere damage (for AD patients see Amanzio, Torta, Sacco, Cauda, D'Agata, Duca et al.; in press). Both of these structures do indeed have numerous subcortical connections (Leritz, Loftis, Crucian, Friedman & Bowers; 2004). Leritz and colleagues thus underlined the need for further studies on unawareness in PD patients with a long history of the disease. On the other hand, it should be stressed that the patients included in this study did not undergo a different evaluation for the *on* and *off* states. Differences in the *on* and *off* states have been found in relation to behavior (Torta, Castelli, Latini-Corazzini, Banche, Lopiano & Geminiani; 2010; Torta et al., 2009). Indeed patients *on* medication have shown to be less able to postpone the possibility of a reward (delay aversion) (Torta, Castelli, Zibetti, Lopiano & Geminiani; 2009) and this incapacity has been found to be related to the therapy dose (the higher the dose, the greater the impulsivity: Torta, Castelli, Zibetti, Lopiano & Geminiani; 2009). This finding suggests the possibility of a motivational account for the unawareness of symptoms in PD patients on medication: the "reward" given by the medication is too high and immediate for patients to renounce it, in order to have a subsequent advantage such as the reduction of dyskinesias. Furthermore, in a previous study we suggested that notwithstanding the patients' lack of awareness in the medication phase (see next paragraph), they can also be scarcely aware of their motor abilities in the *off* phase (Torta, Castelli, Latini-Corazzini, Banche, Lopiano & Geminiani; 2010).

5. Impaired Awareness of Movement Disorders in Parkinson's Disease (See Tables 1-6)

We adopted an innovative approach to study unawareness of motor symptoms in cognitively unaffected PD patients (Amanzio, Monteverdi, Giordano, Soliveri, Filippi & Geminiani; 2010). We recently investigated unawareness of dyskinesias in twenty-five patients (thirteen women) suffering from idiophatic PD, under L-dopa and dopamine-agonist treatment who presented motor fluctuation and peak-dose dyskinesias (Amanzio, Monteverdi, Giordano, Soliveri, Filippi & Geminiani; 2010; see table 1). PD patients were excluded if they had hedonistic homeostatic dysregulation, HHD (Pezzella, Di Rezze, Chianese, Fabbrini, Vanacore, Colosimo et al.; 2003; Giovannoni, O'Sullivan, Turner, Manson, & Lees; 2000).

Patients were tested twice: first in the *off state*, with no medication coverage and then in the *on* state, under the effect of medication. This allowed us to evaluate awareness not only for hyperkinesias (dyskinesias) typical of the *on* state, but also awareness of hypo- and bradykinesia typical of the *off* state, when symptoms are not controlled. The evaluation concerned motor, as well as cognitive and neuropsychiatric aspects (see table 2). Motor evaluation was carried out using the *Unified Parkinson's Disease Rating Scale* (UPDRS, Fahn & Elton; 1987). Lack of awareness was evaluated using: the "Global Awareness of Movement" (GAM) disorders scale, the "Dyskinesias Rating Scale" and the Hypo-bradykinesia Rating Scale (see tables 5 and 6).

Data showed that PD patients had greater awareness and psychological suffering in the *off* state than in the *on* state. Indeed, unawareness scores varied significantly between the two phases, as reported in table 3: In the *on* state patients showed poor awareness of dyskinesias as measured on the *Global Awareness Movement Disorders Scale* (GAM) and on the *Dyskinesias Rating Scale* (DS-I), whereas in the *off* condition awareness of hypokinesias and bradykinesia appeared well preserved.

Table 1. Demographic and clinical measures expressed by mean (± SD). [Adapted from Amanzio, Monteverdi, Giordano, Soliveri, Filippi & Geminiani; 2010].

PD patients N=25	Mean (± SD) Min-Max
Age (years)	59.12 (8.98) 39-74
Sex (f/m)	13/12
Education (years)	10 (4.90) 5-18
Duration of disease (months)	137.60 (42.03) 84-240
Duration of motor fluctuations (months)	52.48 (36.19) 6-156
Duration of levodopa pharmacological treatment (months)	114.32 (44.05) 48-228
Dose of levodopa (mg per day)	845.0 (359.92) 400-1500

Table 2. Clinical, neuropsychological and neuropsychiatric measures expressed by mean (± SD). [Adapted from Amanzio, Monteverdi, Giordano, Soliveri, Filippi & Geminiani; 2010].

PD patients N=25 [$p < 0.03$ *]	*On* state	*Off* state
Unified Parkinson Disease Rating Scale, UPDRS III *	17.36 (7.46)	46.72 (8.80)
MMSE	27.80 (2.04)	27.50 (2.32)
Claridge modified Test * -Total score	4.60 (3.04)	3.08 (3.03)
Wechsler Memory Scale -Subtest IV -Subtest VII	6.76 (4.81) 11.70 (4.07)	6.65 (4.65) 10.65 (4.51)
WCST, modified version -Total score	36.48(11.61)	36.20 (12.14)
Phonemic Fluency Test	30.72 (11.24)	29.92 (10.87)
Brief Psychiatric Rating Scale *	29.60 (4.17)	35.76 (5.75)
Hamilton Anxiety Scale *	17.96 (6.34)	24.96 (9.02)
Hamilton Depression Scale *	14.04 (2.71)	19.28 (3.45)

In detail, twenty-two patients out of twenty-five showed a lack of awareness of their dyskinesias, whereas only six out of twenty-five patients were unaware of their motor disturbances in the *off* state (bradykinesia and hypokinesia). Unawareness thus emerged from neurological evaluations, from the comparison between patients' and neuropsychologists' evaluations and from the comparison between indexes of awareness of motor symptoms (see table 3).

Table 3. Global Awareness of Movements (GAM) scale of dyskinesias and hypo-bradykinesia on each patient in the *on* and *off* states. Higher scores indicate more severe impairment in terms of reduced awareness of movement disorders. Awareness measures of each PD patient also considering dyskinesias (DS-I) and hypo-bradykinesia (HS-I) motor symptoms. In most cases, considering DS-I, patients evaluate their symptoms as less serious. DS-I=Dyskinesias Subtracted Index; HS-I=Hypo-bradykinesia Subtracted Index. [Adapted from Amanzio, Monteverdi, Giordano, Soliveri, Filippi & Geminiani; 2010].

Patient code	GAM dyskinesias	GAM hypo-bradykinesia	*On* state DS-I	Examiner	Patient	*Off* state HS-I	Examiner	Patient
1	0	0	0	2	2	0	3	3
2	1	0	0	2	2	-1	1	2
3	1	0	1	1	0	1	3	2
4	1	0	1	3	2	0	2	2
5	1	1	1	3	2	0	2	2
6	2	0	0	1	1	0	2	2
7	2	0	0	2	2	-1	1	2
8	3	0	2	3	1	0	2	2
9	2	0	0	2	2	0	3	3
10	2	0	1	1	0	0	2	2
11	1	0	-1	2	3	0	3	3
12	2	1	1	3	2	0	3	3
13	2	1	1	2	1	0	3	3
14	2	1	1	3	2	0	2	2
15	1	0	0	3	3	0	3	3
16	1	0	1	2	1	0	3	3
17	1	0	1	2	1	0	2	2
18	2	0	1	3	2	0	3	3
19	2	0	1	3	2	-1	2	3
20	1	1	0	2	2	0	3	3
21	1	1	1	2	1	0	3	3
22	0	0	1	3	2	0	3	3
23	2	0	1	3	2	0	3	3
24	1	0	1	3	2	0	3	3
25	0	0	-1	1	2	0	2	2
M (±SD)	1.36 (0.76)	0.24 (0.43)	0.60 (0.71)	2.28 (0.74)	1.68 (0.75)	-0.08 (0.40)	2.48 (0.65)	2.56 (0.51)

The neuropsychiatric evaluation was performed by administering the *Hamilton Anxiety Rating Scale* (HAM-A), the *Hamilton Depression Rating Scale* (HAM-D) and the *Brief Psychiatric Rating Scale* (BPRS). Patients obtained higher scores in the *off* phase than in the *on* phase, especially on items concerning anxiety and apathetic-depressive symptomatology.

PD patients were also more troubled by motor disabilities related to hypokinesias and had mood-related symptoms and a perception of disability in activities of daily living in the *off* state. The results obtained with the *North University Disability Scale* (NUDS, Canter, De Latorre & Mier; 1961), used to evaluate the degree of disability in carrying out instrumental activities of daily living, showed that patients reported more severe disability during the *off* condition than in the *on* condition (see table 4).

Table 4. Awareness of disabilities in activities of daily living and autonomy level on the NUDS scale in the on and off states. NUDS-I: NUDS Subtracted Index. [Adapted from Amanzio, Monteverdi, Giordano, Soliveri, Filippi & Geminiani; 2010].

Patient	<<<<<<<<<<<*On* state>>>>>>>>>>			<<<<<<<<<<<*Off* state>>>>>>>>>>		
code	Patient	Caregiver	NUDS-I	Patient	Caregiver	NUDS-I
1	10	13	-3	35	37	-2
2	11	6	5	24	25	-1
3	2	7	-5	4	12	-8
4	11	20	-9	33	37	-4
5	5	9	-4	11	16	-5
6	1	11	-10	23	26	-3
7	2	5	-3	37	40	-3
8	14	12	2	41	42	-1
9	5	6	-1	32	37	-5
10	4	11	-7	22	35	-13
11	27	27	0	42	42	0
12	12	15	-3	38	38	0
13	11	12	-1	20	31	-11
14	13	13	0	19	32	-13
15	9	12	3	36	36	0
16	7	10	-3	31	32	-1
17	2	7	-5	28	28	0
18	22	23	-1	34	36	-2
19	20	27	-7	35	35	0
20	15	15	0	31	30	1
21	14	20	-6	33	33	0
22	13	13	0	42	42	0
23	14	21	-7	19	44	-25
24	35	35	0	40	40	0
25	5	6	-1	32	32	0
M (±SD)	11.36 (8.17)	14.24 (7.71)	-2.64 (3.73)	29.68 (9.75)	33.52 (7.74)	-3.84 (6.04)

Interestingly, patients only showed a selective reduction of awareness of movement disorders associated with executive functions - on the *Wisconsin Card Sorting Test* (WCST, Nelson; 1976) - and related to dyskinesias in the *on* state, compared to a preserved awareness of hypokinesias in the *off* state. On the contrary, no association with executive functions was found in the *off* state.

Table 5. Assessment of awareness of movement disorders: The Global Awareness of Movement (GAM) Disorders scale (Amanzio, Monteverdi, Giordano, Soliveri, Filippi & Geminiani; 2010), adapted from the scale of Bisiach, Vallar, Perani, Papagno & Berti; (1986).

The Global Awareness of Movement (GAM) Disorders scale	Score: [N]
When questioned by the examiner, about his/her state of health, the patient spontaneously reported the presence of involuntary movements (in the on state if present) or motor hindrance (in the off state if present)	[0]
The patient reported the presence of involuntary movements (in-on) and motor hindrance (in-off), but only after an explicit request by the examiner concerning those motor disturbances	[1]
The patient only admitted the presence of involuntary movements and motor hindrance after focusing attention on his/her evident dyskinesias on any part of the body and after a request to perform fine movements (i.e. a pronation/-supination hand task), which was done with evident difficulty or slowness (not due to his/her dyskinesias)	[2]
The patient did not admit the presence of his/her evident motor disturbances, even after the above mentioned demonstrations	[3]

Table 6. Assessment of awareness of movement disorders: The Dyskinesias Rating Scale and the Hypo-bradykinesia Rating Scale (Amanzio, Monteverdi, Giordano, Soliveri, Filippi & Geminiani; 2010).

The patient was requested to perform the following three simple actions:

- Write down a sentence: "*Oggi e' una bella giornata di primavera*" (*Today is a lovely spring day*).
- Hold a half-full glass in his/her hands, bring it up to the mouth and put it down again (patient is sitting at the table).
- Stand up from a chair, walk for two meters, go back to the chair and sit down again.

The actions were rated using the following scales of dyskinesias and hypo-bradykinesias.

Dyskinesias Rating Scale	**Hypo-bradykinesias Rating Scale**	Score: [N]
Absence of dyskinesias (unusual and involuntary movements)	Absence of hypo-bradykinesias (difficulty or slowness of movements)	[0]
Slight dyskinesias (slightly visible)	Slight hypo-bradykinesias (slightly evident, only during the execution of fine movements, such as writing)	[1]
Moderate dyskinesias (clearly evident but without significant impact on the result of the execution of the actions, except in particularly fine tasks)	Moderate hypo-bradykinesias (clearly evident but without impact on the execution of actions except in fine movements)	[2]
Severe dyskinesias (clearly evident and with a negative impact in the result of the execution of the actions)	Severe hypo-bradykinesias (clearly evident and impacting on the execution of actions)	[3]

The results of the cognitive evaluation indicated no difference in patients' performance on the *Mini Mental State Examination* (MMSE, Folstein, Folstein & McHugh; 1975), used to screen for dementia and on the WCST, used to evaluate executive functions, during the *off* condition in relation to the *on* condition. A similar result was obtained for their ability to access the internal lexicon (phonemic fluency: Novelli, Papagno, Capitani, Laiacona, Vallar & Cappa; 1986) and for the short-term memory, evaluated using subscale IV of the *Wechsler Memory Scale* (WMS, Wechsler; 1987). In contrast, in the *on* condition patients performed better on the *Claridge Test* (Claridge; 1967), used to evaluate selective attention and cognitive switching and on subscale VII of the *Wechsler Memory Scale,* which assesses associative learning abilities.

These results may depend on several factors: in particular, discrepancies may be explained by the complex influence of dopaminergic therapy on behavioral and cognitive dysfunctions. One hypothesis is that L-dopa treatment may produce a detrimental effect on the functions of the cingulate cortex, where lesions are often associated with emotional disturbances such as fear, irritability and depression and of the orbitofrontal cortex, where lesions appear to be associated with reduced attention and self-monitoring abilities, disinhibition, stereotyped behavior and lack of empathy (Miller & Cummings; 2007). In PD patients the progression of dopaminergic depletion can involve the dorsal striatum sooner and more severely than the ventral striatum (Agid, Ruberg, Javoy-Agid, Hirsch, Raisman-Vozari, Vyas et al.; 1993; Kish, Shannak & Hornykiewicz; 1988), also in situations complicated by motor fluctuations. Levodopa therapy limits motor dysfunctions, associated with the dorsal striatum. However, high doses of Levodopa may indeed improve motor symptoms, but at the same time, they can 'overdose' the ventral striatum. The relationship between awareness disturbances and dyskinesias in the *on* state (GAM scale) supports this hypothesis.

Poor performance on memory tests and on the *WCST* can also be explained in the same way, as can patients' lack of awareness of involuntary movements in the *on* state, which does not seem to be related to cognitive impairment. Rather, such inability appears to be more closely related to metacognitive deficits in the self-monitoring systems. A similar hypothesis was suggested by Jenkinson, Edelstyn, Stephens & Ellis (2009). These authors elaborated a model according to which the reduced awareness may result from a discrepancy between the planned and the actual movement, due to an inability to correct mistakes. Thus, metacognitive abilities may be necessary in order to be aware of the on-going movement. Such metacognitive abilities are also involved in monitoring activities of daily living. The comparison of the results on the NUDS-I[1] revealed no significant difference between the two states. This would suggest that levodopa acts not on the global system of awareness, but rather only on the specific system which monitors motor behavior in case of motor deficits. As yet there is no significant evidence in the literature to support this explicative hypothesis.

Conversely, L-dopa administration exerts a good effect at motor level and similarly stimulates all the dopamine-depleted systems, thus improving all tasks that depend upon proper functioning of those circuits. For instance, dopamine stimulates the subcortical circuit that connects the dorsolateral-prefrontal cortex and nuclei of the dorsal caudatus. This explains the improved performance on the attentional and switching abilities, measured using

[1] The awareness index was obtained by subtracting patients' evaluations of level of autonomy from caregivers' evaluations of the patients' level of disability, and labeled the NUDS Subtracted Index (NUDS-I) for the on and off states.

the *Claridge Test*. Similarly, dopaminergic therapy acts on the frontal-subcortical circuits so as also to improve the psychiatric aspects of PD, with patients being less depressed, less anxious and less apathetic after dopaminergic stimulation. In particular, it has to be underlined that notwithstanding the fact that patients with depression or dysthymia were excluded (according to DSM-IV criteria; 2000), the use of psychiatric scales still revealed that patients are more depressed when they are not under the effect of therapy. This has a deep impact on the diagnosis of lack of awareness: indeed depression may alter patients' perception of their problems, so that they overstate them. This may represent a confounding variable in the study of unawareness of illness (Clare; 2004).

Besides depressive and anxious symptoms, evaluation in the *off* condition showed signs of apathy. In particular, patients showed a general reduction in emotional responses, interest and initiative. Importantly, these results suggest that an early mild change in behavior occurs in patients, and that this is not to be considered as relevant from a psychopathological point of view.

In the literature, the presence of apathy has often been reported in PD patients (Pluck & Brown; 2002; Aarsland, Litvan & Larsen; 2001; Starkstein, Fedoroff, Price, Leiguarda & Robinson; 1992), as well as anxiety and depression (Leentjens, 2004; Slaughter, Slaughter, Nichols, Holmes & Martens; 2001). These aspects may be related to physical disability, which is obviously greater in the *off* phase. According to our results, dopaminergic therapy seems to have the effect of reducing apathy. Indeed, alterations to the frontal cortex follow basal ganglia dysfunctions; for this reason patients show loss of initiative and interest and difficulty in elaborating and keeping a precise strategy (Levy & Dubois; 2006). Thus both the cognitive deficits and affective-motivational problems that characterize parkinsonian patients during the *off* state are correlated with dysfunctions in the frontal-subcortical structures and may increase as a result of dopaminergic treatment.

Conclusions

There is still only a limited amount of research investigating unawareness of dyskinesias in PD. We believe our studies add important elements to the literature on neuropsychological impairments observed in unaware patients with PD in terms of executive dysfunctions and has important implications for managing this particular class of pathology. In particular, we hypothesize that the disruption of prefrontal subcortical connections may cause impaired insight, irrespective of cognitive deterioration.

Further studies are therefore needed to better understand the phenomenon of unawareness of illness and in particular, unawareness of dyskinesias in PD patients.

References

Aarsland, D., Litvan, I. & Larsen, J.P. (2001). Neuropsychiatric symptoms of patients with progressive supranuclear palsy and parkinson's disease. *J Neuropsychiatry Clin Neurosci, 13*, 42-49.

Agid, Y., Ruberg, M., Javoy-Agid, F., Hirsch, E., Raisman-Vozari, R., Vyas, S., et al. (1993). Are dopaminergic neurons selectively vulnerable to Parkinson's disease. *Adv Neurol, 60,* 148-164.

Albin, R.L., Young, A.B. & Penney, J.B. (1989). The functional anatomy of basal ganglia disorders. *Trends Neurosci*, *12*, 366 –375.

Amanzio, M. & Torta, D.M.E. (2009). *Unawareness of deficits in Alzheimer's disease through a biopsychosocial perspective:* In Clayton B. Larson (Ed). Metacognition: New Research Developments. Nova Science Publishers, New York. Chapter 14, pp. 239-253.

Amanzio, M., Monteverdi, S., Giordano, A., Soliveri, P., Filippi, P. & Geminiani, G. (2010). Impaired awareness of movement disorders in Parkinson's Disease. *Brain Cogn*, *72*, 337-346.

Amanzio, M., Torta, D.M.E., Sacco, K., Cauda, F., D'Agata, F., Duca, S.,et al. Unawareness of deficits in Alzheimer's disease: Role of the Cingulate Cortex. *Brain*. In press.

American Psychiatric Association (2000). *Diagnostic and Statistical Manual of Mental Disorders,* 4th Edition, Text Revision. Washington, Dc.

Antoine, C., Antoine, P., Guermonprez, P. & Frigard, B. (2004). Awareness of deficit and anosognosia in Alzheimer disease. *Encephale*, *30*, 570-577.

Beck, A.T, Brown, G., Steer, R.A., Eidelson, J.I. & Riskin, J.H. (1987). Differentiating anxiety and depression: a test of the cognitive content-specificity hypothesis. *J Abnorm Psychol*, *96,* 179- 183.

Bisiach, E., Vallar, G., Perani, D., Papagno, C. & Berti, A. (1986). Unawareness of disease following lesions of the right hemisphere: Anosognosia for hemiplegia and anosognosia for hemianopsia. *Neuropsychologia*, *24*, 471-482.

Braak, H. & Braak, E. (1991). Neuropathological staging of Alzheimer's-related changes. *Acta Neuropathol*, *82*, 239-259.

Burns, A., Jacoby, R. & Levy, R. (1990). Psychiatric phenomena in Alzheimer's disease. II: Disorders of perception. *Br J Psychiatry*, *157*, 76-81.

Canter, G.J., De Latorre, R. & Mier, M. (1961). A method for evaluating disability in 829 patients with Parkinson's disease. *J Nervous Mental Dis*, *133*, 143–152.

Clare, L. (2004). Awareness in early stage Alzheimer's disease: a review of methods and evidence. *Br J Clin Psychol*, *43*, 177–196.

Claridge, G.S. (1967). *Personality and arousal. A psychophysiological study of 836 psychiatric disorders.* Pergamon Press, Oxford.

Colosimo, C., Martinez-Martin, P., Fabbrini, G., Hauser, R. A., Merello, M., Miyasaki, J., et al. (2010). Task force on scales to assess dyskinesia in Parkinson's Disease: critique and recommendation. *Mov Disord*, *9*, 1131-1142.

DeBettignies, B.H., Mahurin, R.K. & Pirozzolo, F.J. (1990). Insight for impairment in independent living skills in Alzheimer's disease and multi-infarct dementia. *J Clin Exp Neuropsychol, 12*, 355–363.

Defer, G.L., Widner, H., Marie, R.M., Remy, P. & Levivier, M (1999). Core assessment program for surgical interventional therapies in Parkinson's disease (CAPSIT-PD). *Mov Disord*, *14*, 572–584.

Derouesne, C., Thibault, S., Lagha-Petrucci, S., Baudouin-Madec, V., Ancri, D. & Lacomblez, L. (1999). Decreased awareness of cognitive deficits in patients with mild dementia of the Alzheimer type. *Int J Geriatr Psychiatr*, *14*, 1019-1030.

Fahn, S. & Elton, R.L. (1987). *The UPDRS Development Committee. Unified Parkinson'sDisease Rating Scale*: Fahn S., Marsden C.D., Calne D. & Goldstein M. (Eds.). Recent developments in Parkinson's disease. Macmillan Health Care Information, Florham Park, New York.

Folstein, M.F., Folstein, S.E. & McHugh, P.R. (1975). Mini- Mental State: a practical method for grading the cognitive state of patients for the clinician. *J Psychiatr Res*, *12*, 189-198.

Folstein, M.F., Folstein, S.E. & Brandt, J. (1990). *Huntington's disease*: Cummings J.L. (Ed.). Subcortical dementia. Oxford University Press, New York.

Gharabawi, G.M., Bossie, C.A., Lasser, R.A., Turkoz, I., Rodriguez, S. & Chouinard, G. (2005). Abnormal Involuntary Movement Scale (AIMS) and Extrapyramidal Symptom Rating Scale (ESRS): Cross scale comparison in assessing tardive dyskinesia. *Schizophrenia Res*, *77*, 119–128.

Giovannoni, G., O'Sullivan, J.D., Turner, K., Manson, A.J. & Lees, A.J. (2000). Hedonistic homeostatic dysregulation in patients with Parkinson's disease on dopamine replacement therapies. *J Neurol Neurosurg Psychiatry*, *68*, 423– 428.

Goetz, C.G., Stebbins, G.T., Shale, H.M., Lang, A.E., Chemik, D.A., Chmura, T.A., et al. (1994). Utility of an objective dyskinesia rating scale for Parkinson's disease: inter-and intra-rater reliability assessment. *Mov Disord*, *9*, 390-394.

Goetz, C.G. (1999). Rating scales for dyskinesias in Parkinson's disease. *Mov Disord*, *14*, 48–53.

Goetz, C.G., Nutt, J.G. & Stebbins, G.T. (2008). The unified dyskinesias rating scale: presentation and clinimetric profile. *Mov Disord*, *23*, 2398–2403.

Guy, W.A. (1976). *Abnormal Involuntary Movement Scale (AIMS) ECDEU Assessment Manual for Psychopharmacology*. U.S. Department of Health Education and Welfare, Washington, DC.

Hauser, R.A., Friedlander, J., Zesiewicz, T.A., Adler, C.H., Seeberger, L.C., O'Brien, C.F. (2000). A home diary to assess functional status in patients with Parkinson's disease with motor fluctations and dyskinesia. *Clin Neuropharmacol*, *2*, 75-81.

Hillis, A.E., Lenz, F.A., Zirth, T.A., Dougherty, P.M., Exkel, T.S. & Jackson, K. (1998). Hemispatial somatosensory and motor extinction after stereotactic thalamic lesions. *Neurocase*, *4*, 21-34.

Hoff, J.I., van Hilten, B.J., & Roos, R.A. (1999). A review of the assessment of dyskinesias. *Mov Disord, 14*, 737-743.

Hung, S.W., Adeli, G.M., Arenovich, T., Fox, S.H. & Lang, A.E. (2010). Patients perception of dyskinesia in Parkinson's disease. *J Neurol Neurosurg Psychiatry*, 81, 1112-1115.

Jankovic, J. (2005). Motor fluctuations and dyskinesia in Parkinson's disease: clinical manifestation. *Mov Disord*, *20*, S11-S16.

Jenkinson, P.M., Edelstyn, N.M.J, Stephens, R. & Ellis, S.J. (2009). Why are some Parkinson disease patients unaware of their dyskinesia? *Cog Behav Neurol*, *22*, 117-121.

Kaszniak, A.W. & Zak, M.G. (1996). On the neuropsychology of metamemory: Contributions from the study of amnesia and dementia. *Learning and Individual Differences, 8,* 355-381.

Kish, S.J., Shannak, K. & Hornykiewicz, O. (1988). Uneven pattern of dopamine loss in the striatum of patient with idiopathic Parkinson's disease. Pathophysiologic and clinical implication. *N Engl J Med, 318,* 876-880.

Kral, V. (1983). The relationship between senile dementia (Alzheimer type) and depression. *Can J Psychiatry, 28*, 304-6.

Kumral, E., Kocaer, T., Ertubey, N. & Kumral, K. (1995). Thalamic hemorrhage: A prospective study of 100 patients. *Stroke, 26*, 964-970.

Langston, J.W., Widner, H., Goetz, C.G., Brooks, D., Fahn, S. & Freeman, T. (1992). Core assessment program for intracerebral transplantations (CAPIT). *Mov Disord, 7*, 2–13.

Lazzarino, L.G., & Nicolai, A. (1991). Hemichorea-hemiballism and anosognosia following a contralateral infarction of the caudate nucleus and anterior limb of the internal capsule. *Rivista di Neurologia, 61*, 9–11.

Leentjens, A.F.G. (2004). Depression in Parkinson's disease: conceptual issues and clinical challenges. *J Geriatr Psychiatry Neurol, 17*, 120–126.

Leritz, E., Loftis, C., Crucian, G., Friedman, W. & Bowers D. (2004). Self awareness of deficits in Parkinson disease. *Clinical Neuropsychologist, 18*, 352-361.

Levy, R. & Dubois, B. (2006). Apathy and the prefrontal cortex-basal ganglia circuits. *Cerebral Cortex, 15*, 1064-1074.

Lopez, O.L., Becker, J.T., Somsak, D., Dew, M.A. & DeKosky, S.T. (1994). Awareness of cognitive deficits and anosognosia in probable Alzheimer's disease. *Eur Neurol, 34*, 277-282.

Mangone, C.A., Hier, D.B., Gorelick, P.B., Ganellen, R.J., Langenberg, P., Boarman, R., et al. (2003). Measuring motor complications in clinical trials for early Parkinson's disease. *J Neurol Neurosurg Psychiatry, 74*, 143-146.

Martınez-Martın, P., Gil-Nagel, A., Gracia, L.M., Gomez, J.B., Martınez-Sarries, J. & Bermejo, F. (1994). Unified Parkinson's Disease Rating Scale characteristics and structure. The Cooperative Multicentric Group. *Mov Disord, 9*, 76–83.

Martinez-Martin, P. & Cubo, E. (2007). Scales to measure parkinsonism. *Handb Clin Neurol, 83*, 289-327.

Michon, A., Deweer, B., Pillon, B., Agid, Y. & Dubois, B. (1994). Relation of anosognosia to frontal lobe dysfunction in Alzheimer's disease. *J Neurol Neurosurg Psychiatry, 57*, 805–809.

Migliorelli, R., Teson, A., Sabe, L., Petracca, G., Petracchi, M., Leiguarda, R. et al. (1995). Anosognosia in Alzheimer's disease: A study of associated factors. *J Neuropsychiatry Clin Neurosci, 7*, 338–344.

Mikos, A.E., Springer, U.S., Nisenzon, A.N., Kellison, I.L., Fernandez, H.H, Okun, M.S. et al. (2009). Awareness of expressivity deficits in non-demented parkinson disease. *The Clinical Neuropsychologist, 23*, 805-817.

Miller, B.L. & Cummings, J.L. (2007). *The human frontal lobes: functions and disorders*. 2nd ed. The Guilford Press, New York.

Nelson, H. E. (1976). A modified Card Sorting Test sensitive to frontal lobe defects. *Cortex, 12*, 13–24.

Newcombe, F., (1969). *Missile wounds of the brain: A study of psychological deficits*. Oxford University Press, London.

Novelli, G., Papagno, C., Capitani, E., Laiacona, M., Vallar, G. & Cappa, S.F. (1986). Three clinical tests for the assessment of lexical retrieval and production from 320 normal subjects. *Archivio di Psicologia, Neurologia e Psichiatria, 47*, 477–506.

Ott, B.R., Lafleche, G., Whellihan, W.M., Buongiorno, G.W., Albert, M.S. & Fogel B.S. (1996). Impaired awareness of deficits in Alzheimer disease. *Alzheimer Dis Assoc Disord, 10*, 68-76.

Pearson, J., Teri, L., Reifler, B. & Raskind, M. (1989). Functional status and cognitive impairment in Alzheimer patients with and without depression. *J Am Ger Soc*, *37*, 1117-1121.

Pezzella, F.R., Di Rezze, M., Chianese, M., Fabbrini, G., Vanacore, N., Colosimo, C. et al. (2003). Hedonistic homeostatic dysregulation in Parkinson's disease: A short screening questionnaire. *Neurol Sci*, *24*, 205–206.

Pezzella, F.R., Colosimo, C., Vanacore, N., Di Rezze, S., Chianese, M., Fabbrini, G. et al. (2005). Prevalence and clinical features of hedonistic homeostatic dysregulation in Parkinson's disease. *Mov Disord, 20*, 77– 81.

Pluck, G.C. & Brown, R.G. (2002). Apathy in Parkinson's disease. *J Neurol Neurosurg Psychiatry, 73*, 636–642.

Reitan, R.M. (1958). Validity of the Trail making Test as an indicator of organic brain damage. *Percept Mot Skills*, *8,* 271–276.

Rosenblatt, A. & Leroi, I. (2000). Neuropsychiatry of Huntington's Disease and Other Basal Ganglia Disorders. *Psychosomatics*, *41*, 24-30.

Schacter, D.L. (1990). Towards a cognitive neuropsychology of awareness: Implicit knowledge and anosognosia. *J Clin Exp Neuropsychol, 12*, 155–178.

Seltzer, B., Vasterling, J.J., Yoder, J. & Thompson, K. (1997). Awareness of deficit in Alzheimer's disease: Relation to caregiver burden. *Gerontologist, 37*: 20–24.

Seltzer, B., Vasterling, J.J., Mathias, C.W. & Brennan, A. (2001). Clinical and neuropsychological correlates of impaired awareness of deficits in Alzheimer disease and Parkinson disease: A comparative study. *Neuropsychiatry Neuropsychol Beh Neurol, 14*, 122–129.

Sevush, S. & Leve, N. (1993). Denial of memory deficit in Alzheimer's disease. *Am J Psychiatry, 150*, 748–751.

Slaughter, J.R., Slaughter, K.A., Nichols, D., Holmes, S.E., & Martens, M.P. (2001). Prevalence, clinical manifestations, etiology, and treatment of depression in Parkinson's Disease. J Neuropsychiatry Clin Neurosci, *13*, 187–196.

Spielberger, C.D. (1983). *State-Trait Anxiety Inventory*. Mind Garden: Palo Alto, CA.

Stacy M. & Galbreath, A. (2008). Optimizing long-term therapy for Parkinson disease: options for treatment-associated dyskinesia. *Clin Neuropharmacol, 31*, 120-125.

Starkstein, S.E., Fedoroff, J.P., Price, T.R., Leiguarda, R. & Robinson R.G. (1992). Anosognosia in patients with cerebrovascular lesions: a study of causative factors. *Stroke, 23*, 1446-1453.

Starkstein, S.E., Sabe, L., Vazquez, S., Teson, A., Petracca, G., & Chemerinski, E., et al. (1996). Neuropsychological, psychiatric and cerebral blood flow findings in vascular dementia and Alzheimer's disease. *Stroke*, *27*, 408-414.

Stein, S. & Volpe, B.T. (1983). Classic parietal neglect syndrome after subcortical right frontal lobe infarction. *Neurology*, *33,* 797-799.

Tonelli, H., Tonelli, D., Poiani, G.R., Vital, M.A. & Andreatini, R. (2003). Reliability and clinical utility of a Portuguese version of the Abnormal Involuntary Movements Scale (AIMS) for tardive dyskinesia in Brazilian patients. *Braz J Med Biol Res*, *36*, 511–514.

Torta, D.M.E. & Castelli, L. (2008). Reward pathways in Parkinson's disease: clinical and theoretical implications. *Psychiatry Clin Neurosci, 62,* 203-213.

Torta, D.M.E., Castelli, L., Zibetti, M., Lopiano, L., & Geminiani, G.C. (2009). On the role of dopamine replacement therapy in decision-making, working memory and reward in Parkinson's disease: does the therapy dose matter? *Brain Cogn, 71,* 84-91.

Torta, D.M.E., Castelli, L., Latini-Corazzini, L., Banche, A., Lopiano, L., & Geminiani, G. (2010). Dissociation between time reproduction of actions and of intervals in Parkinson's disease. *Journal of Neurology, 257,* 1356-1361.

Verhagen, M.L, Myre, B., Verwey, N., Hassin-Baer, S., Arzbaecher, J., Sierens D., et al. (2004). Test–Retest Reliability of UPDRS-III, Dyskinesia Scales, and Timed Motor Tests in Patients With Advanced Parkinson's Disease: An Argument Against Multiple Baseline Assessments. *Mov Disorders, 19*, 1079- 1084.

Vitale, C., Pellecchia, M.T., Grossi, D., Fragassi, N., Cuomo, T., Di Maio, L., et al. (2001). Unawareness of dyskinesias in Parkinson's and Huntington's diseases. *Neurol Sci, 22,* 105–106.

Wechsler, D. (1987) *Manual for the Wechsler Memory Scale-Revised. Psychological Corporation: New York.*

Weinstein, E.A., Friedland, R.P. & Wagner, E.E. (1994). Denial/unawareness of impairment and symbolic behavior in Alzheimer's disease. *Neuropsychiatry Neuropsychol Behav Neurol, 7*, 176–184.

Wragg, R. & Jeste, D. (1989). Overview of depression and psychosis in Alzheimer's disease, *Am J Psychiatry, 146,* 577-87.

Yesavage, J.A., Brink, T.L., Rose, T.L., Lum, O., Huang, V., Adey, M.B. et al. (1983). Development and validation of a geriatric depression rating scale: a preliminary report. *J Psychiatric res, 17*, 37-49.

In: Movement Disorders: Causes, Diagnoses and Treatments ISBN: 978-1-61209-200-3
Editor: Barbara J. Larsen

Chapter VII

Traditional Mirror Therapy (TMT) in the Physical Therapy Management of Movement and Postural Control Problems*

Martin J. Watson
School of Allied Health Professions (AHP) & Health and Social Sciences Research Institute, Faculty of Health,
University of East Anglia (UEA), Norwich NR4 7TJ, UK

Introduction

Mirrors have a long history as an 'essential' piece of rehabilitation equipment, and can be found in many physical therapy treatment areas. Traditionally one of their main uses is to provide patients with a reflected body image of themselves, usually as (a component of) a therapeutic strategy aimed at retraining movement control and posture. For example, when as a result of central nervous system (CNS) damage such as stroke, people have impaired postural control, then therapists might provide them with a reflected mirror image of themselves to deliver augmented visual feedback during treatment sessions where motor training is occurring.

There has recently been much interest in the therapeutic use of mirrors placed perpendicular to the patient's coronal plane; i.e mirrors able to reflect an image of one limb onto the limb of the opposite body side. Recent works by researchers such as Ramachandran [1-4], and Sutbeyaz and Yavuzer [5, 6], have indicated that this may be a useful therapeutic strategy in instances where CNS pathology has resulted in unilateral instances of paresis, neglect or phantom pain. So for example, a mirror might be used to reflect the left (sound) arm onto the right (paralysed) arm following a stroke, as part of a therapeutic strategy aiming

---

* A version of this chapter was also published in *Handbook of Motor Skills: Development, Impairment and Therapy*, edited by Lucian T. Pelligrino published by Nova Science Publishers, Inc. It was submitted for appropriate modifications in an effort to encourage wider dissemination of research.

to rehabilitate movement on the affected side. One proposed mechanism is that reflection creates an illusion of normal movement/sensation on the affected side of the body, thus facilitating voluntary production of movement and/or normal sensory processing on that side.

Whilst this newer work, now often referred to as 'mirror therapy', is advancing, the original more traditional and (possibly) simpler therapeutic use of mirrors described at the start appears to be being somewhat overlooked and neglected. In this more traditional context (hereafter referred to as 'Traditional Mirror Therapy' or TMT), a full length body mirror is typically placed in front of the person (i.e. parallel to their coronal plane), thus providing them with a full frontal image of their body and its movements. In this way the person is provided with augmented (visual) feedback of their postural alignment and/or bodily movement. This might typically be carried out in conjunction with corrective instructions from the therapist.

One of the puzzles regarding TMT is the apparent absence of any evidence base or instructional advice for what is in effect a fairly simple and straightforward training strategy with a seemingly long history. The notion of therapist/educator-provided augmented feedback during (motor) learning is a well established one; in a recent narrative review for example, van Vliet and Wulf identified a reasonably substantial (albeit nascent) evidence base for this general strategy for motor skills training following stroke [7]. They identified verbal, visual, video and kinematic feedback strategies as the main ones which have been used and evaluated by therapists working with this very common patient group. Interestingly however, this overview did not identify any literature relating to TMT. Similarly, if one accesses key physical therapy instructional texts, there is usually a very limited amount of information on TMT. For example, in a fairly seminal UK text, Howe and Oldham [8] state that "*Full length mirrors are frequently used in physiotherapy departments to make patients more aware of their static posture either in sitting or standing and dynamic posture during movement. Mirrors are also employed in gait retraining...*" (p.237). Howevere no further details are provided.

It is perhaps not difficult to explain this dearth of information regarding TMT. Despite its longstanding presence in the physical therapist's armamentarium, it is easily conceivable that the approach has yet to receive the level of investigation and exploration which it deserves. The physical therapy evidence base is still in its relative infancy and the majority of existing therapeutic strategies await appropriate formal evaluation; TMT is probably no exception in this respect.

The aim of this chapter is to provide an overview of several aspects of TMT. Specifically, the chapter covers 3 topics, these being:

- Literature: what is known about TMT from published peer-reviewed reports of formal investigations of this strategy
- Recent research: an overview of 3 pilot projects conducted by the author and colleagues which each evaluate an aspect of TMT
- Clinical perspectives: a report of a pilot evaluation of how practising UK clinicians utilise TMT

What Is Known About TMT: Existing Scientific Studies

As stated in the introduction to this chapter, there appears to be a dearth of evaluative studies into the effectiveness of TMT in motor skill acquisition training. The author is currently undertaking a systematic review of the literature, and this has so far identified a (limited) number of studies of this topic. Of those published in peer-reviewed English language journals, the following are amonst the main studies which have so far been identified and stand out as representative examples of this limited knowledge base. These studies identify that there is in fact an evidence base in existence, although this does so far appear to be fairly limited.

Ross et al's 1991 study [9] was an evaluation of the use of mirror feedback as a component of treatment for long-standing facial nerve palsy. Subjects were engaged in daily practice of facial muscle exercises, using their reflected mirror image to obtain feedback during this process. The wider remit of this project was to evaluate whether electromyographic feedback, in combination with a mirror-based facial exercise regime, was any more advantageous than mirror-based exercises alone. A third group of subjects who received neither form of intervention acted as controls. Overall, treatment of either form appeared to confer benefits on subjects in terms of improvements in facial muscle control, facial symmetry and electrical measurements of facial nerve responses, in comparison with control subjects who received no therapy. There were no differences in outcome between the two intervention groups.

Gauthier-Gagnon et al's 1986 study [10] compared the effects of two different forms of training in the rehabilitation of standing postural control in two groups of unilateral below-knee amputees. The "traditional approach" treatment group received weight-shifting and balance exercises, combined with therapist provided verbal instructions and manual correction, but also utilising visual feedback via mirror. The experimental group received this same training, but augmented by the addition of auditory feedback generated and delivered by a pressure sensitive Limb Load Monitor placed beneath the prosthetic limb. The study reported that "both treatment modalities were shown to be equally effective in the early retraining of stance" (p.137); i.e. outcomes were comparable in both groups. This study clearly does not permit an evaluation of the effects of mirror feedback in isolation, although it might be argued that it suggests that this modality cannot be 'bettered' by the addition of augmented auditory feedback. it is also interesting to note from the graphical displays of some of the results that the 'mirror only' group appeared to demonstrate a higher level of postural control post-treatment.

Sewall et al's 1988 study [11] analysed the use of concurrent mirror feedback in a sports performance context, namely when young men learn a weightlifting technique (the 'power clean movement'). Eighteen college students participated in this study. Half of the group practised the technique with the use of mirrors whilst the other half did this without, both groups having first received standardised training in the specific weightlifting method via an instructional videotape. All subjects were assessed at the start and end of the study according to quality of technique, using a recognised weightlifting scoring system administered by a blinded assessor. Both groups showed improvements in technique by the end of the trial ($p<0.01$), but there were also differences in performance between the two in favour of mirror use ($p<0.05$). Whilst this study appears to support mirror feedback, the researchers made the significant point that they may have provided demonstration of the axiom that "subjects perform best under the condition in which they practice" (p.717), insofar as the best post-test results were obtained when subjects were assessed whilst using a mirror. It was apparent however that even without mirror feedback at assessment, the group which had used reflected body image to learn the technique were better performers by the end of the trial.

Radell et al's 2003 study [12] attempted to evaluate the effects of mirror feedback when female dance students were learning new ballet skills. One group of 14 students learned without the use of mirrors whilst another group of 13 students used mirrors. When students were assessed at the end of the semester it was found that dancers who had not used mirror feedback generally achieved better scores than those who had. Therefore in this instance mirror feedback appeared to have had a deleterious effect on motor skill acquisition. The authors reflect on how, in this specific context, such a result might come about because "the use of the mirror was distracting and inhibited the dancers' ability to focus more internally on the performance" (p.963). In other words, this is a group whose members have the potential to become overly focused on the aesthetics of personal body form and function, and that mirror use might potentially aggravate this effect, to the detriment of skill acquisition.

Vaillant et al's 2004 study [13] looked at the effects of simple mirror feedback on standing postural stability in healthy elderly people. A group consisting of 11 subjects with a mean age of approximately 70 years had their postural sway assessed whilst stood on a force platform. Subjects were assessed in two separate conditions: with and without mirror feedback. Perhaps unsurprisingly their postural sway appeared to be reduced when mirror feedback was available to subjects. The nature of the evaluation system permitted a somewhat more complex analysis: medio-lateral postural sway (i.e. side-to-side movement) was more significantly reduced when using the mirror than was antero-posterior (backwards-forwards) movement. This finding was attributed to the fact that subjects' sensory systems were better able to detect the latter than the former whilst viewing their reflected body image.

With the exception of Radell's work, all of the preceding studies appear to provide some support for the notion that TMT can contribute to the control and/or training of movement and posture. Two of the five studies appeared to find in clear favour of mirror useage [11, 13], with a third being cautiously favourable when results were looked at in more detail [10]; a fourth study could be interpreted as showing that the benefits conferred by mirror useage could not be improved upon when augmented by additional EMG-based input [10]. The study by Radell et al [12] could perhaps be considered as a special case, looking at a healthy subject group (dancers) for whom mirror use is apparently counter-productive. Three of these five studies were of course looking at normal as opposed to impaired study groups, hence having limited implications for neurological rehabilitation. Conversely the Ross et al study at least concerned a peripheral nervous lesion, whilst Gauthier-Gagnon et al provide some sense of the intervention's worth in a scenario of potentially gross postural/control problems; i.e. unilateral loss of structural and sensory integrity following limb amputation. Furthermore the Vaillant study indicates this therapy's potential worth in a predominantly aging population. Overall therefore the existing evidence base, whilst somewhat limited in amount and nature, does provide some support for the effectiveness of TMT in a skill (re)learning context.

Three Recent Projects

UK undergraduate students on honours degree courses typically undertake final year projects which may involve carrying out small scale empirical research. There is debate in some quarters regarding the extent to which work of this sort can contribute significantly to an existing evidence base – such projects are after all intended primarily as an opportunity for students to develop their skills of enquiry. Nonetheless useful work can be and is sometimes undertaken by pre-registration undergraduate physical therapy students which is worthy of dissemination. In this section a brief overview of 3 pertinent student projects is provided, each of which was supervised by the writer. All of these studies aimed to identify the extent to which a reflected body image provides useful visual feedback during some form of movement/postural control.

Study 1: The Effect of Simple Mirror Feedback on Limb Position Sense

This study set out to evaluate the effects of mirror feedback on the abilities of subjects to replicate joint angles [14]. The premise of this study was that a reflected body image confers on subjects an enhanced awareness of limb/body spatial positioning. Eighteen healthy subjects were each asked to replicate 3 pre-determined angles of shoulder joint abduction (50°, 110° and 140°), the precise amplitudes of which they were blind to. Each angle was first passively demonstrated to the subject, following which the arm was lowered, and then the subject was asked to actively replicate the initial limb position. Accuracy of joint angle replication was measured by the experimenter using a plurimeter, according to standardised criteria. Order of testing for the 3 pre-determined joint angles was counterbalanced across subjects, as were the conditions of testing, these being 1) visual feedback via mirror only, 2) visual feedback via direct sight of arm only, and 3) visual feedback by mirror and direct sight of arm. For condition 1, a cardboard blinker was used to prevent subjects from seeing sideways, thus preventing direct (lateral) sight of arm whilst permitting straight-ahead view of a reflected image of the limb. For the mirror conditions (1 and 3), subjects were presented with a frontal body image reflection, provided using a full length mirror placed directly in front of them. Data on accuracy of joint angle replication were analysed using a one factor within subjects ANOVA test. This identified that any differences occurring between the conditions did not reach statistical significance ($F=0.444$, $p=0.590$). The 95% confidence intervals for accuracy of replication did however suggest that condition 1 showed the best results, with condition 2 showing the worst. These results therefore suggested some support for the notion that mirror reflection confers benefits rearding limb position awareness.

Study 2: The Effect of Simple Mirror Feedback on Sitting Postural Control

This study aimed to evaluate how providing subjects with their reflected body image influences their sitting postural control [15]. This is a pertinent context for physical therapists, who might for example use mirrors to help patients to relearn their sitting postural control abilities when these are impaired say following stroke. Eighteen healthy female undergraduate students (mean age 20.8 years) had their postural sway evaluated in two standardised experimental conditions; with and without mirror feedback. Subjects were tested three times under each condition (hence 6 tests in total), with a mean performance value for each of the two conditions then being derived. Order of testing across the 6 tests was varied for each subject using a Latin Square procedure, to control for a learning effect. As these were subjects with intact neuromuscular systems, they were asked to maintain a complex (standardised) sitting position during each test, thus challenging their postural control abiliites. (Subjects were asked to perform balanced sitting, with knees extended so that their legs were held out straight in front of them; both arms were held out to their sides.) Subjects were evaluated by requiring them to sit on the seat plate sensor of a Balance Performance Monitor (BPM) [16, 17]. This was used to generate values for the amount of postural sway occurring, measured as length of sway path (mm) during a 30 second sampling period. Group mean sway path with mirror feedback was lower (i.e. better) than without, with values of 165.72mm [SD 40.52mm] versus 244.74mm [SD 68.48mm]. This difference was statistically significant (related t test, $t = 4.873$, $p<0.001$, 95% CI 44.80mm – 113.23mm). This suggested that mirror feedback had an immediate effect on postural control ability, with subjects apparently being more stable when able to view their reflected body image when adopting a complex sitting position.

Study 3: The Effect of Simple Mirror Feedback on Standing Postural Control

A similar study to the previous one was undertaken, but evaluating the extent to which the availability of a reflected image influences *standing* postural control [18]. Twenty healthy subjects were used in this evaluation. A similar protocol to the previously described study was used, wherein all subjects were tested under two conditions; i.e. standing 1) *with* and 2) *without* the availability of a reflected body image. As with the previous study, subjects were tested 3 times in each of the two conditions, with order of testing across these 6 trials being varied between subjects to control for systematic bias due to a learning effect. To make the test position more challenging for these healthy young subjects, they were each asked to maintain a standardised one-legged balanced standing position during all tests. Postural stability was ascertained by evaluating subjects whilst stood on a single foot plate sensor connected to a BPM, monitoring postural sway (sway path, measured in mm). Group mean sway path with mirror feedback was lower (i.e. better) than without, with values of 178.67mm [SD 41.13mm] versus 229.04mm [SD 38.21mm]. This difference was statistically significant (related t test, $t = 7.350$, $p<0.001$, 95% CI 36.02mm – 64.71mm). This suggested that mirror feedback had an immediate effect on standing postural control ability, with subjects apparently being more stable when able to view their reflected body image.

Overall, all 3 of these studies appeared to find support for the notion that, in normal subjects, a simple reflected mirror image enables improved postural control. Two of these studies presented statistically significant results, suggesting perhaps a relatively strong effect, albeit in a sample of healthy subjects. All of these studies had positive finding regarding the *immediate* effect of mirror feedback, suggesting that once subjects have a mirror image available then there is an instant alteration in control abilities. The mechanisms of this effect, and its ability to carry over during a movement training situation, requires investigation. Finally, the extent to (and means by) which the effects revealed in these studies are transferable to a patient population needs to be elaborated.

Assaying UK Clinicians' Viewpoints and Perceptions Regarding TMT

What do physiotherapists actually do with mirrors during routine clinical practice? Most UK physiotherapy departments appear to own a mirror. Furthermore the author observes that, when asked, most clinicians working in relevant clinical areas will profess to using mirrors during clinical practice. Yet it seems difficult to pinpoint what it is that therapists actually do with them. As indicated earlier, there is a shortage of texts discussing specifically how TMT should be carried out, and investigative research still appears to be in its relative infancy. An additional source of confusion is that anecdotally some clinicians appear to dislike TMT, claiming that it is counterproductive, unuseful, or indeed contra-indicated.

A strategy recently adopted by the author has been to undertake a preliminary assessment of how UK clinicians typically using TMT in everyday clinical practice. This is in preparation for a more substantial and formal survey of national practice. The recent evolution of internet-based information sharing brought about by Web 2.0 innovations has begun to impinge positively on physiotherapy practice [19], and in the UK this has occurred primarily by way of the Chartered Society of Physiotherapy's (CSP's) Interactive CSP (iCSP) initiative. This facility enables practicing clinicians, as well as physiotherapy academics and researchers, to pose questions online to all registered CSP colleagues. In March 2008 a query regarding TMT was posed by the author to the neurology section of iCSP. After first explaining that comments were being saught regarding the more traditional form of mirror usage, the 'question' posed was as follows:

To inform some ongoing research work, I am very keen to gauge clinicians' opinions of the usefulness or otherwise of this therapeutic strategy. Have you had some positive experiences of the use of mirror feedback for postural/movement training? Are you aware of situations where it is unwise to use this form of training feedback? Do you feel that this is an outdated or useless strategy? I would be very interested to see colleagues' comments, whilst hopefully also encouraging a discussion of the topic.

A small number of responses were initially received regarding this query, albeit similar in number to those shared for other queries posed to this site. (Busy clinicians are perhaps still somewhat reluctant to engage in web initiatives like this, except in instances where the queries being posed/discussed are of very specific and immediate relevance to contributors/respondents.) A reminder was posted after several weeks, to attempt to ensure that an extensive as possible online discussion had been undertaken on the topic. Eleven experienced clinicians eventually participated in this electronic forum. This relatively small group appeared to offer a rich diversity of views and contributions. Some of their responses appeared either explicitly or implicitly related to movement relabilitation following stroke, although some broader views were also shared. An attempt was made to theme and sub-categorise all of the contributions, and this resulted in the following summary of findings. (All of these appeared to relate to situations where the subject looks ahead into a mirror placed directly in front of them, unless otherwise stated.)

- Specific strategies. A number of successful strategies were specifically identified, including:
    - The 'cover my body' strategy, where, to encourage normal postural control in sitting, the therapist sits behind the subject and encourages him/her to align themselves in the mirror so that their reflected body image 'covers' the reflected body image of the therapist who is sat behind them;
    - Using the mirror to simply provide a 'snap-shot' of progress for the patient; i.e. showing them their reflected body image, as occasional feedback regarding success during postural control training. The mirror is taken away again once it has been used for this purpose. (It was suggested that mirror feedback is something which some of us are accustomed to using anyway for certain everyday functional tasks, but that it is otherwise confusing if used to excess and out of personal context);
    - Placing the mirror behind the patient. This reputably enables the therapist (who is in front of the patient, giving administering postural/ movement training) to gain an 'all round' picture of the patient's postural alignment whilst they are providing them with therapy.
- Specific scenarios where mirror use is found to be useful and successful. These scenarios included:
    - Working with patients with so called 'pusher' syndrome. This is a situation where subjects with stroke have problems recognising that they are actively moving away from midline, pushing themselves excessively towards the affected side when either sat or stood, in an erroneous effort to self-correct their postural alignment [20]. A mirror image apparently enables some people with this problem to identify what it is they are doing wrong and thus helps them to correct the problem;
    - Subjects who require help to find their midline alignment. (This includes the above 'pusher' type patients, but appeared to extend beyond that group also);
    - As a therapeutic adjunct when encouraging patients to hold their heads up; i.e. facilitation of active neck/cervical extension/retraction and head elevation in instances where poor head/neck control results in the head falling forward onto the chest. A corrective effect apparently occurs

when the subject is asked to "look up and look at yourself in the mirror";
  - Walking training, in instances where there is poor side-to-side weight transfer; i.e. subjects are encouraged to move their body (image) from side to side whilst walking "so that it touches each lateral edge of the mirror";
  - Patients with good problem-solving abilities, but who have impaired sensation/proprioception, who are instantly able to perceive (via reflected body image) the deficiencies of their postural alignment/ control and are hence able to do something actively about this;
  - During dressing training, particularly where this is occurring in the bathroom and there are bathroom mirrors available. This was presumed by respondents to be helpful as this is a natural environment and setting for such activity (and for mirrors to be present) for some patients.

- Specific reflections and advice on mirror use. This included:

  - To progress with mirror usage during movement/posture training by later working without a mirror; i.e. its use should be withdrawn as movement control improves;
  - To always ask the patient first before using a mirror in therapy, primarily in case patients are concerned regarding seeing their own image;
  - That mirror use can be useful to restore self-esteem, providing subjects with the opportunity to see how successful therapy has been;
  - That therapists will often know instantly whether mirror feedback is going to be useful or not with a particular patient, as soon as it is tried with a particular individual;
  - That there may be specific time-limited periods during rehabilitation where mirror use appears to be useful, before/after which this strategy does not work as well.

- Adverse effects of mirror use. The following suggestions were made:

  - That right/left reversal seen in the reflected body image is simply too confusing for some people (including sometimes therapists too) and that clinicians therefore need to be on the lookout for this. It was noted that mirrors can sometimes exaccerbate or cause left/right confusion;
  - That some people do not like/wish to see themselves in a mirror. One therapist reported an extreme adverse reaction following mirror use, when a patient was very shocked to see how they looked as a result of illness, and became incapacitated for several days as a result;
  - That some of the stroke patients who have cognitive attentional/ neglect problems don't respond well to mirror use because they cannot attend properly to a reflected mirror image.

more extensive survey (and possibly structured interview and observational) work might enable elaboration regarding the general procedures adopted by therapists when carrying out TMT. There is obviously a need to identify the frequency of this strategy's use, as well as the specific clinicial diagnoses and functional problems for which it is optimally useful for. Finally the notion that there are circumstances where TMT might be contra-indicated requries further exploration. The views and insights of the recipients of TMT, as well its users, obviously need to be taken into account.

Concluding Comments

Traditional mirror therapy (TMT) does appear to have a significant role to play in providing augmented feedback during the remediation of movement and postural control problems. Physical therapists have probably been aware of the benefits of this strategy since the very early days of the profession, although evaluations and elaborations of its utilisation have so far had limited presence. Formal scientific studies of this strategy are limited in number, although some useful evaluations nonetheless exist. These provide pointers for the types of clinical/educational roles which mirrors might provide, as well as giving some indications of the further research which needs to be conducted. The writer has facilitated pertinent small scale student research projects which also identify how a simple reflected image may immediately enhance the movement and postural control abilities of subjects. Whilst these projects have all involved normal healthy subjects, they all suggest that mirror reflections can easily improve subjects' motor abilities. Finally, although only preliminary in nature, a survey of clinicians has produced some very useful insights into the probable uses (and limitations) of this therapeutic strategy. As with many of the therapeutic modalities currently used by physical therapists, there therefore appears to be much to support the continued and extended use of this approach, pending further evaluations and evaluations.

References

[1] Ramachandran, V.S. and D. Rogers-Ramachandran, *Synaesthesia in phantom limbs induced with mirrors. Proc. Biol. Sci.* 1996. 263(1369): p. 377-86.

[2] Ramachandran, V.S., E.L. Altschuler, and S. Hillyer, *Mirror agnosia. Proc. Biol. Sci.*, 1997. 264(1382): p. 645-647.

[3] Ramachandran, V.S., et al., Can mirrors alleviate visual hemineglect? Med. Hypothes es. 1999. 52(4): p. 303-305.

[4] Altschuler, E.L., et al., Rehabilitation of hemiparesis after stroke with a mirror. Lancet. 1999. 353(9169): p. 2035-6.

[5] Sutbeyaz, S., et al., Mirror therapy enhances lower-extremity motor recovery and motor functioning after stroke: a randomized controlled trial. Archives of Physical Medicine and Rehabilitation. 2007. 88(5): p. 555-9.

[6] Yavuzer, G., et al., Mirror Therapy Improves Hand Function in Subacute Stroke: A Randomized Controlled Trial. Archives of Physical Medicine and Rehabilitation. 2008. 89(3): p. 393-398.

[7] van Vliet, P.M. and G. Wulf, Extrinsic feedback for motor learning after stroke: what is the evidence? Disability & Rehabilitation. 2006. 28(13-14): p. 831-840.

[8] Howe, T. and J. Oldham, *Posture and balance*, in *Human movement: an introductory text*, M. Trew and T. Everett, Editors. 2001, Churchill Livingstone: Edinburgh. p. 225-239.

[9] Ross, B., J.M. Nedzelski, and J.A. McLean, Efficacy of feedback training in long-standing facial nerve paresis. Laryngoscope. 1991. 101(7 Pt 1): p. 744-50.

[10] Gauthier-Gagnon, C., et al., Augmented sensory feedback in the early training of standing balance of below-knee amputees. Physiotherapy Canada, 1986. 38(3): p. 137-142.

[11] Sewall, L.P., T.G. Reeve, and R.A. Day, Effect of concurrent visual feedback on acquisition of a weightlifting skill. Perceptual and Motor Skills. 1988. 67: p. 715-718.

[12] Radell, S.A., D.D. Adame, and S.P. Cole, Effect of teaching with mirrors on ballet dance performance. Perceptual and Motor Skills. 2003. 97(3 Pt 1): p. 960-4.

[13] Vaillant, J., et al., Mirror versus stationary cross feedback in controlling the center of foot pressure displacement in quiet standing in elderly subjects. Archives of Physical Medicine and Rehabilitation. 2004. 85(12): p. 1962-5.

[14] Tuff, N. and M.J. Watson, The effect of visual feedback via mirror on immediate performance of an upper limb positioning task. Physiotherapy. 2005. 91(1): p. 56.

[15] Watson, M.J., Peck, M., A pilot study investigating the immediate effects of mirror feedback on sitting postural control in normal healthy adults. Physiotherapy Research International, 2008. 13(4): p. 204.

[16] Haas, B.M. and T.E. Whitmarsh, Inter- and intra-tester reliability of the Balance Performance Monitor in a non-patient population. Physiotherapy Research International. 1998. 3(2): p. 135-147.

[17] Haas, B.M. and A.M. Burden, Validity of weight distribution and sway measurements of the Balance Performance Monitor. Physiotherapy Reearch International. 2000. 5(1): p. 19 32.

[18] Watson, M.J. and May, A., An investigation of the immediate effects of mirror feedback on standing postural control in normal healthy adults. Clinical Rehabilitation. (in press)

[19] Barsky, E. and D. Giustini, Web 2.0 in physical therapy: a practical overview. Physiotherapy Canada, 2008. 60(3): p. 207-210.

[20] Perennou, D.A., et al., Lateropulsion, pushing and verticality perception in hemisphere stroke: a causal relationship? Brain. 2008. 131(Pt 9): p. 2401-13.

Index

B

C

D

E

F

G

H

I

N

O

P

Q

R

S

T

U

V

W

X

Y

Z